MEDICAL CULTURES OF THE EARLY MODERN SPANISH EMPIRE

Early modern Spain was a global empire in which a startling variety of medical cultures came into contact, and occasionally conflict, with one another. Spanish soldiers, ambassadors, missionaries, sailors, and emigrants of all sorts carried with them to the farthest reaches of the monarchy their own ideas about sickness and health. These ideas were, in turn, influenced by local cultures. This volume tells the story of encounters among medical cultures in the early modern Spanish empire.

The 12 chapters draw upon a wide variety of sources, ranging from drama, poetry, and sermons to broadsheets, travel accounts, chronicles, and Inquisitorial documents; and it surveys a tremendous regional scope, from Mexico, to the Canary Islands, the Iberian Peninsula, Italy, and Germany. Together, these essays propose a new interpretation of the circulation, reception, appropriation, and elaboration of ideas and practices related to sickness and health, sex, monstrosity, and death, in a historical moment marked by continuous cross-pollination among institutions and populations with a decided stake in the functioning and control of the human body.

Ultimately, the volume discloses how medical cultures provided demographic, analytical, and even geographic tools that constituted a particular kind of map of knowledge and practice, upon which were plotted: the local utilities of pharmacological discoveries; cures for social unrest or decline; spaces for political and institutional struggle; and evolving understandings of monstrousness and normativity. *Medical Cultures of the Early Modern Spanish Empire* puts the history of early modern Spanish medicine on a new footing in the English-speaking world.

New Hispanisms
Cultural and Literary Studies

Series editor: Anne J. Cruz

New Hispanisms: Literary and Cultural Studies presents innovative studies that seek to understand how the cultural production of the Hispanic world is generated, disseminated, and consumed. Ranging from the Spanish Middle Ages to modern Spain and Latin America, this series offers a forum for various critical and disciplinary approaches to cultural texts, including literature and other artifacts of Hispanic culture. Queries and proposals for single author volumes and collections of original essays are welcome.

Medical Cultures of the Early Modern Spanish Empire

Edited by

JOHN SLATER,

MARÍALUZ LÓPEZ-TERRADA,

and JOSÉ PARDO-TOMÁS

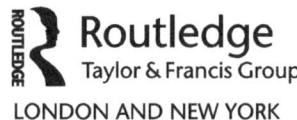

LONDON AND NEW YORK

First published 2014 by Ashgate Publishing

2 Park Square, Milton Park, Abingdon, Oxfordshire OX14 4RN
52 Vanderbilt Avenue, New York, NY 10017

Routledge is an imprint of the Taylor & Francis Group, an informa business

First issued in paperback 2020

British Library Cataloguing in Publication Data
A catalogue record for this book is available from the British Library

The Library of Congress has cataloged the printed edition as follows:
Medical cultures of the Early modern Spanish empire / edited by John Slater, Maríaluz López-Terrada, and José Pardo-Tomás.
    p. cm.—(New hispanisms: cultural and literary studies)
    Includes bibliographical references and index.
    ISBN 978-1-4724-2813-4 (hardback: alk. paper)
    I. Slater, John, 1972– editor. II. López-Terrada, Maríaluz, editor. III. Pardo-Tomás, José, editor. IV. Series: New hispanisms.
    [DNLM: 1. Medicine in Literature—Spain. 2. History of Medicine—Spain. 3. History, Early Modern 1451–1600—Spain. WZ 330]

    R555
    610.946—dc23

                                                                            2014017438

ISBN 978-1-4724-2813-4 (hbk)
ISBN 978-0-367-66922-5 (pbk)

To José María López Piñero

Contents

List of Figures and Tables

Figures

Tables

List of Contributors

Elisa Andretta is associate research scholar at the Institut d'Histoire de la Médecine et de la Santé (University of Geneva). She is the author of Roma medica. Anatomie d'un systeme medical au XVIe siècle (Rome, 2011), as well as several essays on the social and cultural history of medicine in early modern Rome. Her current research concerns medical practices and natural history in papal and Spanish courts in the early modern period.

Ralph Bauer is an associate professor of English and Comparative Literature at the University of Maryland, College Park, where he teaches courses on the literatures of the Americas, including Anglo, Spanish, and Native American literatures. His research interests include the literatures and cultures of the colonial Americas, early modern studies, hemispheric studies, and the history of science. His publications include *The Cultural Geography of Colonial American Literatures: Empire, Travel, Modernity* (Cambridge University Press, 2003, 2008); *An Inca Account of the Conquest of Peru* (University Press of Colorado, 2005); and (co-edited with José Antonio Mazzotti) *Creole Subjects in the Colonial Americas: Empires, Texts, Identities* (UNC Press, 2009), as well as articles in collections and journals such as *American Literary History, American Literature, Early American Literature, PMLA, Revista Iberoamericana, Colonial Latin American Review, Dieciocho,* and *Latin American Research Review.* He is currently completing a monograph entitled "The Alchemy of Conquest: Discovery, Prophecy, and the Secrets of the New World."

William Eamon is Regents Professor of History, Distinguished Achievement Professor, and Dean of the Honors College at New Mexico State University. He is the author *Science and the Secrets of Nature: Books of Secrets in Medieval and Early Modern Europe; The Professor of Secrets: Mystery, Medicine, and Alchemy in Renaissance Italy;* and over 50 articles and book chapters on various aspects of early modern science and medicine. He is also the co-editor of *Más allá de la Leyenda Negra: España y la Revolución Científica.* He is currently at work on two book projects: *Science and Everyday Life in Early Modern Europe, 1500–1750;* and *The Discovery of Nature and the Origins of Modern Science.*

Enrique García Santo-Tomás is Professor of Spanish Literature at the University of Michigan, Ann Arbor, and Elected Senior Fellow at the Michigan Society of Fellows. He is the author of over 120 publications on early modern Spanish literature and culture. He has received numerous awards for his research, including the Premio L. F. de Moratín de Ensayo a la Investigación Teatral, the Premio de Investigación Villa de Madrid, a Guggenheim Memorial Foundation Fellowship, the 2009 William Riley Parker Prize for an Outstanding Article in *PMLA*, and the Michigan Humanities Award. His most recent book is *La musa refractada: literatura y óptica en la España del Barroco*.

M. A. Katritzky is the Barbara Wilkes Research Fellow in Theatre Studies in the English Department of The Open University, Milton Keynes, UK. Recent books include: *The Art of Commedia: A Study in the commedia dell'arte 1560–1620* (Rodopi, 2006); *Women, Medicine and Theatre 1500–1750: Literary Mountebanks and Performing Quacks* (Ashgate, 2007); *Healing, Performance and Ceremony in the Writings of Three Early Modern Physicians: Hippolytus Guarinonius and the Brothers Felix and Thomas Platter* (Ashgate, 2012); and (co-authored with colleagues in The Open University English Department) *The Handbook to Literary Research* (Routledge, 2010).

Tayra M. C. Lanuza-Navarro is a post-doctoral researcher at the Institut d'Història de la Medicina i de la Ciència "López Piñero" in Valencia, Spain. Her research concerns the history of early modern science and medicine with a focus on early modern astronomy and astrology. She has previously been a fellow at the Chemical Heritage Foundation in Philadelphia (S. Edelstein Fellow 2010–2011), as well as at the European University Institute, Florence, Italy; at Bath Spa University, UK (2007); and at the Dibner Library for the History of Science at the Smithsonian Institution in Washington, DC (2005). In addition to articles on the history of science, she is co-editor of the books *Beyond Borders: Fresh Perspectives in History of Science* (Cambridge Scholars, 2008) and *Synergia: Jóvenes Investigadores en Historia de la Ciencia* (CSIC, 2007).

Maríaluz López-Terrada is Senior Researcher (*Investigadora científica*) at the Instituto de Historia de la Medicina y de la Ciencia López Piñero, of the Spanish National Research Council (CSIC). She has published more than 100 books, articles, and book chapters on the history of science. Her research has three foci. The first is the social history of medicine in early modern Spain, particularly hospitals, medical practice, medical pluralism, and popular practices related to health and disease, and the representation of medicine in the early modern Spanish drama. The second is the natural history of the same period, especially the introduction of American plants into Europe. Lastly, she is director of the database *Historical Bibliography of Science and Technology in Spain* (http://www.ihmc. uv-csic.es/buscador.php).

Angélica Morales Sarabia is associate investigator in the History of Science program at the Center for Interdisciplinary Research in Science and the Humanities (CEIICH) at the National Autonomous University of Mexico (UNAM). Her research analyzes cultural ignorance (agnotology) and the revalorization of Mexican medicine (XVI–XIX). She is the author of articles on natural history and the history of medicine, and is currently working on a book entitled *A Journey through the Works of the Naturalist José Ramírez, 1879–1904.*

José Pardo-Tomás is Senior Researcher at the Department of History of Science in the Institute "Milà i Fontanals" (CSIC, Barcelona, Spain). He has been a visiting scholar at the universities of Padua (Italy), Humboldt (Berlin, Germany), Bordeaux (France), and UNAM (México). His research is focused on the social and cultural history of medicine, natural history, and scientific books in the early modern period. His books include *Ciencia y censura* (CSIC, 1991), *El tesoro natural de América* (Nivola, 2002), *El médico en la palestra* (Marcial Pons, 2004), and *Un lugar para la ciencia* (Fundación Canaria Orotava, 2006), among others. He has co-authored books with Maríaluz López-Terrada—*Las primeras noticias sobre plantas americanas* (CSIC, 1993)—and José María López Piñero—*Nuevos materiales y noticias* sobre la *Historia natural de Nueva España* (CSIC, 1994) and *La influencia de Francisco Hernández* (CSIC, 1996).

Mauricio Sánchez Menchero is researcher at the Center for Interdisciplinary Research in Science and Humanities (CEIICH) of the National Autonomous University of Mexico (UNAM) and a member of the National System of Researchers. He is author of *En el centro de los Prodigios* (2010) and many articles on historiography. He is currently working on the research project "Culture in the medical periphery of colonial New Spain, 1521–1621," funded by the Ministry of Science and Innovation of Spain.

John Slater is Associate Professor in the Department of Spanish and Portuguese at the University of California, Davis. His research examines the early modern textual genres that represent human beings' experience of the natural world, from natural history to religious drama. In addition to numerous articles, he is the author of *Todos son hojas: Literatura e historia natural en el barroco español* (CSIC, 2010) and is completing a second book on the politics of natural history in early modern Spain entitled *Momentary Monuments: The Vegetable Kingdom and the Reign of the Spanish Hapsburgs.*

Acknowledgements

This book is the fruit of years of conversation, conference panels, and correspondence among scholars who were not only willing to collaborate but also eager to learn from one another. We are indebted to the many friends and colleagues who were our interlocutors, proofreaders, and sources of counsel. We would especially like to thank Àlvar Martínez Vidal, James Amelang, and Charles Davis for moderating panels and listening to us pitch ideas as the plan for this book was just coming together. Felipe Jerez Moliner helped us select the cover image. Vicente Zorrilla and Julio Ferrer provided excellent input, aesthetic and otherwise. Katherine Meis, Caitlin Brady, and Harrison Meadows graciously read complete drafts of the manuscript.

This book was also conceived and written during a time of economic crisis, when institutional budgets were tight. For this reason we would especially like to thank the Spanish Ministry of Science and Innovation's Dirección General de Investigación for two grants: *Cultura médica en la periferia colonial: Nueva España 1521–1621* [HAR2009-11030-CO201] and *La cultura médica ante su público: la representación de la medicina en el teatro del Siglo de Oro* [HAR2009-11030-C02-02]; in addition, the University of Colorado's Center for the Humanities and the Arts provided fellowship funds, and the Office of Research of the Division of Humanities, Arts, and Cultural Studies of the University of California, Davis offered publication assistance.

Introduction

John Slater, José Pardo-Tomás, and Maríaluz López-Terrada[1]

The history of early modern Spanish medicine, when told in English, has long been recounted with some measure of aversion. Spanish medicine would seem to have been, at turns, backward and insular, parasitic and largely derivative of developments elsewhere in Europe, sinisterly effective, or condemnably disorganized. The Inquisition is often invoked as if the word itself had talismanic power, capable of resolving doubts and squelching debate with a simple utterance. If, as Paul Julian Smith noted, Spain was the "'woman' of European culture," it continues to be Europe's medical Other (204). Spain's medical history has frequently served scholars as a bizarre, negative example or a story of missed opportunities, callous disregard for the health of indigenous peoples, and great power squandered to some dark purpose. In short, the history of Spanish medicine often includes a great deal of nonsense.[2]

William Eamon, explaining related problems, has called politically motivated accounts of Spanish science flatly "racist" ("Nuestros males" 13), and Richard Kagan shows that American histories that characterized Spain as spectrally despotic, bigoted, and decadent served a particular purpose, making possible a narrative of "Western" enlightenment and progress ("Prescott's Paradigm"). But the situation described by Eamon and Kagan is changing, and it is finally possible to tell the story of Spanish medical cultures without using them as a foil for French or English medical triumphs. Recent books on the history of science—such as Víctor Navarro Brotons and William Eamon's *Beyond the Black Legend: Spain and the Scientific Revolution* or Daniela Bleichmar, Paula De Vos, Kristin Huffine, and Kevin Sheehan's *Science in the Spanish and Portuguese Empires, 1500–1800*—and the history of medicine—for example, *Health and Medicine in Hapsburg Spain: Agents, Practices, Representations*, edited by Teresa Huguet-Termes, Jon Arrizabalaga, and Harold Cook—have made important progress in this area.[3] There still remain a number of challenges, however. It is not clear

---

[1] Research for this chapter was funded by the projects entitled *Cultura médica en la periferia colonial: Nueva España 1521–1621* [HAR2009-11030-CO201] and *La cultura médica ante su público: la representación de la medicina en el teatro del Siglo de Oro* [HAR2009-11030-C02-02], underwritten by the Dirección General de Investigación of the Spanish Ministry of Science and Innovation.

[2] Some of the myths about Spanish medicine are nearly 500 years old and continue to shape current historiography (Slater, "The Green Gold Falacies").

[3] A decade ago, in 2004, Jorge Cañizares Esguerra posed a question in volume 12 of *Perspectives on Science* that has come to characterize a historiographic limitation: "Iberian

to many scholars whether Antwerp and Naples were "Spanish" in the way that Manila and Lima were. Even astute historians considering Peru and Flanders in 1570 may tend to think that Peru—a kingdom that was sparsely populated with Spaniards, not primarily Spanish speaking, only nominally Roman Catholic, and had been held for only a few decades—can be considered more properly Spanish than Flanders, which was awash in Spaniards, had been subject to a the Spanish monarchy for almost two decades longer than Peru, and shared Spain's Roman Catholicism. Clearly, the reason that we believe some regions of the Hapsburg empire to have been more impervious to Spanish rule and culture than others has a great deal to do with entrenched ideas about European cultural superiority. But this, too, is changing, if slowly.

Medical Cultures of the Early Modern Spanish Empire shows that during the sixteenth and seventeenth centuries, Spain was a global empire in which a startling variety of medical cultures came into contact, and occasionally conflict, with one another. For this reason the methodological and theoretical point of departure for all of the essays in this volume is the understanding that medicine constitutes, on the one hand, a varied form of cultural practice and production, and on the other, a significant matrix for the intersection of a wide range of cultural phenomena (political, literary, religious, or otherwise). Most familiar to many readers are the conflicts that arose when academic medicine—and its ideas about sickness and health, therapy and cures—came in contact with Amerindian systems of belief about the body. But it is also the case that academic medicine had its own representational strategies that were in dialogue with developments in literature and the visual arts, both in Spain's European territories and in the colonies. The medicine that was taught in European universities, oftentimes rooted in classical values and practices, was always subject to debate and challenge within the academy itself. During the sixteenth and seventeenth centuries, however, the culture of academic medicine was increasingly brought into contact with other cultures, medical and otherwise. Spanish soldiers, ambassadors, missionaries, sailors, and emigrants of all sorts carried with them to the courts of Europe and the farthest reaches of the monarchy their own ideas about sickness and health. These ideas were, in turn, influenced by autochthonous medical cultures.

In the early modern world of the Hapsburg empire, medical cultures proved powerful tools for imagining the spaces of the body politic and for extending the ideologies of the Spanish state. But they were also interrogated, transformed, subverted, and willfully misunderstood. Both afar and at court, medical cultures provided new means of understanding the past (e.g. the collapse of indigenous

---

Science in the Renaissance: Ignored How Much Longer?" Since that time, there has been a marked increase in scholarly interest in the histories of Spanish medicine and science. Recently, particular attention has been paid to the history of medicine during the reign of Philip II (1556–1598); see, for example, Alexandra Parma Cook and Noble David Cook's excellent *The Plague Files: Crisis Management in Sixteenth-Century Seville* or Michele L. Clouse's *Medicine, Government and Public Health in Philip II's Spain.*

populations), of representing a worrisome present (lending the broader culture an idiom to speak about generation and succession), and of imagining an often uncertain future (through practices of prognostication). In short, medical cultures provided demographic, analytical, and even geographic tools that constituted a particular kind of map of knowledge and practice, upon which were plotted the local utilities of pharmacological discoveries; cures for social unrest or decline; spaces for political and institutional struggle; and evolving understandings of monstrousness and normativity.

Across Europe, economic and social upheaval frequently altered the nature of interaction among university-trained physicians, surgeons, apothecaries, and extra-academic practitioners.[4] And within Spain, newly popularized forms of representation—particularly the theater and the novel—threatened to control the public face of medical practice. Like any culture or system of beliefs, customs, and practices, medical culture was forced to change after contact with other cultures. These interactions occasionally gave way to confrontation and rivalry; more often, however, the upshot of these cultural encounters was more subtle forms of negotiation and the circulation of knowledge, even when there were significant inequalities of power. This volume tells the story of some of these cultural encounters in the early modern Spanish empire.

The empire itself was not simply the product of military conquest or religious evangelization. The extension of Hapsburg imperial power was based on the expatiation, in a literal sense, of Spanish institutions, including medical institutions. Following upon the notion that the proper seat of the House of Austria was the Spanish throne, imperial Spain was made possible by the belief that the proper scope of Spanish laws, sovereignty, religion, and bureaucratic practices was everywhere in the world. It was the realization of the amplest conception of Catholicism. The promise of eternal life in Christ was spread with the same innocence with which Western democracies export their values in our own time: through war, commerce, science, music, and so on. Medicine, like its university rivals—canon law and civil law—played an important role in the attempt to make global rule possible; in a monarchy that did not regard geographic limitations to its power as natural, Spanish medical practitioners were, to be playfully anachronistic, the first modern *médecins sans frontières*. At least in theory. The problem was to find enough of them, and the lack of suitable practitioners capable of extending the reach of Spanish medical institutions is a recurring subject in this book.

The power of a monarch such as Philip II, who ruled from 1556 to 1598, may have been conceived of as universal in the ideal, but it was far from absolute in practice, whether on the Iberian Peninsula or elsewhere. Particular institutions

---

[4] Since the 1980s there have been significant considerations of the complicated interactions among different kinds of medical practitioners; notable in this respect is Bynum and Porter's *Medical Fringe and Medical Orthodoxy: 1750–1850*. Also significant are Brockliss and Jones's *The Medical World of Early Modern France* and Pelling and Mandelbrote's *The Practice of Reform in Health, Medicine, and Science, 1500–2000*.

had their own successes and failures, and the amplification of political influence and power did not imply the uniform extension of institutional practices. This is especially true of medicine.[5] People will sometimes worship a new god before they abandon the hot toddy they take for a head cold. And to consider only the institutional manifestations of medicine within the broad scope of the Hapsburg empire, such as academic medicine, is essentially to limit discussions to the least successful product of Spanish universities. Academic medicine did not always take root the way Spanish jurisprudence did, as we discuss below.

One might think of the spread of the movement of medical cultures from the Iberian Peninsula to other parts of the world as akin to the spread of the Spanish language. Some territories of the monarchy, such as Flanders, Naples, or the Philippines, never became entirely or lastingly Spanish speaking, despite centuries of Iberian rule; other territories (such as the American colonies) developed their own regional and later national linguistic characteristics while maintaining indigenous languages to a lesser or greater degree. Not even the Hapsburg's Iberian kingdoms became exclusively Spanish speaking. Similarly, the medical cultures of some Hapsburg territories were more influenced by Iberia than others, but rarely in predictable ways. There is no single mechanism or process to explain the acceptance or rejection of particular elements of medical cultures within the vast empire of the Hapsburgs. This is true despite the many similarities among the political institutions—royal audiences and viceregal courts—set up to govern the kingdoms, duchies, counties, "colonies" (a term even scholars persist in using, although the Spanish almost never did), and other lands of the Hapsburgs.

The often contradictory set of circumstances described to this point plainly suggests a number of issues that could only be addressed by the collaborative work of scholars representing a variety of disciplines. This book is the result of that work; it provides a range of case histories that draw upon different textual genres, social milieus, institutional contexts, and locations that span from New Spain (Mexico) to Italy, Germany, and, of course, the Iberian Peninsula. We have not tried to establish a grand, totalizing narrative, which would necessarily obscure nuance. Instead, our attempt has been to apply a single methodological approach to a variety of practices and beliefs related to medicine—broadly construed—in early modern Spain in order to open up new avenues of research. The concept of "medical cultures" provides coherence to what can seem to be disparate phenomena by demonstrating how experiences and beliefs related to medicine were reflected

---

[5]   Representative of the conflict between the aspirations of the monarch and the realities of political negotiation and resistance at the local level is the medical tribunal known as the Tribunal del Protomedicato. The "Protomédico" (royal first physician) and the tribunal, in theory, were to create normative standards for the practice of medicine kingdom-wide and oversee everything having to do with medicine. In practice, this power was very limited, particularly within municipalities. See Lanning's *The Royal Protomedicato: The Regulation of Medical Professions in the Spanish Empire*; Campos's *El Real Tribunal del Protomedicato castellano, siglos XI–XIX*; and the studies collected in López-Terrada and Martínez-Vidal's "El Tribunal del Protomedicato en la Monarquía Hispánica."

in discourses, practices, and politics. This means that our questions are not limited to the perspectives and beliefs of physicians and other medical practitioners, but include those of patients (even those who, without seeking medical assistance, were diagnosed, classified, or criticized by medical practitioners). "Medicine," as Maarten Bode explains, "is culture dependent, not culture independent. We look upon medical systems as social systems when we take the broader cultural and political context in which medical theories are constructed and medicine is practiced into account" (Bode 14). Still further, medicine is not only culture dependent, but is a *constituent* of culture; medicine is shaped by, and is an index of, the culture of the early modern Spanish empire.

Whether we consider medicine to be primarily a body of texts with its own genres and conventions, a system of beliefs and practices, a mechanism that abets the political control of human bodies, or a system for the classification and study of natural phenomena (*materia medica*, etc.), medicine presupposes a number of cultural negotiations in our volume. These negotiations frequently impinge upon the realms of religion, politics, and jurisprudence: What and how much should one consume? When, how, and how often should one have sex? What are the causes of disease, affliction, and death? What is the normal or ideal state of bodies? The answers to these and other questions provide tools with which to consider the constitution of the body politic, human beings' place in the universe, and the appositeness of rules governing a broad array of human impulses. In almost every case, the cultural negotiations presupposed by medicine are conducted at the local level within a broader framework of institutional practices and specific ideologies.

The term "medical cultures" is drawn from anthropology and is, to a certain extent, a synonym of "medical systems," particularly when speaking of traditional or folk medicine.[6] At its most basic, a medical culture is a shared system of beliefs and practices associated with health and sickness. Medical cultures entail concepts of clothing, diet, work, sex, what is natural or unnatural, what is beneficial or harmful, the way that one's own body or the bodies of others are to be brought to order, and so on. These dimensions of medical culture are constantly in contact with other systems of belief and practice—religious, political, and otherwise— that have their own ideas about how and what to consume, or the behaviors and comportments that lead to positive outcomes (be they health, salvation, security, or happiness).

It is possible to organize the beliefs and practices of a medical culture according to modern categories (nosology, etiology, therapy), or label some practices superstitious or rational, retrograde, or modern. The hierarchies implicit in such attempts, however, tend to distort the historical interactions of medical cultures.

---

[6] For example, the term "medical cultures" is often used to refer to the traditional medicine of Latin America and Japan or Ayurveda. On the other hand, the term has been used extensively in gender studies to analyze "masculine" or "masculinist" medical cultures, the cultural regime to which women have historically been forced to adapt in order to become medical professionals (More, Fee, and Parry).

The intersections of medical cultures and other cultural practices are almost always productive of something that does not pertain exclusively to either culture. Intersection, of course, does not imply equality or fairness, but this does not mean that influence moved only from the powerful to the powerless. In order to explain the dynamics of cultural exchange in the context of the experience of sickness and health, we have been careful to select transatlantic interactions, European encounters, and meetings within the world of Spanish letters. On the other hand, we have included a variety of kinds of interaction from each of these contexts. Some of the contributors to our volume work within a framework that is national in scope, others examine variability among communities as small as a village, and still others look at the experience of individual observers or the rhetorical devices of particular texts. The results of this approach are to demonstrate that Spain may have been an empire, but it was anything but monolithic. The tremendous expansion of Spanish influence did little to consolidate ideologies and practices; on the contrary, it multiplied the spaces and venues for cultural interplay. This growth in the number and kind of encounters among medical cultures, as well as between medical cultures and other forms of cultural expression, made negotiation the only constant in the early modern experience of sickness and health.

Despite the undeniable transformation that the history of medicine has undergone over the last three or four decades—a transformation made possible by the influence of the cultural history of science, which has dominated recent approaches to science and medicine—our feeling is that many historians continue to construct medicine too narrowly. Sometimes, historical phenomena related to medicine are not considered in their medical dimension.[7] At other times, the history of medicine ignores larger cultural influences that may shape or condition the experience of health and sickness. Many historians tend to use (and impose) disconcertingly limiting definitions of what is "medical" and what is not when it comes to analyzing and interpreting past events related to health, sickness, and the control of human bodies (one's own or that of another) by social actors. We would think it absurd if we limited the history of religion to events such as "going to church" or "talking about God." In the same way, limiting the history of medicine to the study of medical textbooks or trips to the physician makes no sense.[8] Doing so causes us to lose sight of how medicine is often in competition and/or negotiation with a wide array of forms of cultural production and practice. The competition, rivalry, collaboration, and other forms of intersection between

---

[7]   Robert A. McGuire and Philip R. P. Coelho demonstrate the benefits of examining economic history in light of the medical challenges faced by different ethnic groups in *Parasites, Pathogens, and Progress*.

[8]   Within Spain, there is a long tradition of defining medicine broadly and considering a variety of cultural phenomena from the standpoint of the history of medicine. Notable studies in this vein include the extraordinary works of Luis García Ballester—works devoted to medical pluralism, such as the 2002 special issue of *Dynamis* edited by Ballester; López-Terrada and Martínez Vidal; and gender studies of medical history, for example, Cabré i Pairet and Ortiz Gómez's *Sanadoras, matronas y médicas en Europa, siglos XII–XX*.

medicine, law, religion, politics, and so on—all of which seek to provide basic answers to questions surrounding the status of human bodies and the natural order—shape each of these fields.

The modern predilection for linear, historiographic narration—we are people of prose, not lyric—means that historians tend to prize narrative sources that can be most easily assimilated into a master account. The results of this are often very pleasing. But while structured narration is one form of medical signification (examination, diagnosis, prognosis, outcome), it is far from the only, and perhaps not even the predominant form. Changing the methodological framework and opening up narrow definitions of medicine permits us to utilize new sources (textual, visual, and otherwise) that have not played a significant role in traditional narratives of the history of medicine. More sources means, logically, more voices and more actors, but also more questions that demand a fresh approach. Thus, in this volume we show how the inclusion of new sources permits the incorporation of new voices into the history of medicine: from the pulpits of preachers and the stages of playwrights, to the participants in the Council of Trent, to travelers to America and indigenous Mesoamericans, all of whom deploy particular discursive tools to represent sickness and health. Whether historical actors deploy these tools on their own behalf or to represent the experience of another (real or fictional), the voices that reach us from the past evidence the intersections of diverse medical cultures, as well as the relationships among these cultures.

In fact, the first conclusion that emerges from our approach to medical cultures and their social ordering has to do with the academic medicine of university-trained practitioners, which has long been the focus of the history of medicine. Readers may be surprised to find that academic medicine is not the predominant voice in this volume. This is neither a mistake nor an oversight. Academic medicine was not the predominant or most pervasive medical culture in the early modern Spanish empire. In light of this, we believe it to be necessary to interrogate the way historians have generally constructed medical hegemonies and hierarchies in order to make room for conceptualizations of order that may be non-hegemonic, temporary, fluid, and even unstable. Reducing early modern Spanish medical history to an oscillating binary (academic medicine falls while extra-academic medicine rises) is not the answer. Instead, it is necessary to have a broad understanding of the medical cultures operative in specific locales at particular times—the means of perception, interpretation, and explanation of a given community—including but not limited to academic medicine, in order to understand responses to disease, infertility, pain, and so on. Almost all of our studies illustrate the need to examine very specific situations: a particular book, the flow of information from one locality to another, a particular genre or author. None of these articles suggests that it is possible to make a grand, overarching statement that could summarize the character of medicine during the two centuries of Hapsburg rule.

Despite our granular approach, the articles share methodological premises. The most important of these is that medicine in early modern Spain was produced at the local confluence of practices and beliefs concerning the human body; the more varied the localities, the less uniform the response. In other words, medicine in its simplest terms involved local negotiations—on the page, in the home, in a specific city or region during a particular moment—that occurred within a broader context of beliefs and practices. The early modern Spanish empire was much larger than other states at the time and the stages of medical negotiation were amplified and multiplied accordingly. Just as we do not expect folk medicine to have been the same in Antwerp and Manila, we cannot expect that medicine, as a cultural phenomenon, was in any way uniform. We have long assumed that the expansion of Spanish influence involved the attempt to impose beliefs and practices of religion and law to varying degrees of success. Over the last several decades, scholars have studied the ways in which this attempt transformed the metropolis in the process. For whatever reason, medicine is not generally considered alongside religion and jurisprudence, despite the fact that we think of religion and jurisprudence as means of understanding health and the control of bodies. Our volume, we hope, will help correct this blindness.

Each of the 10 chapters in this volume focuses on a particular context for the meeting and production of medical cultures in early modern Spain. The first section, made up of three articles, deals with New Spain. The chapter by José Pardo-Tomás contains surprising findings about the ways in which the colonial bureaucracy collected information about epidemics and how, through new formats for acquiring information, new ways to construct medical authority were generated. In their respective chapters, Angélica Morales Sarabia and Ralph Bauer take a fresh look at the obstacles to and contexts for the reception of new medicinal plants and New World drugs. Between them, Bauer and Pardo-Tomás subtly reframe questions about how Spaniards understood the New World, demonstrating that Spaniards were not as quick to label New World nature "demonic" or indigenous Americans "sinful" as has sometimes been claimed.

The reason we begin with a section dedicated to the Americas is not simply to reflect the authors' belief that New Spain was not peripheral or marginal to the production of medical cultures, but because many of the dynamics that are at play throughout the volume are made especially plain there. Looking at the ways in which European academic medicine came into contact with American healing practices, the administrative realities of colonial life, and so on clarifies the nature of meetings between medical cultures and other forms of cultural expression or practice. Three axes of analysis predominate in the first section.

The first of these axes is the idea that New Spain represented something genuinely new in the Spanish experience (Gruzinski, "Les mondes mêlés"). New Spain was home to indigenous peoples, Asians, Africans, mestizos, mulattos, native-born Spaniards, and creoles, all of whom were organized into socioeconomic strata of varying rigidity. To some extent, a similar ethnic and social mix might be found in places such as Seville, but the difference was this: the demographic weight of each group in New Spain was almost completely reversed in the metropolis. Added to this, the structure of guilds, colleges, and universities that served to control medical knowledge and practice on the Iberian Peninsula was not lacking in New

Spain but was very weak; still further, there were very few university-trained physicians (Martínez Hernández). This meant that academic medicine did not come to predominate or characterize the array of medical cultures in New Spain.

Another factor that affected the differential configuration of medical cultures in New Spain and on the Iberian Peninsula had to do with the particularities of the public-health challenges faced in each. Both regions suffered from war, hunger, and epidemics during the early modern period; but they did not suffer from the same diseases, and hunger was due to very different causes. The acuteness of the suffering attributable to epidemics in New Spain obliged medical cultures to incorporate new strategies, practices, and explanations concerning the health of the population (N. D. Cook, *Born to Die*). This prompted an enormous growth in the circulation, exchange, and appropriation of ideas and practices among medical cultures.

The second axis of analysis, related to the first, has to do with the interaction of medical and religious cultures. One the one hand, medicine had a *regimen sanitatis* or "rule of health," which encompassed a spectrum of issues, from procreation to the handling of bodies before burial, sickness and its conceptualization, legislative action, and the construction of spaces designated for medical intervention. On the other hand, religious cultures had a frequently overlapping and sometimes conflicting rule of spiritual health—a *regimen christianum* or *regimen reipublicae christianae*—for the salvation of souls and of the body politic. The professional ethics of physicians and other medical practitioners provided guidance as to what pertained to medicine and what was due religion. Such guidance was often missing in New Spain, meaning that medicine might take on an increasingly spiritual dimension and religion might concern itself with what had, in the Old World, been medicine's purview.

New Spain was, of course, immersed in an ongoing and complex process of religious conversion (Ricard). But there was a parallel process of what we might call medical conversion (Pardo-Tomás, "Conversion Medicine"). By medical conversion we mean that one might reasonably identify with a particular medical culture—feel some sense of ownership of it, understand it as a cultural inheritance, or feel that it was appropriate to one's station—but seek assistance and comfort in another.[9] This could lead to a new identification with what had formerly been a "foreign" medical culture. In New Spain, someone seeking medical attention had available a range of therapeutic options, curative approaches, invocations in familiar and unfamiliar languages that promised the restoration of health or protection against the trials of disease, and so on. Indigenous peoples borrowed from the "friars' medicine" brought from Europe, Europeans and Indians alike appropriated animist medical concepts that arrived with African slaves, and nearly everyone had to rely to some degree on indigenous knowledge (radically

---

[9] Morales's chapter in this volume contains a marvelous example of the medical conversion of Petrona Babtista.

transformed by conquest) of native medicines.[10] The contributions by Morales and Pardo-Tomás in this volume demonstrate that the extent to which colonial subjects drew on any of these bodies of knowledge to explain public health crises or for their own treatment depended a great deal on the demographic composition of the location; distance from or proximity to what was familiar or recognizable; the ecology of the area and the availability of particular medicines at market; and the way political authority was exercised, among other factors. In short, medical conversion was frequently the product of necessity, but rarely involved a wholesale abandonment of one culture for another.

The third axis of this section has to do with the circulation of practices and knowledge of medical cultures within the empire of the Hapsburgs. Here, we pay special attention to the flow of cultural practices from the colonies to the metropolis.[11] While it has become a commonplace in most fields to recognize that the meeting of Amerindian and European cultures caused changes in each—just as courtly cultures influenced one another—there is still a tendency in the history of medicine to fixate on the ways in which the colonies were transformed through subjugation. This is not *de facto* wrongheaded unless it leads to a misunderstanding of the colonial reality or a study of the "deficits" and "backwardness" of the imperial periphery. Ralph Bauer's article demonstrates that scholars have tended to misunderstand the intellectual and ideological framework that conditioned the European acceptance and dissemination of knowledge of New World medicines. The colonies were not dependant on novel medical ideas or treatments that might or might not arrive from the Iberian Peninsula, and were not awaiting medical modernization that could only radiate from the imperial court and the king's physicians.

The second section of this volume is composed of three chapters about the movement of Spain's medical cultures, tracing itineraries across medical geographies westward from Spain to the New World, eastward from the Canary Islands to Germany, and back and forth among centers of ecclesiastic power. Its spaces include not only the hospitals and places in which patients were examined, but also churches and pulpits, academies, and the courtly environments where "monstrous" humans were put on display. The contributions of Mauricio Sánchez-Menchero, M. A. Katritzky, and Elisa Andretta rarely overlap geographically, but they all situate the circulation of medical knowledge in complex social and representational contexts. Katritzky and Andretta focus on Europe, but the New World is a large presence throughout this section. With the invention of America

---

[10]   African contributions to the medicine of New Spain have received considerable attention, beginning with the classic study by Gonzalo Aguirre Beltrán. More recent works include Laura A. Lewis's *Hall of Mirrors*. Among the studies of colonial Mexico, however, none is comparable to Laura de Mello Souza's study of Brazil, *The Devil and the Land of the Holy Cross*.

[11]   In this sense, our approach is not dissimilar to that taken by Marcy Norton in *Sacred Gifts, Profane Pleasures: A History of Tobacco and Chocolate in the Atlantic World*, although the spectrum of sources we consider is somewhat wider.

came the invention of new demographic and anthropological categories, new epidemiological models, new conceptions of health and sickness, and new means to comprehend and measure well-being and public health. There were new bodies and new strategies to represent them. As the means of apprehension changed, so did medical notions of community, place, and even forlornness, as Sánchez-Menchero shows; the correspondence he examines provides powerful accounts of the unwelcome novelty of being sick in a new world. Katritzky's chapter on Pedro González, the "Wild Man" of Tenerife, reconstructs González's journeys from court to court, from Spain to the Alps, to show how the "literary anthropologies" associated with "congenitally physically exceptional human beings" help us understand the development of humanness as a medical and biological category. Much of the religious language that would condition the way Roman Catholics experienced sin and sickness, salvation and cure was negotiated at the Council of Trent; but as Andretta shows, the Council was also a base of intellectual operations from which men like Juan Páez de Castro could cultivate relationships with famous physicians, found academies, and exchange information with illustrious men. Andretta's work is not a study of Spaniards abroad, but an illustration of how medical cultures spread and changed with the extension of Spanish ecclesiastical influence at Trent and in Rome.

Ricardo Padrón has pointed out the similarities between historiographic emplotment and geographic description, between the representational regimes that organize time and space (21). Left out of Padrón's discussion, and other considerations of early modern cosmography, is the extent to which a new demographic imagination and new medical epistemologies shaped notions of scale, proportion, balance, and symmetry. The Galenic *complexio* one of the most important classical models for the description of symmetry as an anthropocentric value, came under systematic attack. The alchemical or chymical world of transmutation and change was no longer scaled to human bodies; one of the hallmarks of early modern chymical medicine was a rejection of the relationship between micro- and macrocosm. The Hapsburg monarchy, for the first time in history, attempted to manage epidemics that occurred on nearly a hemispheric scale. What it meant for an empire to occupy space, what distance felt like, what sublimity looked like, all of these things were questioned. And all of these experiences were tied, explicitly and materially, to the possession of bodies that could be claimed as the domain of medicine.

The stage was a tool that early modern Spaniards used in order to make space comprehensible and to make the placement of bodies meaningful; the stage and dramatic representation are the principal foci of the third section.[12] Theater, like medicine, is at least partly a discursive system for the control of bodies. Albeit for different reasons, both early modern medical and dramatic texts served to govern the propriety and the expression of particular emotions, indicate the proper

---

[12] On the philosophical and ideological implications of theatrical organizations of space, or "spatiality," see Egginton.

movement and use of bodies, as well as describe the most advantageous conditions for procreation. Beyond this, theater and medicine were cultures of spectacle.[13] Tayra Lanuza-Navarro explores dramatic representations of astrological medicine, focusing on the ways that plays eroticized or otherwise distorted medical and scientific concepts while at the same time reinforcing commonly held ideas about astrology. In her study of early modern Spanish theater, Maríaluz López-Terrada finds that the language associated with sicknesses—much of it drawn from academic medicine—and the ways in which illness is represented in plays demonstrate that drama and medicine share a vocabulary of word and gesture.

But different dramatic genres represent medicine differently; in fact, each genre, as López-Terrada shows, tends to represent a different medical culture. The three-act *comedia* tends to draw on the Galenism of academic medicine; the dialogues of the *comedia* tend to reproduce the terminology and subtle reasoning of medical textbooks. Reflecting the ways in which medical knowledge was disseminated through books, the *comedia* is a drama of transmission. Quite differently, the farcical *entremés* tends to represent the reception, rather than the transmission, of medical ideas; the entremés often pokes fun at medical language by demonstrating how absurd or incomprehensible medical terminology seemed to lay folk. Thus the variation among dramatic genres demonstrates what we find more broadly: that in particular contexts, different aspects of a medical culture or various cultures may be more salient. The chapters by Lanuza-Navarro and López-Terrada are illuminating because they deal largely with the literary production of the first half of the seventeenth century, a time when much of the innovation related to textual strategies for the representation of medical knowledge could be found in sources other than medical textbooks. In other words, dramatic texts are often more daring, experimental, and flexible when it comes to the means of representing sickness and disseminating ideas about therapies than many of the medical textbooks of the period, including works of academic medicine in the vernacular.

Literary genre is not only a system of textual conventions, but also, if more narrowly, a means to classify medical subjects. Pregnancy and childbirth are rarely dramatized in the plays of the seventeenth century; mothers rarely appear and midwives are even scarcer (Díez Borque 96; McKendrick 4). The prose fiction of the period, as Enrique García Santo Tomás shows in his chapter, is less hesitant to represent childbirth. This does not mean that novelists, such as Francisco Santos, portray it sympathetically. Instead, Santos's novels reflect both the widespread concern about Spain's political decline and men's anxieties about women's agency through images of monstrous childbirths and negative portrayals of midwives. John Slater examines another religious and political context for the development of a new medical culture, suggesting that the reception and practice of chemical or chymical medicine (sometimes attributed to French influences) was made possible

---

[13]   The body of scholarship on the spectacular or theatrical dimensions of medicine is substantial, but M. A. Katritzky, a contributor to this volume, provides a helpful introduction in *Healing, Performance and Ceremony in the Writings of Three Early Modern Physicians*.

by the theological preoccupations of powerful preachers. Both Andretta and Slater take aim at the timeworn contention that the Spanish Church was uniformly opposed to medical and scientific innovation. Furthermore, they show that international ecclesiastical networks played an important role in the development of Spanish medical cultures.

Interdisciplinary studies that examine literature and medicine jointly are useful in part because literary history has a more developed lexicon for describing the degrees and effects of influence—whether we speak of allusiveness, intertextuality, or competition (agon, paragone, etc.)—than the history of medicine. Literary history is not immune to the rhetoric of innovation and backwardness, cultural richness or impoverishment, but the politics play out somewhat differently in literary and medical histories. No one hesitates to note the influence of early modern Italian theater on its Spanish counterpart or the influence of Spanish playwrights on the theater of Restoration England, not to mention Molière or Corneille.[14] It goes without saying that Sterne and Fielding were influenced by and not derivative of Cervantes, just as Góngora was influenced by Petrarch, without suffering for the influence.[15] The intersections of medical and literary cultures are somewhat clearer during the sixteenth century—when codes and genres (e.g. the Renaissance dialogue) were more often held in common—than during the seventeenth. But as Maravall pointed out, it was during the seventeenth century that medical language became more pervasive in many forms of textual production while, at the same time, the genres of medical writing became hidebound.

In light of the articles collected in this book, we can confidently draw three conclusions about the historical significance of the medical cultures found in the early modern Spanish empire. These conclusions are deceptively simple: there were many medical cultures; these cultures interacted; and they were medical cultures of the early modern Spanish empire.

First, and fundamentally, there were many medical cultures. Some of these were tied to institutional practices, longstanding traditions, or regional and ethnic identities. These cultures were either provisional and temporary or long lasting, but it is generally impossible to predict the conditions that contribute to the longevity or ephemerality of a particular medical culture. Crucially, however, practices related to health and sickness were undertaken to a great extent by people without formal

---

[14]   The influence of Spanish dramatists on the English stage is amply documented in *The Comedia in English Translation and Performance*, edited by Susan Paun de García and Donald R. Larson. The bibliography documenting the influence of Italian *commedia dell'arte* on Spanish is substantial. The classic studies include Falconieri, Shergold, and Arróniz. For more recent explorations, see Oleza, D'Antuono, Oliva, Ojeda Calvo, and Katritzky ("Stefanelo Botarga and Pickelhering").

[15]   The scholarship devoted to Cervantes's influence on the English novel is vast, but two recent collections summarize this research: *The Cervantean Heritage: Reception and Influence of Cervantes in Britain*, edited by J. A. G. Ardila; and *Cervantes in the English-Speaking World*, edited by Darío Fernández-Morera and Michael Hanke. On Góngora and Petrarch, see Navarrete's marvelous *Orphans of Petrarch*.

medical training who did not identify themselves as medical practitioners. This means that medical occupations and medical practices were not always related in discernible ways. The disentangling of practices and occupations helps explain the multiplicity of medical cultures we find.[16]

Second, medical cultures fit within a broader scheme of cultural exchange and appropriation. For the most part, there was no hegemonic medical culture (to the extent that hegemony indicates ideological conformity) and no medical monoculture. There was always a second opinion. And while it might be tempting to establish hierarchies among these cultures, there are so many exceptions to whatever hierarchy we might establish—such as the perceived superiority of expert or academic medicine to folk or lay medicine—that the attempt is nearly meaningless. For nearly every physician who denounced the superstition or *pseudodoxia* of the "vulgar" masses, there was another who believed the origins of authentic experimental medicine lay in popular practices.[17] Even from university to university, there was considerable variability; the traditions and practices of the universities of Alcalá, Valencia, Salamanca, and Zaragoza were all markedly different.[18]

The interactions of medical cultures often produced something new that did not gain currency as an alloy or hybrid, or even as a novelty; so one might associate a medical practice with mestizo people, but not think of the practice

---

[16]   The existence and coexistence of a variety of medical cultures during the early modern period has been studied by Jütte, in the introduction to *Historical Aspects of Unconventional Medicine: Approaches, Concepts, Case Studies*; Gentilcore, in *Healers and Healing in Early Modern Italy* and "Was there a 'Popular Medicine' in Early Modern Europe?"; Gijswijt-Hofstra, Marland, and De Waardt, in *Illness and Healing Alternatives in Western Europe*; and De Blécourt and Usborne, in "Preface: Situating 'alternative medicine' in the modern period." With respect to the Iberian Peninsula, the multiplicity of ideas surrounding illness and healing practices has been studied by Perdiguero Gil, López-Terrada ("Medical Pluralism"), and Zarzoso.

[17]   Juan Sorapán de Rieros was one physician who argued extensively that popular medicine contained in proverbs was superior to what was taught at universities. Sorapán de Rieros made three arguments about the importance of popular sayings: first, that they were the fruit of long experience ("experimentada verdad"); second, that they signified more transparently than medical discourse ("significan en cierto modo naturalmente"); and third, they best preserved ancient, authentically Spanish teachings: "antes que hubiese Philosophos en Grecia, tenia ya España fundada la antiguedad de sus Refranes." On these claims, see the prologue to Sorapán de Rieros's *Medicina Española*, published in two parts in Granada in 1615 by Juan Muñoz and republished in Madrid in 1615 by Martín Fernández Zambrano. The 1616 edition was republished in the nineteenth century, and two more editions followed in the twentieth.

[18]   On university instruction and variability, see Feingold and Navarro. Still the best source for a systematic overview of the institutional cultures of early modern Spain is José María López Piñero's *Ciencia y técnica en la sociedad espaìola de los siglos XVI y XVII*.

itself as mestizo.[19] Conversely, the origins of a practice or explanation might be disguised or unknown; a treatment might circulate as "Indian" or "the Friar's medicine" when it was neither. As in the cases of peyote (studied by Morales), or Dragon's Blood (in Bauer's case), or chymical medicine as it was practiced in Zaragoza (as Slater indicates), it may be easy to identify some of the sources of the practices described in this volume. But the fact remains that these practices are often discontinuous with their distant and even with their immediate antecedents. Morales' article demonstrates this most clearly. The origin of New Spanish uses of peyote was obviously an indigenous practice and the herb was sometimes understood as related to indigenous traditions; but it was harvested by a mulatto woman and used in ways that were not consonant with indigenous practice.

It is also important to note that medical cultures did not interact exclusively with themselves. Medical cultures shaped and were shaped by other cultural and ideological movements, formulations, and products. Medical cultures relied as much upon the construction of a new town square, convent, theater, or market, on the issuance of a new bureaucratic or Inquisitorial decree, on the survivorship of an epidemic, on the publication of a satire or the preaching of a sermon, or on the shifting ethnic demographics of a population on the move as they did on the words and actions of physicians, surgeons, barbers, midwives, and other medical practitioners.

Our third conclusion is that the objects of study in this volume represent the medical cultures of the early modern Spanish empire, whether we speak of Palermo or Pamplona. Medical cultures interacted on a scale that was commensurate with the size and variability of a global empire; we cannot say with any confidence that the characteristics we identify with a particular region or ethnic group were limited to that region or group. This is because one effect of empire was to abstract forms of cultural expression, practice, and production, denature them, and make them available to subjects elsewhere. The movement of Spaniards, the organization of the state, the demographic variability from kingdom to kingdom and continent to continent—all of these are related to the distribution and exercise of political power within a polity that was unique at the time. Some scholars have tended to assume that in some areas (e.g. Naples and Antwerp) there was relatively little relationship between the exercise of political power and the character of medicine and science; the organization of the Spanish state would seem to have no influence on medicine at moments that seem—to our way of thinking—to coincide suspiciously with twenty-first-century geopolitical realities. To say that Joan Baptista Van Helmont simply happened to be a subject of a Spanish king makes as much sense as saying that Titian happened to be Venetian. There is a related tendency to treat "Italy" as if it were a cultural monolith that conforms to the limits of the modern state of

---

[19] A fascinating discussion of hybridization and the controversies surrounding the concept in different disciplines can be found in Dean and Leibsohn. Helpful for clarifying the nature of hybridity in contemporary culture is García Canclini. On mestizo cultures and *mestizaje*, see Gruzinski's *The Mestizo Mind.*

the same name or to pretend that centuries of Iberian rule devastated Mexico but had no effect on Naples. Inexplicably, it is historiographically permissible to act as if Philip II's rule could explain something about the Castilian physician Andrés Laguna but not the Neapolitan Ferrante Imperato.

This tendency persists despite the fact that the political structure of the Hapsburg empire was quite uniform. The system of governance was basically the same in Sicily as it was in New Spain or Peru; both Sicily and Peru, for example, were conventionally called kingdoms (*reinos*) and both were governed through a viceregal system of *cortes* and *audiencias*.[20] In fact, if we look closely at the political realities of the empire, medical cultures all respond in their own ways to the monarch's lack of absolute prerogatives; the exercise of political power at the level of individual kingdoms of the composite monarchy, or even at the level of municipalities, is subject to compromises, pacts, negotiations, subversion, and resistance.[21] The tension between global ambition and local control is one of the most important factors that make the medical cultures we study belong to the early modern Spanish empire.

The consequence of these three conclusions is to place medicine within the growing scholarly consensus about the political, religious, artistic, commercial, and military cultures of early modern Spain. Although it extends the boundaries of the history of medicine, it does not dilute the concept of medicine. In the same way that scholars do not take the differences in the devotional practices associated with the virgin of Guadalupe and the virgin of Pilar, or the differing pronouncements of one metropolitan synod and another, or the disputes between Franciscans and Dominicans to mean that religion is a meaningless category, we do not find that tracing the full dimensions of medical cultures renders the study of early modern medicine less meaningful. Local input and variability indicate the robustness and not the dilution of religious culture.

Knowing what a given physician read or wrote, whether he died with money to leave his children or left this vale a pauper, what therapies he favored or anatomical dissections he witnessed—these will always be important facts to us and to the history of medicine. But they will represent only facets of a specific medical culture that coexists alongside others and is not perhaps even the most widespread or representative medical culture of its time or place. For this reason, we believe it necessary to resituate medicine and medical cultures more broadly within Spanish society. A disciplinary model is ill suited to explain how imperial subjects understood and responded to health and sickness; this book, however, is not "anti-disciplinary" in an antagonistic sense; it is disciplinarily agnostic, eschewing

---

[20] On the political similarities between the viceregal courts of New Spain and Sicily, see Ciaramitaro.

[21] For a lucid and authoritative explanation of composite monarchies and the degree of "disunity" in early modern Europe, see John H. Elliott's "A Europe of Composite Monarchies."

disciplinary limitations when they become a historiographic encumbrance or an anachronistic obstacle.

This book was first conceived of by three scholars—two working in Spain, one in the United States—during a time of economic crisis and deep skepticism about the ability of modern states to address social and cultural problems effectively, and in the shadow of anxieties about worsening economic inequality and environmental degradation. Our countries allow the management of healthcare to be dictated by monetary considerations that are the product of an economy of selfishness that presents itself as the only possible, even the natural solution to suffering. Although we seem to be constantly on the threshold of medical miracles, our grandparents may live longer than we do, thanks to a series of confounding personal decisions regarding our own health and confusing messages from a medical establishment that holds no hegemonic sway over the opinions that multiply in new media. In the United States, we live with outbreaks of disease, some of which have names that sound almost quaintly antiquated (whooping cough, measles) and others that sound improbably exotic (dengue fever, Chagas disease, murine typhus). In Spain, economic turmoil, different kinds of migration and movement, and another Catalonian quest for independence have led to widespread doubts about the configuration and governance of the state. It would seem as if things had changed very little since 1640, when Spain was wracked by instability and questions about its decline. The exercise and experience of global power has changed little; we export our values through military conquest or commerce. Our leaders seem eerily reminiscent of Philip II (philosophical and retiring, but capable of inspiring intense devotion) or Charles II (half-witted, profoundly inarticulate, and self-indulgent). And we live, as the subjects of the Spanish Hapsburgs did, uncertain of the extent to which our communication may be monitored by a grand bureaucracy (will someone be listening if I transmit the word "bomb" electronically?).

It is time that we better understood early modern Spain and its medical cultures.

PART 1
Spain and the New World
of Medical Cultures

Chapter 1
The Culture of Peyote: Between Divination and Disease in Early Modern New Spain[1]

Angélica Morales Sarabia

Introduction

Early in the seventeenth century, Agustín de Albarado believed himself to be bewitched. He was a poor herdsman from Tepecuaculco, New Spain, and as a mulatto he was socially marginalized.[2] With his health deteriorating, due, he believed, to the enchantment, Albarado made a decision that was not uncommon at the time: he consulted an Indian who, by means of a hallucinogenic herb known as *ololiuhqui*, would be able to divine the identity of the enchanter. After taking *ololiuhqui*, the Indian informed Albarado that the spell had been cast by someone named Nicolás, adding that only Nicolás himself could lift the spell.[3] Albarado's condition was worsening, so he went in search of Nicolás, riding more than 20 kilometers on horseback. At this point, Albarado himself began taking *ololiuhqui*, not as a means to learn Nicolás's whereabouts, but rather as medicine for his "malady and sickness."[4] It was this decision, born of sickness and desperation, that got him into trouble. Albarado was soon tried for his use of the hallucinogen by Hernán Ruiz de Alarcón, an implacable foe of all types of quackery (Peña 48). During his interrogation, however, Albarado insisted that he took *ololiuhqui* only as a medicine and not as a part of witchcraft, an account corroborated by the administrator of Peloncico.[5]

---

[1] This study was made possible by two grants: "Medical Geographies: Discourses, Practices and Representations of Medicine in New Spain (16th–18th centuries)," (sponsored by UNAM, PAPIIT IN 400911-3); and *Cultura médica en la periferia colonial: Nueva España, 1521–1621* (sponsored by the Ministerio de Ciencia e Innovación del Gobierno de España, HAR2009-11030-C02-01).
[2] The term "mulatto" was used to differentiate mixed-race persons with African ancestry from mestizos, Africans, Indians, and creoles. I recognize that many modern readers find the word objectionable, but it is unavoidable in discussions of the caste system of early modern New Spain.
[3] Archivo General de la Nación/Inquisición/vol. 303/f. 78. Subsequent references to the Archivo General de la Nación are abbreviated AGN.
[4] AGN/Inquisición/vol. 303/f. 78.
[5] AGN/Inquisición/vol. 303/f. 79.

This story contains a number of elements that became increasingly common in the Inquisitorial prosecution of the use of *ololiuhqui*, peyote, and other hallucinogenic plants. Race, social status, religion, the blurring of physical and emotional disorders, and the use of hallucinogenic herbs in both sorcery and medicine appeared constantly in the Inquisition's attempt to stamp out what we now recognize to be a complex culture of hallucinogens. Some of what we know about the use of peyote in New Spain can be found in erudite works of natural history or medicine. But physicians and naturalists tell us only part of the story.[6] Inquisitorial trials—particularly the trials of women accused of sorcery and witchcraft—constitute a richer and more varied source of information about the practices associated with hallucinogens in the early modern Spanish empire. Near the end of the sixteenth century and during the first half of the seventeenth, the Inquisition (also known as the Holy Office) prosecuted with particular vigor the use of natural and symbolic resources drawn from the indigenous world. The use of peyote and other hallucinogenic plants may have been related to pre-Columbian traditions, but it was alive in colonial homes where women—mothers, daughters, daughters-in-law, mulattoes, slaves, and domestic servants—lived in close-knit communities. By using herbs, women sought to pacify violent husbands or to find lost valuables and missing family members, among other quests. These daily domestic struggles and women's responses to them reflected the complex negotiations and disputes of the society at large.

Although hallucinogenic plants, their life histories, and their medicinal uses seem to have been part of colonial women's daily experience, sixteenth-century books by naturalists, physicians, and ecclesiastics show little interest in peyote and even less in women's use of hallucinogens. This would change in 1620 with an edict prohibiting the use of peyote. Once the use of peyote becomes a crime prosecuted by the Inquisition, women emerge as the central players in the evolving culture of hallucinogens. By looking first at sixteenth-century books that ignored women's participation in this culture, and then examining the Inquisitorial documents that attest to the rich interplay of varied social forces surrounding the use of hallucinogens, we can better understand how peyote functions as a nucleus around which new cultural practices are generated. In particular, the fascinating story of Petrona Babtista—who was tried by the Inquisition for her frequent peyote use—serves as a guide for understanding the confluence of race, gender, religion, and emerging medical cultures in seventeenth-century New Spain.

The problems inherent in using Inquisitorial documents to reconstruct colonial life are well known. Because these documents were generated in an atmosphere of intense social coercion, we must use them with caution, carefully consider

---

[6]   See Hernández, *Obras completas* (1959); Cárdenas, *Problemas y secretos maravillosos de Indias* (1591); Ruiz de Alarcón, *Tratado de las supersticiones y costumbres gentilicias que oy viuen entre los indios naturales desta Nueua España* (1629); Sahagún, *Historia general de las cosas de la Nueva España* (1985); Motolinía, *Historia de los indios de la Nueva España* (2007).

their reliability, and ask to what extent we can treat them as trustworthy (García Cárcel 100). This does not mean, however, that they are not a valuable resource for understanding the culture of New Spain (Jaffary; Perry; Flores and Masera). The Inquisitorial trials to which women were subjected yield a very particular kind of story, one in which women try to control and act upon the reality they experience. The documents these trials produced reveal a great deal about the material conditions of the period, the operative systems of symbolic signification, and ideas about the body in sickness and health. It was often the case that the medical practices Inquisitors did not understand or found unfamiliar were branded heterodox. As Solange Alberro explains in her influential *Inquisición y sociedad en México*, cures of all sorts became conflated with sorcery and witchcraft.[7] This is especially true in the case of peyote.

Antonio García de León maintains that each individual case brought before the Inquisition bears witness to the ways in which different cultures adapted themselves to one another. This adaptation led to the syncretism we find developing at the end of the sixteenth century and the beginning of the seventeenth. Inquisitorial documents or "processes" contain "a register of gods, incantations, healings, prayers, potions, positions and therapeutic methods" (García de León 582). Through these "registers" we can observe a society of hybridism and admixture, in which Europeans, Asians, Africans, and Indians mingle and compete for space and resources. Within this context, domestic spaces function as microcosms of the broader culture, a complete society in miniature that is markedly stratified, both socially and racially.

The domestic sphere could be a place of conflict, disagreement, and dispute, but it was also a place where new practices were generated and subsequently conserved.[8] Whether within the home or at the level of cities and regions, New Spain was not a place of nicely delineated borders where the spaces of indigenous inhabitants could be clearly differentiated from those of the newly arrived. Instead, it was a place of juxtaposition, of "contacts and layering" (Gruzinski, *Las cuatro partes* 44). In other words, New Spain circa 1600 was in the midst of an unfinished—perhaps even interminable—historical process, becoming a liminal space in which Mesoamerican, Spanish, African, and Asian cultures transformed one another.

---

[7]   Alberro notes that Inquisitorial archives tend not to define sorcery or witchcraft. She follows Evans Pritchard, who contends that witchcraft was primarily an imaginary offense, as psychic elements were its prime components.

[8]   Here I turn to David N. Livingstone's belief that spaces are generated and occupied within the mesh of social relations (11). The production of one of these spaces can be seen as the result of social action. According to this point of view, space and time intermingle in complex social processes. This idea enables me to elucidate domestic space as a primary venue for social action and, as such, the place where the new geography of hallucinogenic plants became visible.

Inquisition, Culture, and Witchcraft

It has been over 50 years since Gonzalo Aguirre Beltrán wrote his pioneering *Medicina y magia* (1963), a work that drew heavily on Inquisitorial documents and in so doing transformed scholarship on the medical cultures of New Spain. In his wide-ranging analysis, Aguirre Beltrán concluded that the practices that emerged from the contact between Mesoamerican cultures and the new settlers were distorted iterations of ancestral usages, containing "extraneous," foreign elements that contaminated indigenous traditions (144). He was much more interested in examining how these "original" and "ancestral" traditions were maintained in the face of Inquisitorial coercion than he was in considering how new cultures, symbols, and practices might have been generated through mutual influence. Aguirre Beltrán is not wrongheaded in thinking that Indians resorted to a series of stratagems to hide their ancient beliefs and gods from Catholic priests and tribunals. But he did not consider, for example, how the renaming of the threefold entity of the Huicholes (corn, deer, peyote) in Roman Catholic terms (Jesus, Our Lady, Saint Rosa María, Saint Nicholas, Saint Anthony, etc.) might do something other than simply conserve or fail to conserve preexisting practices (148–9). The same Inquisitorial documents upon which Aguirre Beltrán relied can provide us with a sense of how the act of renaming is not just a symptom of what is lost or saved, but a conceptual map of the new spaces for the intermingling of cultures.

The catalogues of judicial archives are organized according to the misdeeds that, on the authority of the Inquisition, infringed upon faith or morality. Crimes against morality—such as bigamy, solicitation, singing, and dancing—were more common than witchcraft and sorcery (Rodríguez Delgado 115). The most commonly prosecuted acts were, by order of frequency: heresy, religious misdemeanors, solicitation, and sexual transgressions.[9] But it is in the prosecution of witchcraft that we can learn a great deal about how hallucinogenic herbs were used as instruments in the practice of divination and sorcery.

Peyote and *ololiuhqui* are the hallucinogenic herbs mentioned most often in Inquisitorial documents.[10] There is a reason that hallucinogens caught the attention

---

[9]   Alberro (207) mentions two statistics. The first is based on the Riva Palacio collection, Vol. 49 (AGN), and presents 138 cases of sorcery and witchcraft between 1571 and 1700 (7.2 percent of all cases tried). The second statistic is based on the *Abecedario de relaxados, reconciliados y penitenciarios* (Index of the relaxed, the reconciled and the penitentiary), a manuscript to be found in the Huntington Library in San Marino, California. Here, the total is 121 cases for the same period (8.3 percent of all cases tried).

[10]   *Puyomate* is also mentioned, but this plant has not been identified botanically to date. Nohemí Quesada points out that no pre-Hispanic references have been found concerning *puyomate*. Quesada says the plant was used in "love magic" and was required to attract or repel another person. It is described as a root with a pungent smell and a sexual identity (male or female). Enrique Flores and Mariana Masera have found references to *puyomate* in which it is described as hairy and having a feminine or masculine form.

of the Inquisition: the skilled use of specific herbs and roots—particularly those with the dramatic effects of peyote—implied dominion over nature itself. Some of the women on trial knew where the herbs grew or, at least, the parts of the plant that produced the most powerful effect. They knew how the herbs would affect the body and how to prepare them (whether they were to be used fresh or dried, etc.). It is at least conceivable that many of the women accused of witchcraft and sorcery were extra-academic medical practitioners. But there is a great deal that is not immediately apparent about women's knowledge of herbs, including the women's beliefs about the body and disease, their ideas about the particular ailments that afflicted them, and their awareness of any given therapeutic practice.

Although it may be possible to learn, in greater or lesser measure, what women thought about disease by analyzing Inquisitorial documents, we cannot retrospectively diagnose diseases. Such an attempt would be a pointless exercise in anachronism. Jon Arrizabalaga persuasively explains that an insurmountable barrier exists between our present and the past when it comes to finding the biological origins of illness. Disease is multidimensional; it is a biological event, it contributes to the formation of social roles, and it serves as a vehicle for sanctioning cultural norms. In this sense, disease is neither "natural" nor "trans-historical" (Arrizabalaga, "Nuevas tendencias"). Through a careful consideration of Inquisitorial documents, however, we can learn a great deal about how women attempted to treat disease or sought medical remedies to what we might now consider to be non-medical dilemmas.

Hallucinogenic Plants and Sixteenth-Century Natural History

The natural histories and medical texts composed during the sixteenth century contain numerous references to peyote and other hallucinogenic herbs, although they do not associate the use of these plants with women. The physician Francisco Hernández, for example, reported on two different varieties of peyote. One of these he described as the Zacatecan variety:

> [...] which does not sprout rootlets or leaves above ground, but only a sort of fuzz adhering to it, for which reason it is hard to draw properly. They say that there is a male and female variety. It is sweet and moderately warm. When crushed and applied to the skin it is said to cure joint pain. Prodigious things

They state that it was used extensively in the sixteenth century in the context of "erotic magic," but also for casting evil spells (50). I have located two cases where *puyomate* is mentioned. It is described in both as a root, used in love witchcraft. The first took place in Villa de San Miguel de Culiacán (state of Sinaloa) and the other in Cuencame (state of Durango), AGN/Inquisición/vol. 360/exp. 173/f. 517 and AGN/Inquisición/vol. 356/exp. 163/f. 336, respectively. I infer that a third case may deal with *puyomate*, as it describes the same procedures of love witchcraft. The *çacate* is chewed and later spat out upon the clothes of the man to be seduced. The *çacate* grows under mesquite shrubs (AGN/Inquisición/vol. 356/exp. 163/f. 332).

are said about this root (if we are to accept the opinion widely held among the population), such as that those who eat it can foresee and predict all things: whether, for example, an enemy is to attack the next day, or if better times are ahead; the identity of the thief who stole a utensil or any other object; and many other similar things that the Chichimecas try to investigate by means of this drug. Also, when they wish to discover where this root is hidden under the ground, they discover it by eating another. It grows in humid and limy ground.[11]

Hernández says that he could not draw the plant because it had no branches or leaves above ground. This, when combined with his description of the plant as "sweet," probably means that he had dried samples mixed with honey.[12] Hernández also collected information on a type of peyote that he called the Xochimilcan variety. He described it as:

> [...] excellent medicine, with a thick root, cylindrical and covered with down; other roots look like nuts in shape and size that branch off the principal root here and there; the single stalk is green, cylindrical and soft, with scant leaves similar to those of the pear tree, with purple peduncles, and at the end of the stalks yellow flowers contained in a scarious calyx. Its temperament is cold; one dram of the root is taken against fevers, and also against the flux of the belly.[13]

In Hernández's description a terminological problem appears that will continue to plague naturalists, physicians, and pharmacists until well into the nineteenth

---

[11]   "[...] una raíz de mediano tamaño que no echa ninguna ramas ni hojas fuera de la tierra, si no sólo una pelusa adherida a ella, por lo cual no puede dibujarla debidamente. Dicen que hay macho y hembra. Es de gusto dulce y de calor moderado. Machacado y aplicado dicen que cura los dolores de las articulaciones. Cuentan de esta raíz algo maravilloso (si hemos de dar fe a una creencia muy entendida entre ellos), y es que quienes la comen presienten y predicen todas las cosas: si, por ejemplo, han de atacarlos al día siguiente los enemigos, si les esperan tiempos felices, quién robó un utensilio o cualquier otro objeto, y otras cosas semejantes que los chichimecas tratan de investigar por medio de esa droga. También cuando quieren saber dónde se encuentra dicha raíz escondida en la tierra, lo averiguan comiéndose otra. Nace en lugares húmedos y calizos" (Hernández t. III, vol. II: 92).

[12]   Hernández's comment on the difficulty of drawing peyote is very interesting. In the *Florentine Codex* peyote is described; the *tlacuilo* (Indian artist) drew the cactus as such. I can only make out the *ticitl* (Indian doctor) drinking *peiotl*. According to Richard Evans Schultes and Albert Hofmann, the first botanical illustration ever made of *Lophophora wiliamsii* is dated 1847 (134). In Mexico, probably the first botanical illustrations of peyote were the work of Antonio Tenorio. Tenorio was the chief illustrator of the National Medical Institute (Tenorio).

[13]   "[...] medicina brillante, tiene raíz gruesa, cilíndrica y cubierta de pelusa, además de otras semejantes a nueces en forma y tamaño que nacen aquí y allí de la mayor; tallo verde, único cilíndrico y blando, hojas ralas parecidas a las del peral, con pendúnculos purpúreos, y en el extremo de los tallos flores amarillas contenidas en cálices escariosos. Su temperamento es frío, de suerte que la raíz se toma en dosis de una dracma contra las fiebres y también contra el flujo de vientre" (Hernández t. III, vol. II: 92).

century. In Mesoamerican medical practice, it was quite common to give the same name to plants that had no botanical relationship with each other; instead they might have had a similar morphological trait or therapeutic action that caused them to be associated. It is probable that many of the Inquisitorial cases that make up our documentary corpus are related to "false peyotes" (i.e. any number of species that might be called "peyote").[14] These are almost impossible to identify definitively, in part because the transcripts of the trials do not include physical descriptions of the plants. The Inquisitors generally referred to peyote simply as an "herb" or "root."

In addition to Hernández, Toribio Motolinía and Juan de Cárdenas, among others, wrote about peyote during the sixteenth century. Cárdenas was, like Hernández, a physician. In his *Problemas y secretos maravillosos de Indias* (1591), Cárdenas shows himself to be ambivalent about hallucinogenic effects. At times, the vocabulary he uses to make sense of New World drugs is drawn from European flora: mandrake, henbane, and black nightshade enabled him to explain peyote, *puyomate*, and *ololiuhqui*. At other times, however, Cárdenas reproduces discourses about religious heterodoxy: in describing the effects of the plants, he invokes images of witches, potions, and the devil. This is hardly surprising (Viesca Treviño 45). The seventeenth century was a period of intense interest in witchcraft and sorcery (Bel Bravo). It was also a period in which manuscripts on demonology were common.[15]

Cárdenas recognized that peyote, "poyomate," and "hololisque," if administered as drinks, could cause horrific damage, but that they could also be used as beneficial food or medicine when prepared properly (Cárdenas 33–4).

---

[14]   Taking into account the descriptions of peyote made by Hernández in the sixteenth century, Fernando Altamirano and José Ramírez, three centuries later (1889–1915), undertook botanical and pharmacological studies of peyote and false peyotes for the National Medical Institute (209–10). Several decades later, Albert Hofmann and Richard Evans described the species *Aricarpus retusus*, *Coriphantha compacta*, and *Epitelantha micromeris* (from the Tarahumara región), various species of *Mammillaria* (also from the Tarahumara region), and *Pelecyphora aselliformis* and included them among the false peyotes (Schultes and Hofmann 75). They all grow in the north of Mexico and they all have hallucinogenic effects. However, the peyote that has exhibited the greatest psychoactivity is *Lophophora williamsii*, which contains mescaline, one of 30 alkaloids to be found in these cacti, and which is responsible for hallucinogenic activity. But it is not the only cactus with powerful effects; there is also *Lophophora diffusa*, which is simpler in its chemical composition and differs in various morphological traits. Yet both plants grow in stony desert regions, and almost exclusively in limy soil.

[15]   Javier Puerto points out that the *Reprobación de las supersticiones y hechicerías* by Pedro Sánchez Ciruelo (1470–1548) was widely read throughout the sixteenth century (*La leyenda verde* 299). The various editions of the work speak of a reading public deeply interested in these topics and, to a considerable extent, reflect a society in which there was not always a clear difference between superstition and orthodox belief when trying to explain natural phenomena.

The list of plants with this twofold quality is long and not limited to hallucinogenic herbs.[16] As Juan de Cárdenas writes:

> [...] in many torrid lands in New Spain, certain little apples are grown, of which the outside pulp can be eaten (and is quite tasty) but the inside is deadly poison. And it is truly said about peyote and poyomate, and about hololisque, that if taken by mouth they so truly deprive the poor wretch of his wits that he goes out of his mind; he is visited by the devil, among other terrible and dreadful ghosts, who gives him news, so they say, of things to pass, and all this must be appearances and tricks of Satan, whose talent is to mislead, with divine permission, the miserable wretch.[17]

According to the precepts of Hippocrates and Galen, all plants had virtues and acted on the human body. But the effects that could be expected were limited: nature contained medicinal plants to cure, poisons to kill, and food to give sustenance to the body. The appearance of ghosts and dark visions, the capacity to see the past and predict the future, and the other effects that Indians and Africans claimed they could achieve after eating or drinking certain intoxicating plants could only be the work of the devil, never a natural effect caused by the plant (Cárdenas 274–5).

Toribio Motolinía does not mention peyote, but he does write about *octli* (now known as *pulque*, a mildly alcoholic beverage) and *teonanacates* (mushrooms of the psylocibe family). Motolinia explains that the Indians call these mushrooms *teunanacatlth*, which in their language means "the flesh of God" (quickly correcting this to "flesh of the devil"). He says they worship the mushroom and disapproves of the frenzied gatherings where Indians consume it. Specifically, Motolinia claims that the mushrooms make the Indians cruel and soulless:

> They had yet another form of drunkenness that made them more cruel; and it was with certain small mushrooms found in these lands as in Castile; they are eaten raw, and because they are bitter, after eating them they take some honey; but the mushrooms from this land are of a type that they quickly produce a thousand visions, especially snakes, and as [the Indians] are quite out of their senses, they feel that their limbs and body are full of vermin that are eating them alive, and thus half crazed, they go outside hoping that somebody will kill them.[18]

---

[16]   Some of the hallucinogenic plants that appear in the Inquisitorial trials, like *tlapatl*, *toloache*, and *ololiuhqui*, were used topically as poultices for pain, gout, rheumatism, and arthritis.

[17]   "[...] en muchas tierras calientes de la Nueva España, se cogen ciertas mançanillas, que la pulpa de afuera es de comer, (y no poco sabrosa) siendo lo interior veneno mortífero. Cuéntase con verdad del peyote del poyomate, y del Hololisque que, si se toman por la boca, sacan tan deveras de juicio al miserable que las toma que entre otras terribles, y espantosas phantasmas se les representa el demonio, y aun les da noticia según dizen de cosas por venir, y debe ser todo trazas, y embustes de Sathanás, cuya propiedad es engañar con permission divina, al miserable que en semejantes ocasiones le busca" (Cárdenas 11).

[18]   "Tenían otra manera de embriaguez que los hacía más crueles, y era con unos hongos o setas pequeñas, que en esta tierra las hay como en Castilla; mas los de esta tierra

What we now might recognize as the release of pent-up emotions looked like torture to an uninitiated observer. Motolinía found himself forced to conclude that only the devil would submit men and women to such horrors:

> [...] to them [the Indians] it was a great bother to hear the word of God, and they didn't wish to indulge in anything other than their vices and sins, giving themselves to sacrifices and feasts, eating and drinking and getting drunk in these feasts, and feeding their idols with their own blood; this they extracted from their ears, tongues or arms, and other parts of their bodies, [...] some calling upon the devil, others drunk, and still others singing and dancing; they would beat drums, blow horns, trumpets and great seashells, especially in celebrations of their devils. [...] Before they boil their wine with roots, it is clear and sweet like honey and water. After boiling with the roots, it becomes slightly thicker and smells bad, and those who get drunk on it smell even worse. Usually, they would start drinking after vespers [...] and by the time night came, they were passing out, or falling down, or singing, or yelling mightily calling the devil.[19]

For Cárdenas and Motolinía, the use of intoxicating plants by the indigenous peoples of the New World could not be differentiated from superstition, idolatry, and the deceptions of the devil. Neither in the sixteenth-century descriptions of Cárdenas nor in those of Motolinía do women appear as important characters. But women would take on a new centrality during the seventeenth century, especially in the transcripts of Inquisitorial trials.

The first "edict of faith" which forbade the use of "the herb or root called peyote" was published in 1620. The Inquisitors deemed the use of this plant

---

son de tal calidad, que comidos crudos y por ser amargos, beben tras ellos o comen con ellos un poco de miel de abejas; y de allí a poco rato veían mil visiones, en especial culebras, y como salían fuera de todo sentido, parecíales que las piernas y el cuerpo tenían lleno de gusanos que los comían vivos, y así medio rabiado se salían fuera de casa, deseando que alguno los matase" (Motolinía 24).

[19] "[...] a ellos [los indios] les era gran fastidio oír la palabra de Dios, y no querían entender en otra cosa sino en darse a vicios y pecados, dándose a sacrificios y fiestas, comiendo y bebiendo y embeodándose en ellas, y dando de comer a los ídolos de su propia sangre, la cual sacaban de sus propias orejas, lengua y brazos, y de otras partes del cuerpo, ... unos llamando a el demonio, otros borrachos, otros cantando y bailando; tañían atabales, bocinas, cornetas y caracoles grandes, en especial en las fiestas de sus demonios. Las beoderas que hacían muy ordinarias, es increíble el vino que [en] ellas gastaban, y lo que cada uno en el cuerpo metía. Antes que a su vino lo cuezan con unas raíces que le echan, es claro y dulce como aguamiel. Después de cocido hácese algo espeso, y tiene mal olor, y los que con él se embeodan, mucho peor. Comúnmente comenzaban a beber después de vísperas, y dábanse tanta prisa a beber de diez en diez, o quince en quince, y los escanciadores que no cesaban, y la comida que no era mucha, a prima noche ya van perdiendo el sentido, ya cayendo, ya estando cantando y dando voces llamaban al demonio" (Motolinía 24).

contrary to the "purity and sincerity" of the Catholic faith.[20] The Inquisitors could not accept the notion that the herb might possess "the virtue and natural efficacy" that its proponents claimed. Not surprisingly, Inquisitors denied outright the possibility that it had magical properties or could facilitate the apparition of ghosts or spirits in acts of divination.[21] The same edict established that any person who used the plant would be excommunicated and risk further monetary or corporal punishments, to be administered by the Inquisition. It was also strictly forbidden that "any person, of any rank or condition might use peyote or any other herb with similar effects, or any other effect, under any name, or color, or induce Indians or other people to use them with similar intent."[22] Despite the clarity and vehemence of the edict of 1620, the Inquisition did not put a halt to the use of peyote in multiple regions of New Spain.

Upon the request of the commissioner of the Inquisition, the contents of the edict were made public in the cathedral of Guadalajara during Lent of 1619, a year before the edict was published. In 1621, representatives of the Inquisition gathered in Guadalajara to discuss edicts related to sorcery and superstition. Inquisitors summoned Domingo Velasco, prior of the convent of Santo Domingo in the city of Guadalajara, to testify.

Velasco explained that there had been a number of practical problems related to the edict of 1620. Upon the revelation of the contents of the edict, people started to tell their confessors about their experiences with the herbs. And thus the problem: confessors were not sure whether they should refer their parishioners to the commissioner of the Inquisition or take matters into their own hands, because before the publication of the edicts it was common knowledge that:

> [...] in all this kingdom there has been in the past much abuse of strong herbs as well as divination according to the lines of the hands and the features of the face and the use of the herb known as peyote to know about things that have been stolen or other things past and future.[23]

The Inquisitors decided that an admission of past use of hallucinogens could be dealt with locally, but those who persisted in using the plants after the publication of the edict and in defiance of its instructions would be referred to the commissioner of the Inquisition. This decision demonstrates a tacit recognition that the population

---

[20]   AGN/Inquisición/vol. 289/exp. 12/Edicto de fe de 1620 contra "la hierba o raíz del peyote."

[21]   AGN/Inquisición/vol. 289/exp. 12.

[22]   AGN/Inquisición/vol. 289/exp. 12. In an interesting case, Fray Rodrigo Alonso, an officer of the Inquisition in Texcoco, asked for the acquittal of a woman who was obliged to grind peyote for some men who were prospecting for mines. (The pagination is unclear; it may read 3, 31, or 16.) (AGN/Inquisición/vol. 373/exp. 3.)

[23]   AGN/Inquisición/vol. 340/1620/f. 25v. "Porque [existía] en todo este reyno a avido por lo pasado mucho abuso en materia de yerbas fuertes y adivinaçiones por las rayas de las manos y fisionomia de los rostros y uso de la yerba que llaman peyote para saver de las cosas hurtadas y otras cossas passadas y porvenir."

of New Spain—across geographic, ethnic, and religious boundaries—had great faith in these plants and even venerated them.

The publication of the edict was an important event, not only for Inquisitors and confessors, but also for the women who later testified before the religious tribunal. Women's magical practices were of particular concern to the Inquisition. According to the dictionary definition in the *Tesoro de la Lengua Castellana o Española* (1611), sorcery was practiced by men and women alike. It was, however, "more common" in women because the devil always found them easier to beguile; this was due to their nature, which was "insidiously vengeful" and "envious" (544). Some of the women who testified before the Inquisition would "remember," if only vaguely, an encounter with the plant before 1620; confessing to a loose recollection of something in the distant past may have been a ploy to avoid further suspicion. Other women claimed that they had not heard of the edict and never intended to defy the Inquisition through their use of peyote. Still others claimed to have knowledge of such herbs, but knew it to be "a forbidden thing and very weighty."[24]

The Crossroads of Gender and Race: The Territory of Taximaroa

The culture that developed around the use of peyote and other herbs was not just an attempt to preserve the indigenous practices of healers such as the *ticitl* or the *pahini*. A *pahini* is "he who takes the medicine." Inquisitorial documents show that in some cases a petitioner (ready to pay to have her physical, existential, or material problems resolved) would seek the help of a specialist, such as a *pahini* well versed in the knowledge and techniques of magic and the healing arts. The *pahini* himself, not the petitioner, would ingest the plant so that it might reveal to him the origin of the petitioner's malady (López Austin and López Luján 228). In other cases, however, mulattoes, mestizos, and Spanish women ingested the drugs themselves in search of their own answers.

People could acquire peyote in the markets (*tianguis*) of Mexico City, Huequechula, or Taximaroa. There they found vendors who sold herbs, flowers, and roots, along with instructions on how to prepare them, both as food and as

---

[24] AGN/Inquisición/exp. 32/f. 448–50v. Letter against Juana Baptista and her daughter, María Gutiérrez, dated 29 September, 1608. As Juana Baptista testified, Indian women consumed peyote in the still of the night, which was apparently the appropriate way to commune with the plant. One had to take pains to avoid exasperating or annoying it. Juana's husband, Diego, was the watchman of a hermitage and they lived in San Bartolomé. The story of Juana and her daughter, María Gutierrez, who lived in Huaquechula, Puebla, was not uncommon. One of the two women had lost an article of clothing. To find out where it was, Juana and María were responsible for procuring peyote, candles, and a few grains of *quololoche* (probably *ololiuhqui*), so that an Indian woman might eat the peyote and divine the location of the lost object for them. Both spent the night in the home of an Indian woman who ate peyote in an attempt to find a skirt they had lost.

medicines. Peyote was relatively inexpensive, about half the cost of a candle, and the vendors did a brisk trade.[25] These marketplaces were more than places to hawk wares; they were spaces for interaction and cultural negotiation. Like churches, markets functioned as sites of social exchange that left their imprint on everyday life in New Spain.[26]

Some people resorted to peyote when their problem was very grave or when, driven by despair, it seemed there was no alternative. The most common reasons that women took peyote were in order to find lost possessions,[27] to locate missing people,[28] and the infidelity of a partner or spouse.[29] The desire to recover something lost, to peer into the unknown, as well as family squabbles and the complex culture surrounding the procurement and use of peyote, all come together in the story of Petrona Babtista, one of the most fascinating episodes to emerge from the Inquisitorial trials.

In 1630, everyday life in Taximaroa (now Ciudad Hidalgo), in the province of Michoacán, was upended when several of its inhabitants were summoned to testify before Cristóbal Vaz, commissioner of the Inquisition. Whole families appeared to inform on one another for having used forbidden herbs. Once the questioning started, they seemed to pay little heed to the consequences. In order to "keep a clear conscience" it was preferable to tell the truth rather than to cover up crimes against the faith. Many fingers were pointed at a mulatto woman named Petrona Babtista, the wife of an unemployed man named Juan de León (also known as Juan del Monte).

Petrona was the mother of Mariana, who was married to a Spaniard named Juan Bernal. Both mother and daughter were accused before the Holy Office for using herbs. Petrona was not well liked in her family circle; she had been caught up in scandal and showed little interest in "attending mass and other obligatory

---

[25]   AGN/Inquisición/vol. 335/exp. 96/f. 372–3.

[26]   A number of scholars who have studied the barter of plants and animals in the alimentary culture of early modernity agree that syncretism developed more rapidly around the use of medicinal plants than it did with foodstuffs (Domingo).

[27]   AGN/Inquisición/vol. 284/exp. 32/f. 550–55.

[28]   AGN/Inquisición/vol. 335/exp. 96/f. 2. In this case, Ana María de Soria asks an Indian to help her find a young mestizo woman (14 or 15 years old) who lives in Ana María's home. The Indian ingests the peyote, but the herb does not "speak to his heart," so he is unable to tell Ana María where the young woman might be. The story is highly unsettling due to the fear expressed by Ana María concerning reprimands she is likely to receive from her brother or her husband (AGN/Inquisición/vol. 342/exp. 15/f. 356). María de Castro—after ordering masses to pray for finding her daughter and praying to various saints and virgins, without results—resorts to an Indian (she claims she can't recall whether male or female) who takes *ololiuhqui* to try and divine the whereabouts of her daughter.

[29]   AGN/Inquisición/vol. 335/exp. 59/f. 256. In this case, Damiana de Fuentes was on bad terms with her husband, Gaspar Marroquín, because he was chasing after another woman. Acting on the advice of an Indian woman, she bought some peyote, which the Indian woman ate. The plant spoke to the healer, who in turn told Damiana to stop worrying and entrust her husband to God. This set Damiana's mind at ease.

virtuous acts."[30] She regularly used peyote to find out about her husband's acts of unfaithfulness. The transcript does not say how Petrona learned about peyote, where she found it, or how she learned to prepare it. But, clearly, she was well versed in the plant's life cycle and uses. It was an open secret that she knew when to harvest and consume it. Her 18-year-old niece, María de Baldecañas, claimed that Petrona was fond of peyote; María further remembered that about three years before, Petrona had told her that she was still drinking peyote, "sometimes for her health, other times to see who had been stealing things."[31] It was this last claim—that Petrona had used peyote for divination—that the Inquisition pursued insistently during their interrogations.

Isabel Ximénez, the wife of the storekeeper Antonio Díaz de Villa, accused Petrona of taking peyote to find out with whom her husband was flirting. Isabel knew perfectly well that peyote was forbidden.[32] Petrona probably did, too. By 1630, 10 years had passed since the Inquisition published the edict of faith against the "herb or root known as peyote," and it seems unlikely that the prohibition simply slipped Petrona's mind.[33]

The list of accusers against Petrona kept growing. In addition to the names of María de Baldecañas and Isabel Ximénez was added that of Ximénez's sister-in-law María García. García was 34 years old and married to a local landowner. María recounted that seven months previously, one Sunday after mass, she spoke to Petrona's daughter, Mariana, who told María that Petrona was drinking peyote to learn of her husband's dalliances. The last time that Petrona had been under the effects of the herb, she had managed to see the object of her husband's affection, but the experience was so powerful that "the peyote," addressing Petrona directly, "told Petrona to call her daughters so that they could take her (to her husband) because he was in hell." The peyote further instructed that it was only in the presence of his daughters that her husband would decide to change his ways.[34]

Petrona, however, was not on trial simply for using peyote. She was on trial as a mulatto, a term used broadly to refer to many midwives, slaves, and servant women. At the beginning of the seventeenth century there was a sharp increase in the number of free Africans and mulattoes in New Spain.[35] The population was increased in equal measure by the slave trade and births in New Spain. Slave revolts had caused fear in both Spanish and Indian villages. Although Spanish

---

[30] AGN/Inquisición/vol. 340/exp. 28/f. 362.

[31] AGN/Inquisición/vol. 340/exp. 28/f. 362.

[32] AGN/Inquisición/vol. 340/ exp. 28/f. 361.

[33] AGN/Inquisición/vol. 340/ exp. 28/f. 361.

[34] AGN/Inquisición/vol. 340/ exp. 28/f. 363.

[35] Antonio García de León points out that, alongside the consolidation of colonial order, processes linked to the "manumission and social insertion" of free black people were widespread. Freed slaves became more numerous than slaves and came to dominate certain rural and urban venues, even achieving privileged positions. The descendants of these Africans became the second largest population group after Indians and, towards the end of the sixteenth century, were greater in number than the "whites" (538).

mistrust of Africans grew, fear did not put a stop to the slave trade, which reached its peak between 1580 and 1640.[36] Fear and mistrust on the one hand, and a growing mulatto population on the other, may account for the increase in the number of mulatto women and men tried for sorcery, witchcraft, and magic, as well as the social pressure exerted by New Spanish authorities on this specific group.

The efforts of Spanish elites to maintain race- and caste-based stratification were continually resisted by mestizos, Africans, mulattoes, and impoverished Spaniards. Sometimes resistance took the form of open defiance. On other occasions—as Nora Jaffary's study of "false mystics" suggests—forms of resistance were more subtle. Jaffary shows that the "false" mystical visions and ecstasies of poor women wove together daily concerns and direct access to divinity, combining the quotidian and the ethereal so as to make racial and social hierarchies more flexible (Jaffary 62–9). The claim to have seen a world unlike one's own, in which God speaks indiscriminately to poor and rich, black and white, was felt to be socially destabilizing; the visions produced by peyote, when experienced by mulattoes, may have been similarly threatening.

Tempestuous and frequently unpredictable, peyote itself is one of the most interesting characters in Inquisitorial documents. New Spaniards as well as Indians believed the plant took on a life of its own. This, at least, is how Petrona and some of the more veteran colonists in Taximaroa understood it. The more experienced inhabitants claimed that it could be temperamental; it might help when it chose, but it might also decline. Petrona was completely convinced that she could communicate with peyote as she might with a person: "When I drank it in the dry season, the peyote would feel good and thank me."[37] It felt so good that it would tell Petrona who in the community was well or ill disposed towards her, and also who was being unfaithful.[38] However, if she drank it in the wet season, "it would get very angry and tell me that I must be very desperate if I was looking for it then."[39]

Building New Symbolic and Therapeutic Spaces

We have begun to see that economic instability, racial oppression, and cultural hybridity are important factors in Petrona's story. To understand her milieu better, it might be helpful to know more about life in her village, Taximaroa. Although precise data on Taximaroa around 1630 is unavailable, information on the

---

[36]   Jonathan I. Israel underscores that the growth of the slave trade coincided with the dynastic union of Spain and Portugal (1580–1640), when both empires were ruled by a single king. "Portuguese slave traffickers," notes Israel, were in charge of transporting slaves toward New Spain (75).

[37]   The first author who mentions this is Gonzalo Aguirre Beltrán, who confirms that the dry season is the best time for using peyote (151).

[38]   AGN/Inquisición/vol. 340/exp. 28/f. 362.

[39]   AGN/Inquisición/vol. 340/ exp. 28/f. 362.

nearby province of Acámbaro is plentiful. Because both places share common characteristics in terms of settlement, organization of agricultural production, and geography, Acámbaro makes a useful stand-in for Taximaroa (Acuña IX: 59). Acámbaro once belonged to Nuño de Chavez's *encomienda* (land and Indian populations granted to a Spanish lord), and was known for its abundance of mesquite. The fruit of the mesquite was used to feed Indians and livestock, as the region's magistrate, Cristóbal de Vargas Valadés, reported in 1580. That same year, agricultural production included corn, as well as wheat, barley, and fruit trees introduced from Spain. The land was irrigated by two large rivers, so its fertile soil ensured the population plentiful food (Acuña IX: 59). It was not, however, idyllic.

In 1580, Acámbaro had about 2,600 inhabitants, a population that had been culled by a "pestilence" that had spread over all the territory of New Spain over the previous four years (Acuña IX: 60). The magistrate in charge of gathering the information about the epidemic had heard that "in the old days you could see many old people in these lands" (Acuña IX: 64). All this changed drastically with the "pestilences." Disease offered no respite to the indigenous population, and was particularly unforgiving of the elderly and the very young. Nobody seemed to know the cause for certain, and the belief that it was simply "the divine order of things" was widespread (Acuña IX: 64).

Taximaroa, where Petrona lived, and Acámbaro were territories in which African, European, and Mesoamerican cultures intermingled. The Chichimeca, Otomí, Mazahuan, Tarascan, and Spanish languages were spoken. Slaves spoke their own languages, although the "most general" among all of them was the Tarascan (Acuña IX: 64). This Babel was the backdrop against which Petrona "converted" to peyote. It was a venue riddled with misunderstandings and mutual dependencies, in which no inhabitant could survive without the others.

Land in Acámbaro was organized into agricultural dependencies throughout the Colonial period. This was also the case in the neighboring regions of the Bajío, the Central Plateau, and in the south (Tutino 9–372). In the case of Acámbaro, Indians were allowed to keep some land that they probably used for agriculture (mostly corn) during the wet season; they were also employed as day laborers in haciendas owned by Spaniards (Acuña IX: 60). The system by which land was organized was part of a broader effort by Spanish elites to maintain a strictly stratified society.

According to the "Relaciones Geográficas de Nueva Galicia" (Geographic Account of New Galicia), the people of Acámbaro were divided into two groups: the first was Spaniards; the second group was people of "reasonable understanding," shorthand for the Indians believed to be given to drunkenness (Acuña IX: 60).[40] The ritual and profane uses of *octli*—which prior to the Spanish conquest had been closely regulated within Mesoamerican societies—were disrupted, and in just a few decades the thirst for *octli* and other alcoholic beverages became a

---

[40] On the *Relaciones Geográficas de Nueva Galicia*, see the chapter by Pardo-Tomás in this volume.

social and public health problem. For the indigenous cultures of North America and Mesoamerica, the introduction of distilled liquor was just one more step in the domination process set in motion by the colonists (Ginzburg 141–2).

In the case of alcohol, we find that colonization disrupted the traditional means to regulate consumption; subsequently, the Inquisition and civil authorities attempted to impose a new regime of control. Something similar may have happened in the use of hallucinogenic plants. It may be that the effects of these plants were genuinely interpreted as the work of the devil, supernatural influences that had to be suppressed with any and all resources, as Cárdenas and Motolinía claimed. After the edict of 1620, it is also possible that peyote and related herbs were a pretext used by the Catholic Church to bring the local population under more effective control. Yet, regardless of how we interpret the response of the Church, hallucinogenic plants occupied a symbolic and therapeutic space that was constantly under construction. The plants were a powerful palliative agent that imbued individuals with a sense of control over their reality. The plants knew everything and cured everything. This knowledge exerted an undeniable attraction for the inhabitants of the new settlements at the end of the sixteenth and beginning of the seventeenth centuries.

Petrona's jealousy and her concerns about her husband's infidelity also make sense in light of the patriarchal society she inhabited. The constant preoccupation of women about the infidelities of their husbands, and the fact that they turned to peyote—among other means—were symptoms of the vulnerability of women within a patriarchy.[41] The watchful eyes of masculine figures—fathers, brothers, sons, or confessors—in matters of law or faith invariably colored women's experiences (Perry 10). Women's economic stability and social position depended on the support of men. With people relentlessly on the move in search of better living conditions, the family structures upon which women depended were often in a state of flux.

With high degrees of social instability on the one hand and pressures from the Church to conform to sacramental ideas about matrimony on the other, women such as Petrona were often forced to take extraordinary measures to secure their futures in viable social units. Peyote played a role in these attempts. Petrona used peyote to calm and "remove the anger" from her husband. She also used the plants

---

[41]   AGN/Inquisición/vol. 293/f. 422. Isabel de Zúñiga mentioned that once, when suffering severe abdominal pain caused by eating earth, she resorted to the services of María de Espinosa, a mulatto woman who lived next door to her in Mexico City. María was free and unmarried. On that occasion, María told Isabel to try taking peyote, as it was "good for her ailment." Isabel did so and in a short while became "inebriated." At that moment, María began to ask her what she was seeing, and if she, "the mulatto woman, was going to marry a man she had fallen for." María was taking advantage of the situation, and soon made her intentions clear: she was not interested in curing Isabel's stomach ache, but in trying to predict her own amorous and economic future. Isabel spent the whole night "inebriated" in her room, suffering hallucinations. On medical responses to the problems caused by eating dirt and clay, see López-Terrada's article in this volume.

to catch a glimpse of an uncertain future, in the hope of making her precarious situation somewhat more secure. In one sense, sorcery and witchcraft, at least during the period under study, were outgrowths of women's unstable position within society.

Conclusion

The number of trials carried out in many different regions of New Spain is proof of the success and rapid appropriation of the cultures of peyote. The domestic space in which Petrona Babtista lived obliges us to examine in detail the models of family life in New Spain during the sixteenth and seventeenth centuries and reconsider the foundations of the dominant culture in terms of gender. The culture of peyote suggests three things: first, that there was no single model of social organization; second, that Spanish ideology did not take root unconditionally; and third, that indigenous ritual practice was generally not conserved in a "pure" or "primitive" form. Of course, not all of this is new; as Francois Giraud points out, the notion of family was characterized more by its "plurality of models and convictions concerning kinship, alliances and sexual relationships" than by its homogeneity (Giraud). Furthermore, the models that resulted were strongly influenced by immigration and the internal shifting of populations that had a decisive impact on the construction and dissolution of family and affective relationships. This is one reason why illicit cohabitation became one of the Inquisition's main concerns. But by examining the uses of peyote—such as Petrona's attempts to secure her family relationships—we can have a better understanding of the responses to social and cultural instability.

Domestic spaces, as they were configured (and reconfigured) in New Spain, created serious tensions within the old dichotomy between the public and private spheres. Inquisitorial trials, like the judicial processes of the eighteenth century in New Spain studied by Steve Stern, suggest blurring of the lines between public and private rather than strictly defined zones (Stern 25). When Petrona Babtista and Damiana Fuentes resorted to witchcraft, they were not subverting the social order; on the contrary, they claimed to be upholding it. They were making use of their prerogative as wives and mothers in the face of the unfaithfulness of their husbands.

There are many explanations for the proliferation of cultures of peyote in the sixteenth and seventeenth centuries. It may well have been that adhering to old traditions was at times a form of cultural resistance. In other cases, such as that of Petrona, the use of peyote may represent an attempt to comply with the mandates of a patriarchal state. Between resistance and compliance there are doubtless many other reasons that led the inhabitants of New Spain to use hallucinogenic herbs. At the very least, however, mono-causal explanations of peyote use are unlikely to be satisfactory, especially when we are dealing with women's attempts to navigate the impossible demands of patriarchy and defend their positions within the family (Stern).

There can be little doubt that peyote and other herbs were also used for medicinal purposes. But the fact that the medicinal uses of peyote were influenced by the presence of many ethnic and social groups did not guarantee the longevity of these medical cultures. As in all syncretic, cross-pollinating processes, there was considerable asymmetry in the "exchanges" and "interactions" associated with the cultures of peyote. Some values accrued more power or status than others, and consequently the medical uses of peyote fell into decline. The medicinal use of hallucinogenic plants that developed during the sixteenth and seventeenth centuries became associated with magic; with time, peyote was either forced into or subsumed by the world of sorcery and witchcraft, from which it did not emerge until well into the twentieth century.

Among the many things that peyote may have meant to Petrona, it clearly represented a voice that spoke directly to her. As we have seen, social conditions in early modern New Spain—including access to land, poverty, racial discrimination, patriarchy, and religion—may have created conditions in which the voice of peyote was particularly welcome. Peyote was not only capable of seeing the future and supplying answers to difficult questions, it was a cosmic power that knew Petrona personally. For a poor mulatto woman, direct access to cosmic power must have been exhilarating, particularly given her experience at the hands of the Inquisition. She knew things Inquisitors did not.

The existence of the medical culture associated with hallucinogenic plants is a multidimensional phenomenon. We may be quick to account for its existence as an expression of an inevitable syncretism between old and new residents, unique medical practices encrypted in divination, in magic, and in Mesoamerican and Christian sorcery. There may be times when it is valuable to ask to what culture a particular practice pertains. If we set aside our desire to classify practices, however, what emerges from Inquisitorial documents is a polyphony of voices that carry traces of orality. These traces, though often very faint, communicate the physical ailments and emotional needs of women. In some cases, it is possible to recognize a given disease in its biological aspects (childbirth or stomach pain). But in most instances we do not find just a stomach ache; instead we find a complex environment of domestic difficulties and gender dynamics in which human beings struggle to address "medicalized" social problems (whether the "disease" is gender, powerlessness, infidelity, etc.). The boundaries between physical and emotional ailments are not clearly defined.

The intervention of the Inquisition on both sides of the Atlantic was conditioned by the work undertaken at the Council of Trent and the subsequent Catholic Reformation, in which the clarity and observance of Church teachings became a central objective.[42] For the Inquisition, failure to observe the precepts of faith was invariably due to the work of the devil, who was always willing to corrupt the souls of gullible women. The use of peyote and other hallucinogenic herbs recorded in Inquisitorial processes contravened the laws of nature as they were understood

---

[42]   On the Council of Trent, see Andretta's chapter in this volume.

by the Church: no woman could communicate with an animate entity, as this was a prerogative reserved for God. The practice of witchcraft with hallucinogenic plants therefore acquired a specific meaning in the New Spain of the late sixteenth and early seventeenth centuries. Peyote and other plants used in divination were entities charged with a highly symbolic meaning in the period's medical cultures and in Mesoamerican divination. At the same time, peyote gave mulatto, Spanish, and mestizo women a sense of control over aspects of their lives; it gave them a set of therapeutic options with which to treat their physical and emotional ailments.

Chapter 2
"Antiguamente vivían más sanos que ahora": Explanations of Native Mortality in the *Relaciones Geográficas de Indias*

José Pardo-Tomás[1]

Introduction

The medical cultures of New Spain are the result of a particular confluence of discourses. These discourses could, in theory, be mutually illuminating; in practice, the contact of medical cultures sometimes led to confusion and misunderstanding.[2] Whether through mutual comprehension or misinterpretation, however, the meetings of medical cultures almost always created something new: hybrid or mestizo medical knowledge and therapeutic practices.[3] Texts that give us a good sense of the wide variety of beliefs about disease—for example, how diseases were spread and might be prevented—are quite rare. That is why the *Relaciones Geográficas de Indias*—alluded to in the preceding chapter by Morales and examined in greater detail here—are so exciting. The *Relaciones Geográficas* (henceforth RGs) are a corpus of texts generated in New Spain during the second half of the sixteenth century, and they provide a nearly unique glimpse of a cross-section of the society of the period. The RGs not only cause us to reconsider our estimates of the number of medical cultures at work, but also they demand we reexamine our understanding of the hierarchy of medical cultures, as we shall see. But first it will be helpful to get a better understanding of the RGs and their characteristics.

[1] Funding for this research was provided by the Spanish Ministry of Science and Innovation [*Cultura médica en la periferia colonial: Nueva España, 1521–1621, HAR2009-11030-C0201*] and the Charles H. Watts Memorial Fellowship, awarded by the John Carter Brown Library, Providence, RI. My thanks go to Peter Mason for his help with the English version of this text.
[2] The concept of "Double Mistaken Identity" is illuminating in this respect (Lockhart 442–6).
[3] On our use of the terms "hybrid" and "mestizo" as synonyms, see Safier (136); also helpful in this respect are Gruzinski, *La pensée métisse*; Obregón; Dean and Leibsohn; and Young, *Colonial Desire*.

A Privileged Source, a Problematic Source

New Spain, or Mexico, was conquered in 1521, not quite three decades after Columbus's first voyage. The need to organize and govern these vast new territories led to the creation of a government body known as the Consejo de Indias (Council of the Indies), whose task was to centralize, control, and draw up colonial policies for the Spanish Indies. The creation of this Council in 1524 perfectly illustrates how colonial powers, from the very start, needed reliable knowledge of the territory and of the population subject to its control. The most frequent means to obtain this information was through the use of questionnaires, distributed among the different local authorities throughout the colony; authorities were, in turn, expected to complete them and send results back to the Council. After a number of initial attempts to gather information about Spain's new territories (Bustamante), the cosmographer Alonso de Santa Cruz drew up a set of instructions and a questionnaire requesting descriptions of the new territories, their resources, and their inhabitants.[4] These instructions and questions were refined over time and are generally considered to be the direct predecessors of the questionnaires that Juan de Ovando created for the Consejo de Indias in the 1570s.

In 1577 an order was issued to print the *Instrucción y memoria de las relaciones que se han de hacer para la descripción de las Indias*; a translation of the title does little justice to its contents.[5] The text contained approximately 50 questions and was to be distributed throughout the territory of the Spanish Indies. Metropolitan bureaucrats hoped in this way to obtain a systematic body of coherent information about the territory under their control, especially the human, natural, and material resources that they could exploit. The replies to this questionnaire form the basic nucleus of what historians have come to know as the *Relaciones Geográficas de Indias* (henceforth RGs). The most numerous and informative of these to have come down to us are those from New Spain, most of which were completed between 1579 and 1585.[6] They are an exceptional source of information about life in New Spain at a pivotal time in its history: six decades into Spain's monumental

---

[4]   First published by Jiménez de la Espada. For Alonso de Santa Cruz and his instructions, see Portuondo 68–79, 108–15.

[5]   The document has been fully transcribed in various works, such as all the volumes of the edition of the RGs by René Acuña (6: 99–104).

[6]   A total of 167 RGs from New Spain are extant in three repositories: the Archivo General de Indias, Sevilla; the Real Academia de la Historia, Madrid; and the Nettie Lee Benson Library, University of Texas, Austin. With the exception of the 54 RGs from Yucatán, which have a special character and are not considered here, all the RGs have been consulted in Acuña. Occasionally we have also had recourse to the original documents. On the basis of this information we have elaborated the database *Relaciones Geográficas de Indias*, which we hope presently to publish online.

experiment in hemispheric governance and immediately following one of the terrible epidemics that decimated the native population of New Spain (Fields 11).[7]

The experience of this demographic hecatomb clearly shapes the answers to the questionnaires. This is significant, because one thing that has been lacking in our comprehension of the cultural matrix of New Spain is a detailed picture of the interactions among colonial medical cultures; the RGs provide us with an invaluable resource for beginning this work.

Surprisingly, the RGs have received scant attention since Alfredo López Austin published a selection of the questionnaire replies over 40 years ago in his reconstruction of Nahuatl medicine, *Textos de medicina náhuatl*. Notable exceptions to this scholarly oversight are found in the studies that Raquel Álvarez dedicated to the RGs in the late 1980s and early 1990s (215–91).[8] My own attempt to address this unfortunate scholarly lacuna begins with an examination of the fifth and fifteenth questions of the 1577 questionnaire. The fifth question, really a set of questions, asked three things: first, whether the *partido*—the basic unit of territorial division, variable in size and consisting of a main locality (*cabeza de partido*) and its environs—was home to "many or few *indios*"; second, "if there had been more or fewer of them in the past"; and third, the reasons for population changes. The fifteenth question rather leadingly asked whether *indios* "lived healthier lives in the past than today, and the reasons for that," as well as asking about their "current and former means of sustenance." A complete answer to these two questions, however, emerges only after analysis of all the responses to each of the RGs, because other questions deal with the "temperament and quality" of the soil; "the appearance" of the population; whether the settlement was "on salubrious land or in a healthy location"; "common ailments and customary remedies"; and "plants that the *indios* use as remedies, and their medicinal or poisonous properties."

The replies to these questions go beyond demographic and sanitary considerations and cannot be reduced to a simple catalog of data. On the contrary, each RG is actually an attempt to explain and understand what happened and why. In most cases, this is by means of a complex game of negotiation between the different actors involved in the creation of a discourse that was first produced orally, and subsequently recorded in a written text that could be sent to metropolitan authorities. Thus, the RGs are a series of texts that initially arose in response to a questionnaire formulated in the metropolis but had to be interpreted in the colony, at the local level. Of course, these local interpretations depended a great deal on the

---

[7]   Very useful, too, is the contribution by Angélica Mandujano et al., "Historia de las epidemias en el México antiguo." The true scope of the demographic disaster is still a topic for discussion, for which it is still useful to consult the classic studies by Crosby, *The Columbian Exchange;* Florescano and Malvido, *Ensayos sobre la historia de las epidemias en México*; and N. D. Cook, *Born to Die.*

[8]   Other approaches to the colonial medicine in Spanish America, varying in merit and success, have been published in the last three decades, but none of them tackles the analysis of the RGs in a satisfactory way. Risse is among the earliest and Newson among the most recent.

discretion of disparate individuals, making responses multiform and occasionally arbitrary or contradictory. This makes the RGs a source that is both privileged and problematic, presenting considerable interpretative challenges.

Who Is Speaking in the RGs?

The first problem that arises, even before analyzing the information the responses contain, is to identify who is speaking in each of the documents and who can be considered the author(s) of each of the RGs. Attribution and the construction of authority are complex and freighted. In theory, the questionnaires were addressed to the local Spanish authorities—the *corregidor* or *alcalde mayor* of the local administrative center—and the replies had to be put down in writing by a scribe. Both parties attached their signatures at the end of the document. So, the authors of each RG, again in theory, are the *corregidor* or *alcalde* and the scribe. In fact, however, most of the texts are the written records of public events that took place at a specific time and place, during which questions were read aloud and answers were provided orally. Those who replied to each of the 50 questions were generally neither the scribe nor the corregidor. That makes matters extraordinarily complicated when it comes to attributing the authorship of the text to the colonial official, even if he approved the final document.

In practice, therefore, each RG is a world unto itself, a snapshot of a varied community taken at a particular moment. The questionnaires' instructions—composed in the metropolis—did not always make sense in the colony; discretion had to be used in interpreting the instructions. The instructions left plenty of room for deciding who would reply to the questions and how, so each document has to be analyzed with an eye to the enunciating subject of the text.[9] The majority of the texts are polyphonic ones in which the voices of various actors, mediated to a greater or lesser extent, are perceptible.

This is even the case in those that seem to have a single author, like the example of the *corregidor* of Chiconauhtlan (in the bishopric of Mexico), Pedro López de Ribera. His ego clearly predominates in his text, in spite of the fact that, as we shall see, López de Ribera had access to representatives of the native community who might have contributed more directly. He writes in a self-assured first person:

> In this jurisdiction *I have neither seen nor heard* that there are herbs that the natives use as remedies, but they allow themselves to die like animals, without applying any remedy, and *I know nothing else* about this jurisdiction.[10]

---

[9]   For theoretical and methodological considerations regarding the reading of native voices, Lockhart, Sousa, and Wood's *Sources and Methods* has proved extremely useful, even though it does not contain a chapter specifically on the RGs. In particular, see Lockhart's "Introduction: Background and Course of the New Philology."

[10]   "En esta jurisdicción *yo no he visto ni sabido* que haya yerbas con que se curen los naturales, sino que se dejan morir como bestias, sin hacerse remedio. *Y no sé otra cosa* desta

The native community of Chiconauhtlan still had 2,500 tribute-paying *indios*, despite having lost four-fifths of the population in the various epidemics that swept the region in the wake of the Spanish conquest. In fact, López de Ribera wrote that those epidemics were "still circulating among the natives." Although, as the text shows, the *corregidor* himself did not grant them a voice, the silent presence of the community was reflected in the document via the names of its representatives:

> Don Juan Bautista, governor; Miguel Ximénez, Jerónimo de Rojas, Indian magistrates of this village; don Juan, *indio*, governor of the village of Tecama; don Pedro de Aquino, *indio*, governor of the village of Coacalco; don Cristóbal Tlahuizotl, governor of the village of Ecatepec, all native *indios* by blood.[11]

López de Ribera seemed to assume that what he did not know was not to be known at all. He left no discernible traces of having used native informants. But this was not always the case in the RGs. Three RGs of the Coatepec district contain diverse voices even though they purport to be composed by a single author: the scribe and interpreter Francisco de Villacastín. The echoes of these voices resound in the document, which refers to the ancient paintings in the possession of the community as a reliable source of knowledge about the population's past and present:

> As the old people say today and as is known from paintings that their ancestors left to them [...] there were more than ten thousand *indios* in this province of Coatepec [...] the hillsides and valleys of this village were densely populated and full of the farmhouses and farms of the *indios,* and in all the ravines, as can be seen today from the walls and foundations of houses and sanctuaries [...].[12]

Besides containing one of the most beautiful descriptions of the territory's history, Villacastín's text illustrates how the community's past—a life that may have been hard, but was also healthy—might be given voice by the principal members of the community itself:

---

jurisdicción" (Chiconauhtlan, Tecama, Coacalco, Xaltocan, y Ecatepec, México) (emphasis added).

[11] "Don Juan Bautista, gobernador; Miguel Ximénez, Jerónimo de Rojas, alcaldes indios deste pueblo; don Juan, indio, gobernador del pueblo de Tecama; don Pedro de Aquino, indio, gobernador del pueblo de Coacalco; don Cristóbal Tlahuizotl, gobernador del pueblo de Ecatepec, todos indios antiguos y naturales" (Chiconauhtlan, Tecama, Coacalco, Xaltocan, y Ecatepec, México).

[12] "Según dicen los viejos antiguos que hay ahora y tienen por pinturas que les dejaron sus pasados [...] hubo en esta provincia de Coatepec más de diez mil indios [...] las lomas, laderas y valles deste pueblo estaban muy poblados, y llenos de caseríos y estancias de indios, y en todas las quebradas, como parece hoy en día por los paredones, cimientos de casas y cúes [...]" (Coatepec, México).

> The caciques and lords did not allow their subjects to live in leisure, but rather
> kept them continuously toiling in warlike occupations. Nor did they allow them
> to drink the wine of the territory, unless the captain or some other person who
> had done something worthy of note.[13]

Villacastín's text does not contain a single locution such as "the *indios* say
[...]." On the other hand, Villacastín's deep knowledge betrays considerable
intimacy with his subject. What becomes apparent is that some RGs allow us to
overhear arguments and explanations coming from at least two distinct groups: the
caciques and *señores* (e.g., those mentioned in the RG from Coatepec), and the
common people, or *maceuales*. The two voices often fail to concur, and the tension
prompted by differences of opinion at the moment when the replies are being written
is sometimes patent. For example, the 11 RGs from Ichcateupan—undertaken by
Lucas Pinto, the captain and *corregidor*—often allow the elder *indios* to speak.
The *indios* insist that there used to be order, austerity, and a rigid social distinction
between *señores* and *maceuales*, but that they are no longer observed.[14] Relaxation
of austere habits and the disappearance of social distinctions is the cause of all the
troubles, including the high mortality rate:

> In the past people lived very long and were very healthy, because they ate
> little and worked hard, and did not know a woman before the age of thirty [...]
> because the common *indios* could not eat meat or fowl or drink wine, which
> they now do to excess [...] The leading members of the community were free to
> get drunk, but a *macehual* was not free to do so, and if he did, he was punished
> with a whipping.[15]

The RGs do not designate an enunciating subject in cases such as this. There is
not an individual subject (i.e. an *indio*) speaking, but rather a collective ("the
indios"). Like "the Spaniards," the term "the *indios*" comprehends (and conflates)

---

[13]   "Los caciques y señores no consentían que sus súbditos viviesen con ociosidad,
sino que a la contin[u]a los traían ejercitados en cosas de la guerra. Ni menos les consentían
beber vino de la tierra, si no era al capitán u otra persona que hubiese hecho alguna cosa
señalada" (Coatepec, México).

[14]   The reader will not have missed the similarity of this discourse to the contemporary
one of Bernardino de Sahagún in his "Relación del autor digna de ser notada,"written in
1576 and included as Chapter 27 in Book X of his Spanish-language version of the *Historia
general de las cosas de la Nueva España*: "the people of fifty years or less were occupied
in many activities by day and by night, and they were brought up in great austerity, so that
high spirits and carnal inclinations did not gain the upper hand among them, both in the men
and the women," among other passages in the text (158).

[15]   "Vivían antiguamente mucho tiempo, y esto muy sanos, porque comían poco y
trabajaban mucho, y no conocían mujer hasta ser de treinta años [...] porque los indios
comunes no podían comer carne ni gallina ni beber vino, lo cual ahora hacen en gran
demasía [...] y que los principales tenían libertad de emborracharse y, como fuese macehual
no la tenía, si se emborrachaba, tenía pena de azotes" (Ichcateupan, Oztuma, y Teloloapan,
México).

a plurality of voices. The hermeneutic challenge posed by the RGs is to detect those echoes. And in listening for the timbre of *indios'* voices, we come across an additional difficulty: the presence (and thus the agency) of the interpreter(s).[16] The text that we read in the RGs is almost always the result of a tension or negotiation among what was said, what an interpreter understood, and what the person who finally transferred the text to paper thought the speaker wanted to say, or what he decided to say himself.

In one form or another, we find a series of lay discourses (i.e. not claiming medical expertise) that reflect numerous visions of the demographic problems encountered by the native population during the first half-century of the post-conquest period. The lay character of these discourses is important; they form a crucial point of reference for the discourses of the medical practitioners on the same topics.[17]

Only two physicians appear in the RGs under analysis. One of them, Doctor Toro, is mentioned only in passing. The *indios* of Ahuatlan complained that Toro's way of breeding cattle contaminated their water and forced them to move their settlement.[18] The other physician, Alonso Hernández Diosdado, is the author of the RG of Veracruz, the port of entry into New Spain for transatlantic voyagers. Still, the content of his text is not particularly original and is shorter than one would expect for a city of the size and importance of Veracruz. Despite the fact that the author is a physician, he made no special attempt to provide medical explanations in his replies to questions that called for them and used few medical terms. In fact, Hernández Diosdado attributes the decline of the native population to an insalubrious climate and to the mosquitoes,[19] both explanations well within the reach of the most rustic layperson.

---

[16] For an examination of the intersections of translation and power with theoretical affinities to this one, albeit in a very different historical context, see Enrique García Santo Tomás's chapter.

[17] European, creole, or mestizo experts formed what Gruzinski has called "the first globalized élites" (Gruzinski, *Les Quatre parties du monde* 276).

[18] "Y estaban asentados y poblados en otro lugar que asimismo se decía Ahuatlan y lo despoblaron porque las aguas que bebían y de que se sustentaban se las inficionaban y acenegaban ciertos ganados vacunos del doctor Toro, médico vecino de México, que tuvo una estancia en esta jurisdicción" ["And they were settled and organized in another place which was also called Ahuatlan (Ahuatlan, Tlaxcala), and they left it because the water they drank and on which they depended was infected and smeared by some cattle herds of Dr. Toro, a physician from Mexico, who had a farm in this jurisdiction"] (Ahuatlan, Tlaxcala).

[19] "Ha sido muy notable la quiebra y falta que en los indios desta comarca ha habido después que los españoles señorearon la tierra y cada día se van deshaciendo las poblaciones [...] de manera que no se puede esperar sino una total ruina y acabamiento de los que quedan. Porque, sin ocasión particular se entienda, mas de la mala templanza general e inclemencia desta tierra y de la miserable plaga de los mosquitos que hay en ella." ["The decline and drop in numbers that the *indios* of this region have suffered since the Spaniards became lords of the land has been very striking and the depopulation continues every day [...] so that one can only expect the total ruin and extermination of those who remain.

Opinions attributed to natives are almost always the opinions of native laypersons, not native medical experts or healers. One reason for this was that many indigenous medical experts died in the epidemics. The loss of healers is explicitly lamented in Tonameca[20] and Teutitlan;[21] it is likely that the loss of native healers was felt acutely in many more places.

The Causes of the Hecatomb: Laying Blame

The *corregidor* in Citlaltepec, Alonso de Galdo—together with the scribe Alonso de Guzmán and the local priest—begins the following passage by attributing the ideas to natives: "These natives have us understand [...]." But it is unlikely that all of the ideas can be attributed to natives:

> These natives have us understand that the reason why they were healthier when they were pagans is because they have now grown used to the corruption of the air and of the times [...] so that they have almost acquired our complexion and have begun to eat the meat of cattle, pigs and sheep, and to drink wine, and to sleep beneath a roof [...]. As well as other vices and carnal pleasures, in which they still engage, which naturally leads to a shortening of their lives and leads them to contract many contagious illnesses from which they die.[22]

The passage ends with an explanation based on the change in the complexion (*complexio* or humoral balance) obviously influenced by Hippocratic-Galenic notions concerning health and illness; this entailed a regime of health (*regimen sanitatis*) consisting of the practices connected with the six non-naturals (*sex res non naturales*): the air and the environment, sleep and waking, exercise and

---

It cannot be attributed to any particular cause, but rather the general climate and inclemency of this land and the miserable plague of mosquitos in it"] (Veracruz, Tlaxcala).

[20]   "Y dicen que antiguamente solían tener quien los curaba y, después que vinieron los españoles, no han tenido quien los cure [...] y declaran que antiguamente [...] se curaban con zumo de yerbas que los médicos que tenían les daban y que ahora no hay quien conozca ni sepa de yerbas" ["And they say that in the past they had someone to cure them, but after the arrival of the Spaniards they have not had anyone to cure them [...] and they declare that in the past [...] they were healed with herbal juices that their physicians gave them but that now there is no one who had any knowledge or understanding of herbs"] (Tonameca Puerto de Guatulco, Oaxaca).

[21]   "Hácense pocos o ningunos remedios [...] porque no hay entre ellos médico ni quien sepa curar" ["They apply few or no remedies [...] because there is no physician or healer among them"] (Teutitlán, Oaxaca).

[22]   "Quieren estos naturales decir que la causa porque en su gentilidad vivían más sanos, era por estar habituados a las corrupciones de los aires y tiempos [...] que casi se ha convertido su complexión en la que nosotros tenemos, por haberse dado al comer carne de vaca y puerco y carnero, y beber vino, y dormir debajo de techado [...] Amén de otros vicios y carnalidades, en que todavía están, de que, naturalmente, la vida que tienen se les acorta y caen en muchas enfermedades contagiosas, de que mueren" (Citlaltepec, México).

rest, food and drink, evacuation and retention, and finally the "passions of the soul."[23] Immediately after their reference to the Hippocratic-Galenic *complexio*, the authors of the RG of Citlaltepec alleged that moral incontinence, the "vices and carnal pleasures" of the *indios*, led to their ruin. This combination of classical medicine and censoriousness was more often a feature of the discourses of Spaniards; the words were unlikely to have been uttered by *indios*, despite what the RG says.

It is only a short step from criticizing "vices and carnal pleasures" to branding them sins. Bernabé López Ponce, the priest holding the benefice of Tequixquiac, belonging to the same district as Citlaltepec, explained that the *indios* suffered from the same ailments as Spaniards: "pain in the side, abscesses, fevers and *tabardetes* [typhus], which, because of our great sins, God has allowed to continue from last year [1676] to the present."[24] Given the role clergy played in the composition of some of the RGs, one might expect Bernabé López's conviction that sickness was caused by sin to appear frequently in the responses. But this is not the case. Only a few RGs explicitly attribute the demographic hecatomb of the *indios* to anyone's sins. To be fair, Bernabé López is not alone in believing that divine will alone can explain disease; in Pátzcuaro, the main settlement of Michoacán, we find something similar:

> They lived much healthier lives and lived longer and were more populous, and never was any pestilence seen among them as we have seen and still see every day since the conquest; and the number of people in the past was incomparably larger than today. The cause is unknown; it is all attributed to divine will.[25]

But other RGs reject the oversimplification that characterizes the responses of Bernabé and the people of Pátzcuaro. For example, the third RG from the district of Citlaltepec, that of Xilotzingo, lists a fairly complete series of causes to explain "the deaths from pestilence" that had decimated the native population:

---

[23] Lanuza's chapter in this book examines the relationship of the *sex res non naturales* to astrology. On the role of the *sex res non naturales* in the theoretical formulation of Galenism, see Jarcho. For the health regime within that same theoretical framework, see Gil-Sotres, Paniagua, and García-Ballester's "Estudi introductori" (17–24, 88–110). Although it focuses on the *morbo gallico*, a very useful study regarding the revision of the conception of the multiple causes of illness current in Europe at the time is Arrizabalaga's "Medical Responses" (35–42).

[24] "Y al presente [...] padecen otras [enfermedades] como la gente española, como es dolor de costado y postemas y fiebres y tabardetes, lo cual, por nuestros grandes pecados, ha permitido Dios que dure, desde el año pasado de setenta y seis hasta ahora, que no cesa" (Tequixquiac, Citlaltepec, México).

[25] "Vivían mucho más sanos y duraban y se multiplicaban más, y nunca se vio entre ellos pestilencia, como se ha visto y se ve cada día después de que se conquistaron; y sin comparación era mayor el número de gente que había, que ahora. La causa desto no se sabe; todo se atribuye a disposición divina" (Pátzcuaro, Michoacán).

The cause is that they are a disorderly people without any self-control in eating and drinking, because [...] they never stop drinking *pulque* [...] which is bad and pestilential. They go about the countryside without coats, and when they reach their homes all they find there is smoke because they are very small and dark. They throw themselves on the ground and wake up with cuts on their bodies, leading to contagious illnesses from which they die.[26]

As we saw previously in Citlaltepec, the explanation given is based on the *indios'* failure to observe a proper balance in one of the six non-naturals that constitute a healthy way of life (according to Europeans). In this case they cite three non-naturals: the air they breathe; their disorderly eating and excessive drinking; and their refusal to sleep properly.

In almost 20 RGs the respondents claimed to be completely ignorant of the causes that led to the drop in the native population. Mostly, the RGs reflect respondents' varied ideas about the diversity of causes of mortality. If the respondents did not have a clear idea, they tended to say so. In a few cases, however, death was attributed to the "plagues" generally; what was not known was the cause of the plagues themselves. For example, according to Cristobal de Vargas, *corregidor* of Yurirapúndaro in Michoacán, the natives of the village of Acámbaro replied to the question:

In the past they lived very healthy lives and died old, because those who are still alive remember that a very large number of old people could be seen then and now they are few, and that plagues arrive from time to time, which have finished them off; and they do not know the cause of this.[27]

The declaration in this case came directly from the pen of the *corregidor*, but as in the majority of the other cases, it was recorded as being the reply obtained from questioning representatives of the native community. Again, according to the RGs, it is the *indios* themselves who are silent, or declare their ignorance.[28]

---

[26]　"La causa de lo cual es por ser gente desconcertada y sin orden en el comer y beber, porque [...] jamás dejan de beber pulque [...] tan malo y pestilencial. Andan por esos campos desabrigados y, cuando vienen a sus casas, no hallan en ellas otro regalo, sino humo, por ser muy chicas y oscuras. Y échanse en el suelo y así amanecen cortados los cuerpos, de donde les viene a recrecer enfermedades contagiosas de que mueren" (Xilotzingo, Citlaltepec, México).

[27]　"Que antiguamente vivían muy sanos y morían de viejos, porque los que ahora hay se acuerdan que entonces veían grandísima cantidad de viejos y ahora son pocos los que hay, y que acuden de cuando en cuando pestilencias, por ello que los han acabado; y no saben qué sea la causa desto" (Acámbaro, Yurirapúndaro, Michoacán).

[28]　Other declarations are more terse, but no less effective. These two come from Michoacán too, but from the Tuxpan district: in the center of the district, the natives declared that "antiguamente vivían mucho y sanos, y que al presente no viven tanto, y enfermos; no saben decir la causa dello" ["in the past they lived long and healthy lives, but at present they do not live so long and are unhealthy; they do not know what the cause is"]. In Zapotlán, another locality in the same district, the reply was almost a replica of the previous one, but

Table 2.1   Authorship of the *Relaciones Geográficas*, compiled from the
            database "Relaciones Geográficas de Indias.fp7"

Single authorship: 25 (12 with clear presence of native voices)
   17 the *corregidor*
   2 the *alcalde mayo*r
   2 the scribe-interpreter
   1 a friar-interpreter
   1 a physician
   2 single authors: Juan Bautista Pomar and Diego Muñoz Camargo
Double authorship: 38 (26 with clear presence of native voices)
   16 the *corregidor* and the scribe
   13 the *alcalde mayor* and the scribe
   1 the *corregidor* and a friar
   1 the *alcalde* and a friar
   1 the scribe and a friar
   1 the *corregidor* and a priest-interpreter
   2 the scribe and a priest-interpreter
   1 the *corregidor* and a native interpreter
   1 the *alcalde* and a native interpreter
   1 the *alcalde* and a Spanish witness
Triple authorship: 32 (28 with clear presence of native voices)
   14 *corregidor*, scribe and native interpreter
   3 *alcalde*, scribe and native interpreter
   5 *corregidor*, scribe and friar
   1 *corregidor* and two friars, one of whom interpreter
   1 *corregidor*, native interpreter and Spanish witness
   3 *alcalde*, scribe and priest, who is also interpreter in two cases
   1 *corregidor*, scribe and Spanish witness
   2 *alcalde*, scribe and Spanish witness
   2 *alcalde*, scribe and native interpreter
   1 *corregidor*, scribe and a friar who also provides the singing voice
Quadruple or quintuple authorship: 6 (all with clear presence of native voices)
   3 *corregidor*, scribe, priest and native interpreter
   1 *alcalde*, scribe, friar, native interpreter and Spanish witnesses
   2 *corregidor*, scribe, friar, native interpreter and Spanish witnesses

---

However, Table 2.1 leaves a number of questions unanswered: the length and
variability of the discourses of the various speakers; the identities of particular

---

included an interesting slant on the pre-Hispanic era and the cause of death of those long-
lived elders: "antiguamente vivían mucho y sanos [...] y que al presente no viven tanto, y
enfermos; no saben decir la causa dello" ["in the past they lived long and healthy lives and
grew old (...) but today they do not live so long and are unhealthy; they do not know the
cause"] (Tuxpan and Zapotlán, Tuxpan, Michoacán).

respondents; and the contradictions among or even within different versions (because the RGs do not always specify who is speaking). We shall try to fill in these gaps by looking more closely at a few cases that exemplify the various causes adduced in the text.

Contrary to what one would suppose, Spaniards and the *indios* did not tend to blame one another for the demographic catastrophe. In fact, in a significant number of cases we find Spaniards affirming that they themselves were at fault, as well as indigenous participants who insist that it was their own attitudes towards the conquest that led to their virtual extinction. Of course, in such cases it is logical to suppose that there was either selection bias—choosing native informants unlikely to blame Spaniards—or something akin to a measurement bias, in which the testimony of *indios* that was favorable to Spaniards was collected more zealously or overrepresented. Even if this is the case, the nuances and variations with which authors and scribes represented the opinions of the native communities do not suggest the imposition of a univocal formula exclusively elaborated by the colonists. At the very least, authors chose to represent native claims of native responsibility for the demographic collapse as the product of various discourses being synthesized. And it is always possible that this was more than rhetorical savvy on behalf of colonial authorities; that is, it may be that the testimony transcribed had its roots in an environment of disagreement, debate, persuasion, and negotiation, an environment that included vigorous indigenous participation. In Pátzcuaro, for example, we read:

> The old people say that when they were infidels there was less vice and that men did not know a woman until they were thirty or forty years old, nor did they eat and drink as they do now, and they are extremely prone to vice; and their ailments could be attributed to this.[29]

This passage might have originated in the testimony of Don Juan Puruata, a "native of this city and principal and governor in it," as the RG itself states. A likelier source, however, is the Franciscan Diego de Fuenllana, "a person very skilled in the language of this province and very expert in its matters." The emphasis on the past virtues and current vices of the *indios*—now "extremely prone to vice"— would suggest Fuenllana. Ultimately, it is difficult to know for sure; the three parties involved (civic officials, ecclesiastics, and the native community) seem to have shared a consensus about two things: first, that the ailments decimating the population were due to the "vicious" practices that had spread since the arrival of the Spaniards; and second, that this marked a departure from the austerity and composure that had been characteristic in the past, when they always submitted to the authority of the native élite. These two ideas can be found in many RGs;

---

[29] "Dicen los antiguos que en tiempo de su infidelidad el vicio era menos y que de treinta o cuarenta años no conocían los hombres mujer y no comían ni bebían como agora, en que son extremadamente viciosos; y a esto se podrían atribuir sus enfermedades" (Pátzcuaro, Michoacán).

the differences lie in the nuances with which the ideas are expressed in the final document, a document that was the result of negotiation among parties and agents that had unequal access to power.

Without leaving Michoacán, we find the same ideas in Asuchitlán, although the formulation is somewhat different. Although the focus on past virtues and present vices remains, readers will note the emphasis on the "spoilt way of life" of the *indios* in the following passage:

> They are reduced more and more every day by diseases, and there are some who attribute it to laziness, because in the past they were severely downtrodden and forced to work and did not eat or drink nor wear the clothes and shoes that they do today, nor did they have horses for travel, nor rest, nor quiet, and nowadays when they have everything and are spoilt like children they are in decline.[30]

In spite of the reference to a diversity of opinions on the matter, the authorship of the RG of Asuchitlán is clearly in the hands of the *corregidor*, Diego Garcés, assisted by his 30-year-old son of the same name. In fact, when they broached the question of causes, they began by admitting the maltreatment inflicted by the Spaniards, but hastened to express their personal opinion:

> Although at first they were reduced by the wars and maltreatment of the conquest, nowadays they are so relieved and protected by the Viceroy and the other ministers of justice that they can be called spoilt children; and in spite of all that they are disappearing on a large scale; and I believe it is partly due, as I have said, to laziness, because [...] they are very idle and eat a thousand creepy-crawlies such as locusts, snakes, toads, lizards and similar other things, because they like everything; and because they only sow half of what the Viceroy has told them to sow, they suffer shortage and are hungry [...] and so I believe that when they had to work in the past they lived long and healthy lives, while with their leisure today they are short-lived and are frequently ill.[31]

The opinions of father and son were no doubt recorded, but they were not the only voice in Asuchitlán. Antón de Rodas, "more than fifty years old and very expert

---

[30] "Hanse menoscabado y menoscaban cada día con enfermedades y ausencias, y hay pareceres de que con la ociosidad, porque en la antigüedad eran grandemente vejados y trabajados y no comían, ni bebían, ni vestían, ni calzaban como ahora, ni tenían caballos en qué andar, ni reposo, ni quietud, y ahora, con tenello todo y estar regalados como hijos, van disminuyendo" (Asuchitlan, Michoacán).

[31] "Aunque a los principios los disminuyese las guerras y malos tratamientos de la conquista, en estos tiempos son tan sobrellevados y amparados por el Señor Visorrey y por los demás ministros de justicia, que se pueden llamar hijos regalados; y con todo eso, disminuyen grandemente; y creo ser alguna parte, como he dicho, la ociosidad, porque [...] son muy haraganes y comen mil sabandijas como son langosta, culebras, sapos, lagartos y otras cosas semejantes, porque todo les hace buen gusto; y por no sembrar siquiera la mitad de lo que el Señor Visorrey tiene mandado que siembre cada uno, padecen necesidades y hambres [...] y así creo que con los trabajos de su antigüedad vivían mucho y sanos y agora con el ocio viven poco y enferman mucho" (Asuchitlán, Michoacán).

in the *tarasca* and *cuitateca* languages," interpreted the oral testimony of the representatives of the native communities. Their voices reach us, albeit remotely and highly skewed by distrust and denigration; the *corregidor* and his son seem to recoil at the "perversity" and "ignorance" of the natives:

> They have a very perverse custom which is that, when a person is ill he does not want to eat or even to look at food, and not one of them—father to son, son to father, wife to husband, husband to wife, or any other—begs and implores him or her to eat, and so they wane and die like ignorant persons.[32]

Although in the majority of cases it is by no means clear who is saying what, the final result sometimes appears to reflect a consensus. This consensus, perhaps provisional, may have been the product of the environment in which the questions and answers were read.

What happened in the district of Chichicapa in Oaxaca offers a complex panorama of causes and explanations, but at the end of the process there is a shared vision of the disaster and its origin. Five RGs were completed in Chichicapa, all by the scribe Pedro Pérez Bejarano, with the presence of the *cacique* governors and old members of the villages:

> The old natives explain why people live less long now than when they were infidels; it is because in the past they did not sleep in the village and ate nothing but dried tortillas and had a lot of work and worries, and so they lived hardy and healthy lives. But after the arrival of the Spaniards they built houses and had peace and quiet and an abundance of food [...] and they became spoilt, and the boys marry when they are twelve or fifteen years old. And they think that all these things are the cause that they live less long now [...] which seems to be in conformity with reason.[33]

The obsession of the missionaries to promote very early marriages among the *indios* shocked the natives profoundly; in Chichicapa and elsewhere, natives returned to this subject repeatedly, as several RGs record. Other causes of vice and disease mentioned in the RG of Amatlán, in the same district as Chichicapa, reinforce the consensus mentioned above. On the one hand, the decline in terms of culture and life expectancy was the fault of the Spaniards, who expelled natives

---

[32] "Tienen una costumbre perversísima y es que estando uno enfermo no quiere comer ni ver comida, y ni el padre al hijo, ni el hijo al padre, ni mujer a marido, ni marido a mujer, ni ninguno otro les importunan ni ruegan que coman, y así se descaecen y mueren como brutos" (Asuchitlán, Michoacán).

[33] "Dan por razón los naturales antiguos que la causa de vivir ahora menos que en tiempo de su infidelidad es que, antiguamente, no dormían en poblado ni comían si no eran tortillas secas y hechos a mucho trabajo e inquietudes, y así vivían recios y sanos. Y que, después de venidos los españoles, hicieron casas, y tuvieron quietud y sosiego y muchas comidas en abundancia [...] y se hicieron al regalo, y los mozos se casan de doce y quince años. Y todas estas cosas hallan ellos ser parte de vivir menos tiempo ahora [...] que parece ser cosa conforme a razón" (Chichicapa, Oaxaca).

from the highlands and forced them to live together and to change their form of settlement.[34] On the other, the *indios* themselves were responsible for not being good Christians:

> They had been living in some big mountain ranges towards the east, and the Spaniards ejected them from there and, once they had been conquered and pacified, they settled them in the region and place where they are today [...] In the past they lived much longer than today, because they lived for eighty, ninety or a hundred years [...] They attribute it [...] to many ailments that Our Lord has permitted because they were not the good Christians they should have been.[35]

Cracks in this consensus do emerge, however. This is evident enough in a contradictory account from Amatlán, and can be seen even more clearly in the case of Ocelotepeque, another of the five villages of the district of Chichicapa. Apparently, the rejection of the "consensus" view was so strong in these two places that tensions between the two parties could not be resolved. The final result was a polyphonic RG lacking in harmony. In the document, Spaniards denounced the natives who returned to their "idolatrous" rituals as a result of the illness:

> Three months ago the parish priest Esteban Ramos found out that, during an epidemic that struck this village three years earlier [...] the leaders went back to sacrificing to this Petela [...] to make the illness go away.[36]

In Cuautla, another district of Oaxaca with five RGs, documents were compiled by the *corregidor* Melchior Suárez and the scribe Baltasar de Ribera. In this case, typically Spanish ideas about temperateness and climate are attributed to native herbalists:

> As infidels they lived healthier and longer lives than today. After the arrival of the Spaniards, they live less long [...] because this village is hot rather than temperate, it is unhealthy, and it gives the natives fevers and smallpox, and blood

---

[34] According to 17 RGs, *indios'* health deteriorated drastically when they were forced to change their settlement patterns, moving from scattered dwellings in the highlands to concentrated settlements on the plains. Very useful for putting it in context is Ramírez Ruiz and Fernández Christlieb's "La policía de los *indios* y la urbanización del *altepetl.*"

[35] "Y estaban poblados en unas sierras grandes hacia la banda del oriente, y los españoles los echaron de allí y, conquistados y pacíficos, los asentaron en la parte y lugar do ahora están [...] Antiguamente mucho más vivían que ahora, porque vivían ochenta y noventa y cien años [...] Atribúyenlo [...] a muchas enfermedades que ha permitido Nuestro Señor por no ser tan buenos cristianos como debían" (Amatlán, Chichicapa, Oaxaca).

[36] "Habrá tres meses que su beneficiado, Esteban Ramos, averiguó que, en una enfermedad muy grande que hubo en el dicho pueblo habrá tres años [...] volvieron los principales a sacrificar al dicho Petela [... para] que aplacase la enfermedad" (Ocelotepeque, Chichicapa, Oaxaca).

in their stools and urine. They have Indian herbalists to remedy them, who cure them with herbal medicines, which are of great assistance.[37]

The list of causes was shorter in Cuautla than in Chichicapa, but it would appear that there was a lot of exchange between the *indios*, the *corregidor*, and the scribe. The interpreter Bartolomé Pérez must have played an important role in the final document. Otherwise, it is difficult to understand how some "Indian herbalists" might refer to the "temperate" nature of the environment, never mind use terms like "smallpox" or "blood in their stools."

The four towns and seventeen localities of the district of Ihualapa, in the diocese of Oaxaca, produced a single RG in which the voice of the natives seems to dominate those of the *alcalde mayor*, Antonio Sedano, and the scribe, Juan Luis Maldonado. This resulted in a positive vision of the past (including its drinking bouts) that contrasts starkly with a negative vision of the present (for the excess of work):

> The governor of Ayutla, Don Andrés Orejón, declares that there were many people when it was settled and today there are very few [...] who drank the wine of the land and [...] were very content with this [...] and he understands that they lived much healthier lives then than now [...] and that now so many of them are dying because they have a lot of work to do.[38]

This account contradicts previously cited assertions of the natives' now-leisurely lives. The moral charge to be found among the more common causes of disease and hardship in other RGs was reversed in this case. For the people of Ihualpa, represented by their native governor, the drunkenness of the past was good for everybody, and it was the excessive workload of the present that was responsible for the deteriorating situation. Spanish influence not only made their lives worse but also increased mortality. It is thus unjustifiable to try to set up hard and fast oppositions between what "the *indios*" and "the Spaniards" thought, as though the voices on each side were always in unison.

The RG from Nexapa is an example of a very different result. The reason lies in the person who wrote the RG and in the manner in which he did so more than in the content of the document itself. The Dominican friar Bernardo de Santa María, who was entrusted with the task of compiling the RG by the authorities and who

---

[37] "Vivían, en su infidelidad, sanos y más tiempo que ahora. Y, después acá que entraron los españoles, viven menos [...] por ser este pueblo más caliente que templado, es malsano, y a los naturales les da calentura y viruelas, cámaras de sangre y la misma sangre echan por la orina. Y para su remedio tienen indios médicos erbolarios, que los curan con yerbas medicinales, de que reciben mucho remedio" (Xocoticpac, Xaltepetongo, Cuautla, Oaxaca).

[38] "El gobernador de Ayutla, don Andrés Orejón, declara que era mucha gente cuando se pobló y que ahora hay muy pocos [...] que bebían vino de la tierra y [...] con esto vivían muy contentos [...] y que entiende que vivían más sanos entonces que ahora [...] y que ahora se mueren tantos porque trabajan mucho" (Ihualapa, Oaxaca).

put himself forward as the interpreter of the native community, did the whole thing from start to finish. Drawing on the most classic European Hippocratism, he produced a positive vision of life in the past as a sharp criticism of the settlement in the plains that had been imposed by the friars. In other words, he repeated two ideas that had doubtless been convincingly transmitted to him by his interlocutors (even if he did not fail to comment on their "stench"):

> As for the healthiness of the place, or illnesses, they occur every year, but they have not been particularly dangerous. In the past the people lived on the high peaks of this bank and were very healthy, but today they live in the lowlands, though against their will. Many have died since they were crowded together in settlements, because they naturally carry a terrible stench about them, enough in itself to cause any kind of plague.[39]

The four RGs from Puerto de Guatulco, completed by the *alcalde mayor* Gaspar de Vargas and the scribe Pérez de Urribarri, give extensive replies, among which there is a very interesting calling into question of the practice of bleeding:

> Since the arrival of the Spaniards, they know no other remedy for their ailments except bloodletting; and so they have died without knowing how to apply any remedy. In the past they never applied bloodletting, nor did they know this remedy, but only the remedies of herbs and plants [...] that the physicians they used to have knew and applied [...] And they say that in the old days they used to have someone to cure them and, after the arrival of the Spaniards, they no longer have anyone to cure them, except to bleed them.[40]

Native opposition to the practice of bloodletting was to form a part of the expert discourse of the university physicians of New Spain. So, too, did the native belief in the efficacy of therapeutic baths. Friars, surgeons, physicians, and apothecaries who came from the other side of the Atlantic had to struggle against the opposition of the *indios* to having their blood let, to such an extent that the practice ended up as the paradigm of the medicine imported by the Europeans. Bathing, on the other hand, was an essential part of the healing strategy of the Mesoamericans, so that

---

[39] "En cuanto a la sanidad del sitio, o enfermedades, ocurren en cada un año; pero no han sido notablemente peligrosas. En las lomas altas desta ribera vivían los antiguos muy sanos y, ahora, viven en lo bajo; aunque es contra su voluntad. Hanse muerto muchos después que se juntaron en poblaciones formados, porque su natural traen siempre consigo una hedentina pésima, bastante para engendrar en sí cualquiera pestilencia" (Nexapa, Oaxaca).

[40] "Y no saben, después que los españoles vinieron, otro remedio para sus enfermedades sino sangrarse; y así, se han muerto sin que sepan hacer ningún remedio. Y antiguamente jamás se sangraban, ni sabían este remedio, sino solamente los remedios de las yerbas y plantas [...] que los médicos que solía haber entre ellos las conocían y aplicaban [...] Y dicen que antiguamente solían tener quien los curaba y, después que vinieron los españoles, no han tenido quien los cure, mas de quien los sangre" (Pochutla, Tonameca, Guatulco, Puerto de Guatulco, Oaxaca).

their resistance to abandoning the practice was equally tenacious. This led to the Mesoamerican baths being condemned as an erroneous therapeutic practice and even as one of the causes of the deaths among the native population. The RG of Tehuantepec is one of the clearest texts when it comes to putting the blame on the practice of bathing: "They regularly bathe in the rivers, even when they are ill, and thus it is common for many to die in this season when the north winds prevail."[41] In Tepuztlán, *indios'* defense of their bathing practice is eloquent:

> That now they live very short lives and many are dying [...] the cause is taken to be that in the past they went naked and slept on the ground and bathed twice a day and led healthy lives; but now they wear clothes [...] and sleep in beds and with clothes and when they take the air they fall ill and die. They take this and no other to be the cause.[42]

This is not the place to go into the debate on the pros and cons of bathing or bloodletting, although it is important to remember the importance of the debate on these two procedures that set *indios* and Spaniards at loggerheads for decades. For the present it is sufficient to note that there are enough clues in the RGs to gauge the strength and extent of these two controversies in this period that engaged Spaniards, Creoles, mestizos and, no doubt, the surviving *indios* as well.

Anti-Native Diatribes and Voices of Resistance

In the RG of Ameca, in Nueva Galicia, the cause of illness was squarely placed on the forced removal of the *indios* from the highlands. But Antonio de Leyva, *alcalde* of Ameca, who provided the singing voice in the RG, went on to add a long and explicit diatribe against the natives:

> They are of little intelligence and are not inclined to be of any value [...] feeble of faith [...] false and willing to make allegations [...] lovers of novelty, fickle and lacking in honour; all in general great drunkards [...] ungrateful, disgruntled [...] lazy [...] pusillanimous [...].[43]

---

[41]   "Se bañan en los ríos de ordinario, aunque estén con alguna enfermedad; y, ansí, suelen morir muchos en este tiempo que reinan los nortes" (Tehuantepec, Oaxaca).

[42]   "Y que ahora viven muy poco y se mueren muchos y [...] entiende ser la causa que entonces andaban desnudos y dormían en el suelo y se bañaban cada día dos veces y vivían sanos; y que ahora andan vestidos [...] y duermen en camas y con ropa y que, en dándoles el aire, caen malos y se mueren. Y que no entienden que sea otra la causa" (Tepuztlán, México).

[43]   "Son gente de muy bajos entendimientos, no se inclinan a valer ni a ser algo [...] faltos de fe [...] mentirosos y testimonieros [...] amigos de novedades, gente mudable y de poca honra; todos en general grandes borrachos [...] ingratos, desagradecidos [...] perezosos [...] pusilánimes [...]" (Ameca, Nueva Galicia).

A similar case to that of Antonio de Leyva is Diego Muñoz Camargo's *Relación de Tlaxcala*. The author is among the group of mestizo chroniclers of New Spain who tried in their writings to combine a vindication of their respective native traditions with the European Christian culture that they had absorbed from their conquerors (Adorno; Aguilar Moreno). Muñoz Camargo, the son of a conquistador and a native woman, was a member of the governing élite of Tlaxcala, which was an ally of the conquistadores. With the assent of local authorities, Muñoz Camargo assumed responsibility for answering the 1577 questionnaire, resulting in the text known today as the *Relación de Tlaxcala*. The *ladino* chronicler launched a diatribe that assumes special significance:

> As these natives have little intellectual talent or physical strength, but are feeble and of low intelligence, incapable of anything serious that is entrusted to them; and thus the Spaniards who want to equal them in rage and frenzy are as lacking in judgement as they are, because they are so fragile and miserable that it takes little hardship and fear to bring them down, so that to detach them from their habits and native ways and to make them equal with the talent that God gave to the Spaniards goes against all reason. So it can be said that changing their customs is tantamount to death; that even today there are still *indios* so simple and lacking in understanding that they are like irrational animals. These, and the majority of them, should be treated like children, according to their talent and capacity, like a child of eight or ten years old in Spain; so that for their own preservation, they have to be humored and threatened, as their seniors were, so that they feel that they deserve punishment [...]. They are lacking in honor and reason; they are extremely pusillanimous if they do not win favor and, when they feel they have support, they are bold and courageous; they do not preserve themselves from contagious illnesses and fall ill: they are negligent and allow themselves to die like animals. They eat very little and nourish themselves with food of little substance.[44]

---

[44] "Como estos naturales sean de tan bajo talento en sus ánimos y fuerzas corporales, son muy débiles y de bajos pensamientos, incapaces de cualquier cosa grave que se les encarga; y ansí, los españoles que quieren igualar su cólera y furor son tan faltos de juicio como ellos, porque son tan frágiles y miserables que poca tribulación y espanto los acaba, que sacarlos de su paso y bajo ser en su modo natural e igualarlos con el talento que Dios dio a los españoles [es] contra toda razón. Y por esto se puede decir que mudar costumbre es par de muerte; que, aun el día de hoy, hay indios tan simples y de tan poco entendimiento que se pueden comparar a animales irracionales. Y a éstos, y a la mayor parte dellos, se ha de tratar como a niños, según su talento y capacidad, como a un niño de ocho o diez años de los de España; por manera que para la conservación destos, se han de llevar por halagos, mostrándoles mucho con amenazas, de [la] manera que tenían sus mayores, de suerte que sientan que han de ser castigados [...] Carecen de honra y razón; son pusilánimes en extremo grado si no tienen favor y, cuando sienten ayuda, son osados y atrevidos; no se guardan de males contagiosos, enfermando: son dejativos y se dejan morir bestialmente. Son de muy poco comer; susténtanse con comidas de poca sustancia" (Tlaxcala).

Not everyone matched the elegance of Muñoz Camargo's diction. In Chilchota, Michoacán, the scribe Francisco Toscano, whose opinions, as we have seen, prevailed in the corresponding RG, hardly mentioned the epidemics as the cause of the decimation of the population. He instead wrote a short but vehement diatribe against the native population:

> They are as filthy as pigs, idle, lacking in honour; the only work they engage in is to go to the mines and elsewhere to put themselves out for hire; they have little understanding and are inclined to evil; they are very phlegmatic.[45]

The attribution of a phlegmatic temperament to the *indios*, clearly inspired by the Galenic typology, was to be elaborated in a more sophisticated way by several expert authors, especially after the work of Juan de Cárdenas in the 1590s.[46] As in other controversies that we have already seen, the lay voice of Francisco Toscano appropriates this categorization of the temperament of the *indios* to characterize them as evil, stupid idlers.

There is nothing original in the anti-native diatribes we occasionally find in the RGs. They are larded with commonplaces and nearly all repeat the same elements: drunkenness, slovenliness, sloth, a tendency to deceit and make-believe, the weakness of their Christian faith, and ingratitude towards the missionaries and conquistadores. It is not difficult to perceive the fear behind this hostility: fear that a native population much more numerous than their masters would rise up; fear that arose from misunderstanding and mistranslation, in which incomprehension was often interpreted as animosity. This is very clear in one of the most striking anti-native diatribes, to be found in the RG of Asuchitlán, Michoacán:

> They have evil inclinations and love novelty and are exceptionally malicious and deceitful, lazy and not drawn to what is good, but very clever and concerned when it comes to evil; it is very common for them to perjure themselves, whether in prosecution or in defense [...] they will say no more than is called for. And they are clever in this, that unless repeated questions are put, taking great care that the witness who has made the deposition does not talk with the others, it will be difficult to ascertain the truth [...].[47]

---

[45]   "Es gente puerca, haraganes, no tienen honra; no tienen más granjerías que ir a las minas y a otras partes [a] alquilarse porque se lo paguen; tienen poco entendimiento e inclinados a lo malo; son muy flemáticos" (Chilchota, Michoacán).

[46]   See Juan de Cárdenas (1591), especially Chapters 1–12 of Book III, ff. 180r–223v, in which the young physician, who had already trained in the colony, raises the problem of the temperamental differences of the *indios*, Spaniards, and creoles from a perspective that was already favorable to the latter.

[47]   "Son de malas inclinaciones y amigos de novedades y sobre manera maliciosos y mentirosos, torpes y tardos para el bien, muy hábiles y solícitos para el mal; perjúranse muy de ordinario, así demandando como defendiendo [...] no dirán más de lo que la parte quisiere. Y están diestros en esto, que si no es con muchas repreguntas, con que haya gran

As mentioned earlier, the *corregidor* of Asuchitlán, Diego Garcés, and his son of the same name were the only signatories to the RG, but the *indio* Antón de Rodas, "more than fifty years old and very expert in the tarasca and cuytateca languages," acted as interpreter for the oral testimonies of the senior representatives and elders of the native communities when they were questioned. A full reading of the RG makes it clear that neither the natives nor their interpreter said anything about their "evil inclinations." It is also clear that the difficulties that the Garcés father and son had in understanding them belonged to the past. The reference to the repeated questioning required to "ascertain the truth" alludes to frequent cases prior to the arrival of the questionnaire. The anti-native leitmotif of the *corregidor* and his son is fairly standard, even if it appears here in a particularly accentuated form. The noteworthy aspect, at any rate, is the fact that the extensive diatribe was directed above all against the political behavior of the *indios*, which indicates, among other things, the effectiveness of their strategies of resistance or, rather, their unwilling assimilation.

In fact, many representatives of the native communities countered the anti-native diatribes of the colonists with a celebration of the idyllic past. This celebration concealed, though sometimes barely, a vigorous critique of the living conditions imposed by the conquistadores. As we have seen, in some cases the celebration of the idyllic past included the consideration that they did not have to work so hard then. We find the same idea in the RGs of the district of Cuiseo, in Nueva Galicia, where the *indios* openly declared that they had not worked in the past:

> In the past they lived healthier lives [...]. And the reason is that they lived lives of leisure when they were pagans, with little work or concern to seek and acquire goods.[48]

We have already seen how the scribe Francisco Toscano appeared as an active author in the RG corresponding to Chilchota, Michoacán, by repeatedly noting his personal opinions in the official document. Perhaps he understood something rather unusual in the context of the RGs: that the *indios* lived longer and better lives when they were full of vices than now in a regime of virtue.[49] We find an even more radical account in the RG of Tuscacuesco, in the district of Amula, in Nueva Galicia. The *indios* declared that they lived healthier lives when they were

---

vigilancia en que el testigo que ha depuesto no hable con los demás, apenas se podrá aclarar la verdad [...]" (Asuchitlán, Michoacán).

[48] "[...] Antiguamente vivieron más sanos [...] Y la causa de ello es por haber vivido en su gentilidad ociosos, de poco trabajo y cuidado de buscar y adquirir bienes" (Cuiseo, Nueva Galicia).

[49] "En el tiempo antiguo vivían más tiempo los naturales, y había mucha más gente; porque vivían a gusto en los vicios que ellos querían" ("In the past the natives lived longer and were far more numerous; because they lived lives of pleasure in the vices that they enjoyed") (Chilchota, Michoacán).

"idolaters": "They lived healthier lives than today because they were diligent, night and day, in idolatry and worshipping their idols."[50]

A surprising feature of the RG of Puerto de Guatulco, in Oaxaca, is that the colonial authorities responsible for the RG were confronted by an even clearer symptom of native resistance:

> They heard their ancestors say that before the Spaniards arrived they used to live healthy, hardy and longer lives, and that after the arrival of the Spaniards, they all began to die; and that the reason for that was because they abandoned their gods, who told them what to do to heal themselves when they fell ill.[51]

Two things are notable in this passage. First, we see how the source of the collective memory has been introduced during translation: the expression "they heard their ancestors say that [...]" is not usually found in such an explicit form in the other RGs. Second, the self-critical reason adduced for the decline of the population does not coincide at all with the usual attribution to the conquistadores (their contemporary excesses and ill treatment), but with the very opposite: the cause of the demographic catastrophe is attributed to the fact that "they abandoned their gods," which is what made them lose their medical knowledge and remedies.

Another exception to the commonest version among the Spaniards is that presented by "the most senior and elderly *indios*" of Hueytlalpa in the diocese of Tlaxcala:

> And the reason why there were more people in other times was because each *indio* had the women he wanted and therefore had many children; today, as they do not have more than one and live in harmony, reason, justice and marriage, they bear fewer children.[52]

A positive evocation of polygamy like this stands in sharp contrast to the repeated, explicit condemnations of the practice evidenced in many other RGs. However, Hueytlalpa is not an entirely isolated case. Polygamy reappears in the RG of Villa de Purificación as the reason why the population was larger in the past. Behind this defense is it not difficult to see a criticism of Christian marriage

---

[50]   "Vivían más sanos que ahora era porque andaban diligentes, de noche u de día, idolatrando y adorando a sus ídolos" (Tuscacuesco, Amula, Nueva Galicia).

[51]   "Oyeron decir a sus antepasados que antes que los españoles viniesen solían vivir sanos y recios y mucho más tiempo, y que después que vinieron los españoles, comenzaron a morirse todos; y que la causa dello había sido porque los apartaron de sus dioses, que les decían lo que habían de hacer para sanar cuando caían enfermos" (Puerto de Guatulco, Oaxaca).

[52]   "Y la causa porque había más gente en otros tiempos era porque cada un indio tenía a las mujeres que quería y, a esta causa, parían muchas; y ahora, como no tienen más que una y viven con concierto y razón y justicia y matrimonio, no paren tantas" (Hueytlalpa, Tlaxcala).

(monogamous and early) by comparison with the native institution, which is presented time and again as late and polygamous: "The reason why they all perished is that, in the past, each *indio* had three or four women, and thus, they say, they multiplied more."[53] This is what the scribe Alonso Hernández del Cueto recorded, but the RG was signed by the priest holding the benefice of Villa, who would doubtless have been unable to take a positive view of such an explanation. Nevertheless, on this occasion either he or the scribe limited himself to what the *indios* said.[54] Thus, there is cause to suspect that in other RGs where the voice of the natives seems to discuss their past practices, the intermediaries who ended up compiling the text of the RG (interpreters, colonial authorities, scribes) disguised this type of argument, either refusing to transcribe what was said orally or altering it substantially.

In this context, the account of Muñoz Camargo provides a helpful example. Muñoz Camargo supplies a precise and aseptic synthesis of the central argument in favor of polygamy. It may have been proscribed by the missionaries, but it was a means to populate the land and part of a "natural" way of life for the *indios*, in accordance with their temperament:

> [Because] they had many wives, they had more children than nowadays, and because they were in their natural setting and did not abandon their customs [...] nor changed their temperament or moved to other climates [...] they maintained their health by being in their natural surroundings.[55]

There are many RGs in which the native gaze was directed towards an idyllic past, full of advantages when compared with the present hard times. Such claims about the past implied, even if implicitly in most cases, a harsh criticism of the present and the Spaniards responsible for it. But at the same time, such claims left the native community imprisoned within the discourse of its old masters, the autochthonous *señores*, whose nostalgia for their lost power is perhaps the most insistent of the native voices in the RGs. Even though nostalgic idealization of the past was not always reflected explicitly in the RGs, we can hear it behind the insults cast upon the officials and the moralizing friars.

---

[53] "El haberse acabado todos ha sido porque, antiguamente, cada indio tenía tres y cuatro mujeres; y ansí, dicen, multiplicaban más" (Villa de Purificación, Nueva Galicia).

[54] In fact, they do not fail to record the opinion that they hold of the few indios who have survived the catastrophe: "they are poor and very feeble, and most of the time, because they do not work, they live on fruit, especially bananas, from which they make bread. They are fickle in their behavior and contracts, and have little talent" (Villa de Purificación, Nueva Galicia).

[55] "[Porque] tenían muchas mujeres, engendraban más que ahora, y porque estaban en sus naturales y no quebrantaban sus costumbres [...], ni trocaban temples, ni pasaban a otros climas, [...] conservaban su salud con estarse en su natural" (Tlaxcala).

Conclusion

Juan de Castañeda, the *corregidor* of Cazcatlan, wrote that "the variety" of causes that had led to the demographic crisis was "such that it would be rash to pass judgment on the matter."[56] The RGs show that there was a wide-ranging discussion in New Spain during those years concerning the causes of the catastrophe of illnesses and death. The discussion included many participants of many types and was witnessed by even more. The inquiry was precisely targeted to throw light on the demographic and epidemiological effects of the interaction between new and old processes, and did not display a marked tendency to fall back on such simplifications. Few attributed epidemics to divine will or evaded the issue by claiming ignorance.

To sum up, the principal causes raised for discussion were:

1. The concentration of the population in the lowlands. Many attributed the epidemic to the *indios* having been forced to abandon the highlands in order to facilitate the missionary activities within a spatial framework to which they were not accustomed.
2. Prohibitions against marrying later in life and polygamy. Low fertility rates and generalized feebleness were attributed to procreation at a young age and the institution of monogamy, as was an increased rate of mortality for those born under the new matrimonial regime.[57]
3. Drunkenness on wine or *pulque*. It was widely believed that intemperateness was killing the *indios* who, before the conquest, had been accustomed to the sobriety and strict norms that restricted the use of *pulque* to the dominant élites.[58]
4. The movement of large sectors of the population. *Indios* were obliged by Spaniards to move from one part of the territory to another; they were mobilized as freight transport and used as combat troops or to repopulate deserted territories. Being wrenched from their natural habitat gave rise to changes of temper or climate that made them ill and decimated them.

---

[56]   "Es de tanta variedad que es temeridad juzgar la cosa" (Cazcatlan, Tlaxcala). It is almost impossible not to think of a similar, although not identical, response from about the same time: the pronouncement of the dean of the Cathedral of Guatemala that inspired the volume edited by Noble D. Cook and George W. Lovell, *Secret Judgment of God: Old World Disease in Colonial Spanish America*: "As regards the deaths of Indians and their decline, these are the secret judgments of God, which men cannot understand."

[57]   The RG of San Andrés, in Guatemala, records that the natives declare that bringing forward the age of marriage so much has resulted in their sons becoming "small and effeminate" [salen los hijos pequeños y afeminados] (San Andrés, Santiago Atitlán, Guatemala).

[58]   For an essential study of the context of the debate concerning native drunkenness, beginning at the very moment of the conquest and developing during the period prior to the RGs, see Corcuera de Mancera.

The environmental explanation seemed, in its various formulations, to enjoy a relative consensus.

5. Policies surrounding bloodletting, bathing, and purgatives. This appears to have been the subject of a fairly extensive debate; advocates and detractors of bloodletting and bathing elaborated extensive arguments in favor of or against these practices. Spanish support of bloodletting and opposition to bathing was explicit; *indios'* profound distrust of phlebotomy and their insistence on the practice of therapeutic baths appear in the criticisms of Spaniards rather than in defenses put in the mouths of *indios* by their interpreters. All, however, seemed to agree on the virtues of purgatives, which became the key therapeutic strategy in the medicine of New Spain.

One could go on adding causes, but our aim has been to suggest the multiplicity of themes, discourses, and attitudes that a source like the RGs enables us to hear. The crucial factor from our point of view is the attempt to provide an adequate interpretation of this polyphony of reasons and arguments in the face of a problem whose dimensions were completely unknown in any other context at all prior to the "Iberian globalization," with all its effects and consequences (Gruzinski, *Les Quatre parties du monde* 15–84).

That is why we believe that the RGs enable us to go beyond a simple case study. On the one hand, they demonstrate three things about the medical cultures of New Spain. First, these cultures were relatively independent of the metropolitan debates. Second, the medical cultures of early modern New Spain are particular to that time and place, seen nowhere else. Third, these cultures are radically hybrid. At the same time, the RGs allow us to ask to what extent an adequate analysis of the processes of the construction and circulation of knowledge in the colonial context should transcend the concepts of dominion and resistance; the risk of imposing a binary framework is that singular cultural constructions, such as the medical cultures of New Spain, are rendered nearly imperceptible.[59]

In spite of their provisional nature, analysis of the RGs allows us to study the medical cultures of New Spain without making them depend on the vectors of "modernity versus tradition," which all too often is the model employed by Eurocentric historiography. Approaching the production of knowledge and of certain medical practices from the bottom upwards reveals the diversified world of lay folk who were the authors and creators of their own medical cultures, cultures that only entered the discourse of the experts in an impoverished and schematic form.

---

[59] For a similar line of argument, though applied to somewhat different contexts, see the reflections and proposals of Safier regarding the "centrality of the colonial periphery" in "Itineraries of Atlantic science." Regarding the "considerable autonomy of the colonial periphery," though focusing on a later period than the one under review here, see Bleichmar, "Atlantic Competitions."

Chapter 3
The Blood of the Dragon: Alchemy and Natural History in Nicolás Monardes's *Historia medicinal*

Ralph Bauer

Introduction

In 1571 the *sevillano* physician, businessman, and natural historian Nicolás Monardes (c.1512–1588) released the "second part" of his work on New World *materia medica*, the first part of which had appeared six years earlier (in 1565, republished in 1569).[1] In this new volume, Monardes continued the task of describing the "things that are brought out of our Western Indies" ("cosas que se traen de nuestras Indias Occidentales")—the great variety of exotic medicinal resins, gums, oils, stones, nuts, beans, flowers, roots, and woods to be found in the New World. Although Monardes had never himself traveled to the New World, his project was to become one of the most successful publishing ventures in the early modern literature of discovery, his books being translated into virtually all Western European vernaculars, as well as Latin, by the end of the sixteenth century.[2] They were widely cited by the most celebrated men of science from the sixteenth to the eighteenth centuries, including not only the Flemish translator of his works into Latin, Carolus Clusius,[3] but also such prominent Englishmen as Robert Boyle, William Castell, Nicholas Culpepper, Edmund Gardiner, and John Gerard, as well as the famous Swedish botanist Carl Linnaeus, who named the Wild Bergamot *Monarda fistulosa* in Monardes's honor.[4]

---

[1] The complete title of this "second part" was *Segunda parte del libro, de las cosas que se traen de nuestras Indias Occidentales, que sirven al uso de medicina. Do se trata del tabaco, y de la sassafras y del carlo sancto [...] Hecho por el doctor Monardes medico de Sevilla; va añedico [sic] un libro de la nieue. Do veran los q[ue] beven frio conella ... fecho, por el mismo doctor Monardes.*

[2] The Italian translation by Annibale Briganti appeared in Venice in 1576; the English translation by John Frampton appeared in London in 1577.

[3] This translation was entitled *De simplicicibus Medicamentis ex Occidentali India Delatis, quorum in Medicina usus est* (Antwerp, 1574).

[4] For recent assessments of Monardes's significance for the history of science, see José María López Piñero and Maríaluz López-Terrada's *La influencia española* and Pardo-

Some of the New World *materia medica* that Monardes described, like sassafras, had already been familiar to Europeans from their previous contact with the eastern "Indies" (i.e. Africa and Asia); others, like tobacco, were still new and known primarily from Amerindian medical traditions. Apparently of the former category was a certain fruit that had been brought back to Seville by the bishop of Cartagena and which Monardes called "El Dragon" (the dragon). One of the woodcuts included in the 1571 edition depicts several views of the fruit, including one of its inside (see Figures 3.1 and 3.2). Upon opening the fruit, Monardes relates, he and the bishop had made the startling discovery of a miniature dragon. It was "a marvelous thing to behold" ("cosa maravillosa de ver"), he wrote, for it was made

> con tanto artificio, que parescia vivo, el cuello largo, la boca abierta, el cerro enerizado, con espinas, la cola larga, y puesto en sus pies: que cierto, no ay nadie que lo vea, que no se admire de ver su figura, hecha con tanto articifio, que paresce de Marsil. Que no ay artifice tan perfecto, que major lo pueda hazer.[5]

> (with so much art that it appeared to be alive, with a long neck, the mouth open, and bristles standing up like thorns, a long tail, and standing on its feet, so that surely nobody who saw it could help but marvel to see this figure, made with so much art it seemed that it was made of ivory and that no artisan, however accomplished, could have made it better.)

What should we make of Monardes's strange image and account? Some have suggested that the image of the dragon was (as a sort of biblical snake) intended to represent the "imprint of Satan," an instance of a European tendency to associate the unfamiliar aspects of New World nature with the demonic (Jorge Cañizares-Esguerra 130).[6] To be sure, it is true that Monardes occasionally demonizes Native

---

Tomás's *Oviedo, Monardes, Hernández* (77–126); on Spanish natural history writing about the New World more generally, see Pardo-Tomás and López-Terrada's *Las primeras noticias*.

[5]   Nicolás Monardes, *Historia medicinal de las cosas que se traen de nuestras indias occidentals que sirven en medicina* (Seville, 1988), 79r. This edition is a facsimile reproduction of the 1574 edition. Heretofore, all citations to this edition will appear parenthetically in the text. In the 1571 edition (where it appeared for the first time), this passage can be found on page 91r.

[6]   Like Cañizares-Esguerra, Marcia Stephenson, in a recent article especially devoted to Monardes's treatment of the bezoar stone (a calcinated concretion found in the stomach or intestines of certain Andean quadrupeds, including the llama, the alpaca, the vicuna, and the guanaco), has placed Monardes's natural history in the context of the missionary campaigns to extirpate native idolatry—on a trajectory from inquiry to inquisition—and suggested that New World *materia medica* often came to be associated with diabolism in European natural histories. Stephenson, however, distinguishes between Monardes's attitude toward New World *materia medica* per se and Native American medicinal and religious uses of them. On Monardes's treatment of the bezoar stone, see also Miguel de Asúa and Roger French's *A New World of Animals* (106–10).

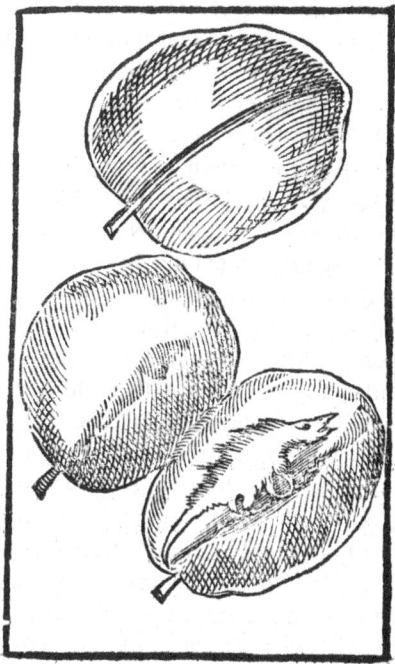

Figure 3.1   Nicolás Monardes, *El Dragon*, woodcut

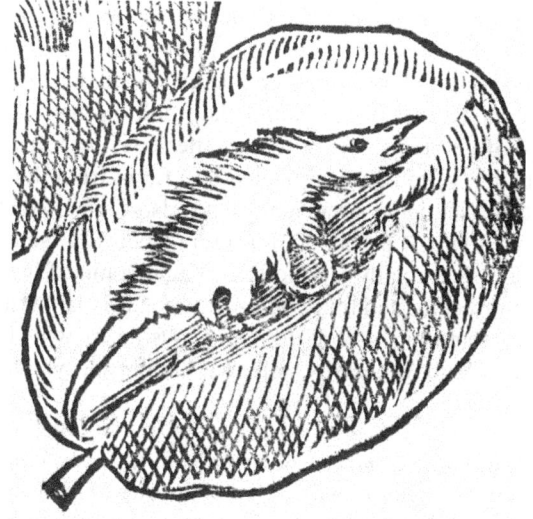

Figure 3.2   Nicolás Monardes, *El Dragon* (detail), woodcut

American uses of medicinal substances. Thus, even though he celebrated the medicinal virtues of tobacco, he claimed that its use in Native American culture was diabolical in origin, writing that "el Demonio ... enseñoles la virtud desta para que mediante ella, viessen aquellas imaginaciones, y fantasmas que se les representan y mediante ella los engañan" ("the Devil ... showed them the virtues of this plant so that through it they might see those imaginings and phantasms that it represents before their eyes and through which they are deceived") (48v–r). Nowhere, however, does Monardes associate New World nature per se with the devil; rather, we find a more likely context in which to read Monardes's dragon in the world of emblems in Renaissance natural history, which drew on a "complex web of associations" linking particular natural "things"—animals, plants, minerals, and metals—with history, mythology, etymology, and the entire cosmos (Ashworth 132–56, 135).[7] In particular, I want to argue that Monardes's "dragon" must be read in the context of Renaissance alchemy and the rich iconographic tradition that this scientific practice had spawned over the course of many centuries.

Based on the general principles of Aristotelian natural philosophy, Western alchemy had developed during the early centuries AD in Hellenistic Egypt and entered the Latin West via translations from the Arabic since the twelfth century. In medieval Christian Europe, however, alchemy was regarded not as an academic branch of its own within natural philosophy but rather as a sort of applied science; and it was practiced primarily as a technical art that explored the practical uses of fire in a number of artisanal fields. Although the attempt to find an artificial way to effect "transmutation" of base metals into gold (chrysopoeia) was always a central aspect of alchemy, its practitioners were engaged in a broad range of experimental activities, including metallurgical essaying, the refining of salts, the manufacture of dye, pigment, glass, and ceramics, artificial gemstones, incendiary weapons, as well as the brewing and distilling of drugs. An artisanal practice whose trade secrets were strictly guarded, alchemy had, over the course of centuries, developed a distinctly esoteric textual tradition that was steeped in the figurative language of emblems, symbols, and allegories. Already in many of the Arabic source texts that were being translated into Latin from the twelfth century on-ward, this esoteric language of alchemy had also teemed with spiritual and prophetic mysticism, some of it Islamic in origin (especially Ismailism), some of it Hellenistic in origin (especially Hermeticism), and some of it a mixture of the two. Likewise, the thirteenth- and fourteenth-century Christian writers on alchemy fused its Aristotelian naturalism and Hermetic mysticism with the language of Christian eschatology and especially millenarian prophecy. During the early

---

[7]　On the continuities of the emblematic tradition in New World natural history, see Andrés Prieto's *Missionary Scientists*, with regard to Counter-Reformation historians; and Christopher Iannini's *Fatal Revolutions*. On early modern natural history more generally, see Brian Ogilvie, *The Science of Describing*; Nicholas Jardine, James Secord, and Emma Spary's *Cultures of Natural History*; Paula Findlen's *Possessing Nature*; and Lorraine Daston and Katherine Park's *Wonders and the Order of Nature*.

modern period, alchemy underwent important changes in its theory and practice, as well as in its status as a 'science' within the order of Western knowledge. Among the most important changes was its move from the artisan's workshop and the monastery into the courts, where its practice enjoyed state sponsorship. Moreover, as I will suggest here, its mixture of scientific empiricism, Hermeticist mysticism, and Christological messianism played an important role also in the European literature of overseas discovery and conquest. In particular, it offered an important rhetorical venue for the apprehension of American exotica by framing the interests in New World *materia medica*, both scientific and commercial, in strongly spiritual and even magical terms. Steeped in the Christological symbolism and the Hermetic mysticism inhering in the recovery of esoteric and arcane knowledge, the language of alchemy synthesized science with religion and hereby not only offered a rhetorical recourse against traditional theological (especially Augustinian) interdiction of *vana curiositas* but also functioned to de- and recontextualize plants used in Native American cultures for their medicinal properties within an Old World providentialist context. In the following section, I place Monardes's New World *materia medica* in the historical context of the sixteenth-century intersecting traditions of humanist medicine and medieval alchemy. In the third section, I discuss the history of the emblem of the dragon in Renaissance alchemy as well as natural history and painting. And in the fourth section, I offer a reading of Monardes's tract *Diálogo del hierro*, which was included (somewhat curiously) beginning with the 1574 expanded edition of the *Historia medicinal* but that has, to date, received little critical attention.[8] I will argue that the inclusion of the *Diálogo del hierro* establishes alchemy as a key but little noted context in which to read Monardes's publications of his *Historia medicinal* and his project in New World natural history generally.

Nicolás Monardes: Commerce, Humanist Medicine, and Vernacular Philosophy

The son of an Italian immigrant from Genoa, Nicolás Monardes had received a humanist education at the Universidad Complutense de Alcalá de Henares, where he obtained, in 1530, a bachelor's degree in Arts and Philosophy as well as, in 1533, a bachelor's degree in medicine.[9] In 1547, he obtained a physician's degree from the Universidad de Santa María de Jesús de Sevilla. During his studies at Alcalá de Henares, he had studied the classics—Hippocrates and Galen—and encountered (and greatly admired) Antonio de Nebrija's 1518 *Lexico artis medicamentae*, an edition that combined the classical *materia medica* of Dioscorides and Pliny.

---

[8]   For some brief discussions of Monardes's treatment of iron, see Javier Lasso de la Vega y Cortezo's *Biografía y estudio crítico de las obras del médico Nicolas Monardes* (40–42) and Raymond Phineas Stearns's *Science in the British Colonies of America* (32).

[9]   On Monardes's life, see Lasso de la Vega y Cortezo; Guerra; Boxer; Rodríguez Marín; Pardo-Tomás, *Oviedo* 77–126; and Torre Revello.

He began writing his own treatises on Spanish, Greek, and Arabic medicines as early as the 1530s;[10] but while, in his early writings, he was dismissive of the medicinal power of New World plants—comparing them unfavorably to the plants of Europe (and of Spain in particular)—he apparently had a change of mind in the course of the following 20 years,[11] when he became increasingly interested in the natural wonders of the New World and their medicinal and economic potential. In 1565, he published the first results of his research on New World plants—the first two "books" of the *Historia medicinal de las cosas que se traen de nuestras Indias Occidentales*, a work that he would continue to revise and expand over the course of the following decade.[12]

Significantly, unlike most of his earlier medical writings—such as the *De secanda vena in pleuriti* (1539), *De rosa et partibus eius* (n.d.), and *De citris, aurantiis, ac limoniis* (n.d.), which manifested a rather conventional Galenism— all of Monardes's editions of *Historia medicinal* about the New World were originally published not in Latin (the language of academic medicine) but rather in the vernacular Spanish. There are a number of reasons for this. For one, as José Pardo-Tomás and Marcy Norton have each pointed out, there were distinctly commercial aspects to Monardes's publications and his interest in New World *materia medica*.[13] Monardes was not only a physician but also a shrewd businessman who published his works not for a professional elite but rather for the general public, hoping to profit from the sale of New World *materia medica* in both sixteenth-century senses of the term—the actual medicinal "things" (*cosas*) imported from the New World (such as tobacco) and their "historia," meaning his treatment of them in writing and print. Thus, he had formed a mercantile enterprise that shipped slaves from Africa and manufactured goods from Spain to be sold in the port cities of the New World, while bringing back precious metals, spices, and other medicinal substances for sale in Spain. For this purpose, he had found a commercial partner on the other side of the Atlantic in Juan Núñez de Herrera, who sent him from Nombre de Dios cochineal as well as seeds and specimens of medicinal New World plants that he cultivated in his garden in Seville.

---

[10] These include the *Diálogo llamado pharmacodilosis o declaración medicinal* (1536), the *De secanda vena in pleuriti* (1539), *De rosa et partibus eius* (n.d.), and *De citris, aurantiis, ac limoniis* (n.d.). For a discussion of the question of authorship surrounding these tracts, see Rodríguez Marín (22–3).

[11] For more on Monardes's apparent change of heart toward exotic plants, see Guerra (87–8), who explains it by the influence of the Portuguese natural historian of India, Garcia d'Orta, and Boxer (20–22), who disagrees with Guerra and explains Monardes's change as a result of his own experience as a collector and cultivator of New World plants in his garden in Seville.

[12] Nicolás de Monardes, *Dos libros: El uno trata de todas las cosas q[ue] trae[n] de n[uest]ras Indias Occide[n]tales, que siruen al uso de medicina [...] El otro libro, trata de dos medicinas maravillosas q[ue] son co[n]tra todo veneno* (1565). This edition was reprinted in 1569 by the publishing house of Hernando Diaz.

[13] See Pardo-Tomás, *Oviedo* 96–103; also Norton, *Sacred Gifts* 107–28.

However, due to some familial and commercial misfortunes involving the marriage of his daughter, he had to declare bankruptcy in 1567 and even seek refuge in a local Sevillian monastery to avoid being jailed by his creditors. When granting him permission to republish his work on New World *materia medica* in 1569, the Royal Council of the Indies noted that Monardes was still living in monastic asylum, and his final release from it was apparently granted so that he could repay his creditors with the profits made from future editions of his medical writings (Pardo-Tomás, *Oviedo* 101–3).

Monardes's books on New World *materia medica* were distinguished not only by their commercial but also by their philosophical character with regard to his practical approach to medicine. Despite his university degrees, Monardes was not an academic with a post at one of the universities but rather a practicing physician who combined his interest in the theory of medicine with its practice at patients' bedsides. This was remarkable in the sixteenth-century context, as the theory and practice of medicine were still generally considered to be separate realms,[14] even though this separation between theory and practice was increasingly being challenged by humanist philosophers such as Juan Luis Vives (1492–1550) and Andreas Vesalius (1514–1564), who demanded that theoretical knowledge be based on an empirical footing. In order to reform knowledge, Vives therefore recommended to scholars that they "should not be ashamed to enter into shops and factories, and to ask questions from craftsmen, and to get to know about the details of their work" (209).[15] The calls by humanist philosophers for a reform of knowledge went hand in hand with the rise of what Pamela Smith has called the "artisanal epistemology" and the "vernacular philosophy" of a new brand of physicians such as Paracelsus and his followers, who stood outside academic culture and were extremely critical of university curricula (especially of Galenism), but who were increasingly gaining self-confidence and influence in the imperial cities and courts of Europe.[16]

These commercial, philosophical, and "artisanal" contexts shed light on many of Monardes's presentations of New World *materia medica* in his *Historia medicinal*, including the plant he called "El Dragon." Modern scholars have ventured several guesses about its identity in modern botanical nomenclature. While some have surmised that it was in fact the South American croton variety *Croton lechleri*, used by native peoples for its wound-healing properties, others have speculated that it was the American cactus variety *Hylocereus*, producing the *pitaya* fruit,

---

[14]   On the distinction between theoria and practica in early modern medicine, see Harold Cook, "Medicine." On Monardes's practices, see Pardo-Tomás, *Oviedo* 86–91.

[15]   On Vives, see also Rossi, *Philosophy, Technology, and the Arts* and Pamela Smith, *The Body of the Artisan* 66–7.

[16]   On "artisanal epistemology," see Pamela Smith, *The Body* 59–93; on "vernacular philosophy," see Pamela Smith, "What is a Secret?" 60. On Paracelsus's challenge to the division of labor between the theory and the practice of medicine, see also Walter Pagel, *Paracelsus: an introduction*; Allen Debus, "Paracelsianism"; and Debus, *Chemistry and medical debate*.

still today available in grocery stores under the popular name of "dragon fruit."[17] Whatever the modern identity of "El Dragon" may be, Monardes's nomenclature, as well as his inclusion of an image and account of a miniature dragon (or lizard), corroborate his attempt to identify and market this New World plant as a source of "Dragon's Blood." Thus, he writes that "henceforth we shall be certified that it [the juice of the fruit] is Dragon's Blood" (Y de aqui adelante, estaremos certificados, que sea sangre de Drago [80v–r]).

"Dragon's Blood" had traditionally been won from a variety of the Old-World "Dragon Tree" (*Dracaena cinnabari*), native to southeastern Africa and India. "Dragon's Blood" (*Sanguis draconis*) was believed to be an antidote with miraculous medicinal efficacy. Since Roman times, it also had been believed to be a source of the bright red mineral known as cinnabar, a mercury-sulfite compound used, in ground form, by painters, goldsmiths, instrument makers, book illustrators, and other artisans as a pigment to produce a deep red. In his *De materia medica*, Dioscorides had written that cinnabar "is brought from Libya. It is very expensive and so scarce that there is hardly enough for painters to variegate lines. It is also of a deep-color, wherefore some people thought that it is dragon's blood" (*De materia medica* 375). Since the late fourteenth century, it also had been harvested from a variety endemic to the Azores and Canary islands (*Dracaena draco*), a specimen of which had been transplanted to Lisbon, where it was, in 1565, admired by the Flemish botanist Carolus Clusius, who later included a discussion of it in his *Rariorum aliquot stirpium per Hispanias observatarum historiae*, published in 1576 (11–12). By the time John Gerard published his monumental *Herbal and General History of Plants* in England in 1597, Monardes's American "El Dragon" had apparently become thoroughly identified with the Old World varieties of the Dracaena genus. In fact, Gerard claimed (wrongly) that some (apparently referring to Monardes) held the opinion that the original dragon tree did not derive from Africa but "was first brought from Carthagena, in Noua orbe, by the bishop of the same prouince" (1340). Although the identity between Monardes's "El dragon" and the Old World "Dragon Tree" would be disproven by the end of the sixteenth century, his nomenclature stuck, and the extract of the American croton variety is still marketed today as "Dragon's Blood," known from Plinean and medieval natural history.

The Blood of the Dragon: The Emblematic Tradition in Art and Alchemy

Much of the mystique surrounding Dragon's Blood derived from the rich web of associations that the substance had acquired in the course of centuries in natural history, art, and alchemy. At least since the thirteenth century, alchemists had been producing an artificial substitute for cinnabar, known as vermilion, by heating

---

[17]   See Cañizares-Esguerra, *Puritan Conquistadors* 130; by contrast, the cataloguer of John Carter Brown's online image collection, Luna, believes that Monardes's "El Dragon" was the *pitaya* cactus.

mercury and sulfur together until they became a black paste which, when further heated and evaporated, condensed in the walls of the crucible as a bright red cake.[18] This red substance—either from natural cinnabar or alchemical vermilion—was used in medieval manuscript illumination, especially to represent the blood of Christ, as it was the product of a "passion" that mercury and sulfur underwent in the crucible analogous to the passion undergone by Christ on the cross (the root of the word "crucible" is "cross"). Blood in general, and Dragon's Blood in particular (as an analogue to Christ's blood), was believed to have efficacious properties in medieval medicine. The dragon tree had therefore enjoyed a rich iconographic tradition, often appearing in Edenic landscapes as the tree of life, as in Michael Wohlgemut's *Liber Chronicarum* (1493) or Hieronymous Bosch's famous *The Garden of Earthly Delights* (c. 1510). It also appears in Martin Schongauer's and Albrecht Dürer's engravings of the story of the holy family's "flight into Egypt," recounted in the Gospel of Matthew, and, especially, in the apocryphal but widely known book of *Pseudo Matthew*, which tells the story of the so-called Dragon Wonder, in which baby Jesus tames wild dragons who subsequently praise and adore him, thus fulfilling the Old Testament prophecy of Psalms 148.7 ("Praise the Lord from the earth, ye dragons; ye dragons, and all ye deeps"). Frequently, the dragon tree is accompanied in this tradition by miniature dragons, or lizards (see Figures 3.3 and 3.4).[19]

The emblematic field of the lizard—dragon—(winged) serpent, associated with the dragon tree and cinnabar in Renaissance iconography, was drawn from the language of medieval alchemy, which had fused Christian with Pagan-Hermetic (i.e. Hellenistic), Arabic-Aristotelian, and Jewish-Cabbalistic elements.[20] Thus, in the New Testament of John (3.14–15), Jesus Christ is compared to a serpent.[21] In the Hellenistic-Hermetic tradition, which entered the Latin West via translations from the Arabic, the image of the winged serpent had been a ubiquitous "sigil" (or seal) that emblematized the eternal circularity of the alchemical opus as an *ouroboros* (a dragon devouring its own tail). But the dragon was also the symbol for the dark

---

[18]   On alchemically produced vermillion, see Pamela Smith, "What is a Secret" 60, "Vermilion."

[19]   On the iconography of the Dragon Tree, see Renée Gicklhorn, Walter Göpfert, Irmgard Müller, and Hans Schadewaldt, "Bemerkungen zur Geschichte"; on the cultural history of the Canary variety, see Jost Casper, *Die Geschichte des Kanarischen Drachenbaumes*; also, Peter Mason ("A dragon tree"), who makes the argument that the iconographic tradition of the Dragon Tree can be seen as a movement from "religious" to a "secular" or "scientific" understanding, although he is aware that such a characterization may be overly schematic. The alchemical treatment of the Dragon Tree in Monardes, however, offers a concrete example of how the religious is not so easily disassociated from the "scientific" in the sixteenth and seventeenth centuries, but rather that the two realms were inextricably interlocked.

[20]   On alchemy, Cabbala, and Christianity, see John Slater's chapter in this volume.

[21]   For an excellent discussion of the history of the symbol of the snake in Western culture, see Charlesworth.

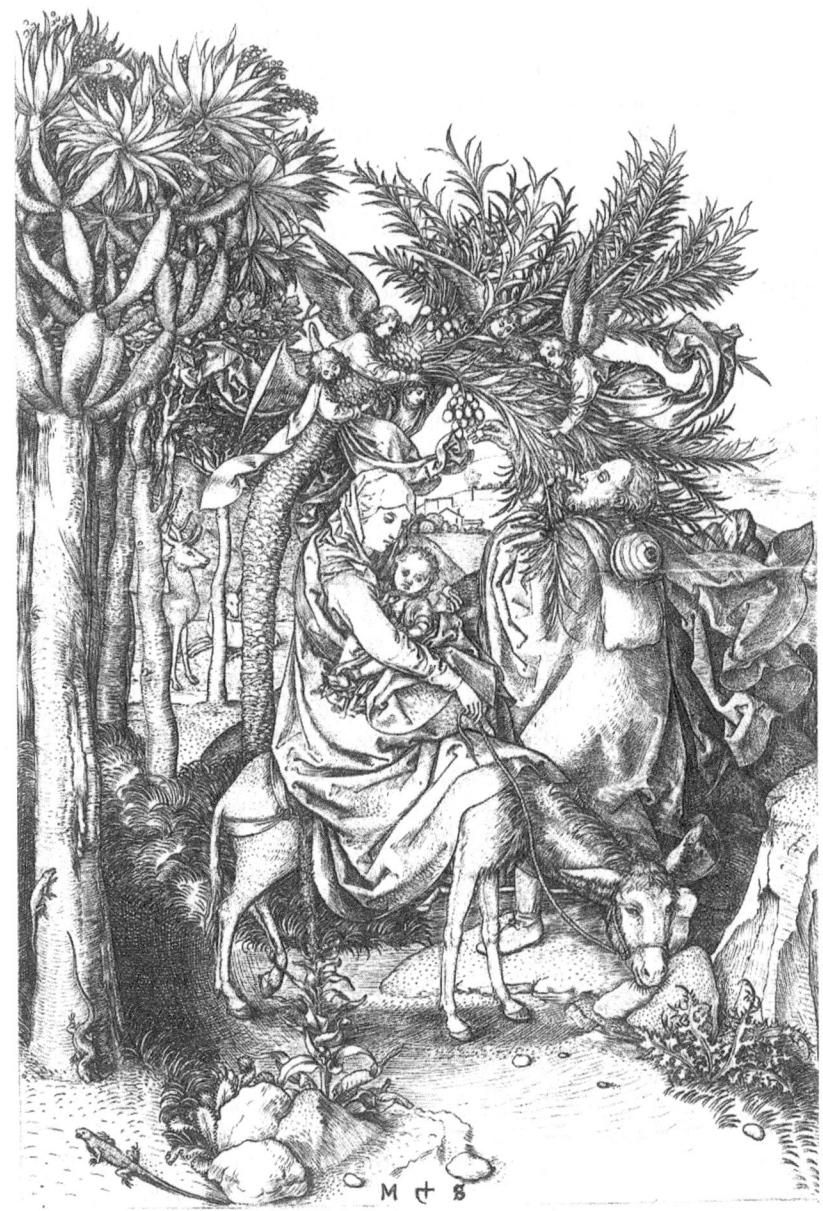

Figure 3.3   Martin Schongauer, *Flight into Egypt*, woodcut

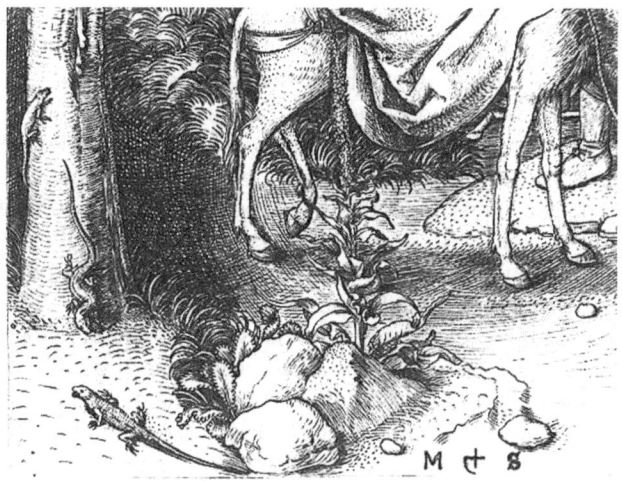

Figure 3.4   Martin Schongauer, *Flight into Egypt* (detail), woodcut

chthonic phase at the beginning of the alchemical opus, in which the alchemist dissolves the base metal or matter into the original stuff of creation, the prima materia, in order to obtain the double seed of metals from which the philosopher's stone is "grown"—philosophical sulfur and philosophical quicksilver, the two "metals," which are compared to two dragons, one male and one female, which are united in a violent copulation to produce the mercurial water (also called "Dragon's Blood") and eventually transformed into the harmonious serpents entwined around the caduceus of Hermes.[22] In medieval Christian alchemy, mercury is often also associated with the lizard, as in a book of secrets attributed to Albertus Magnus. "Take a Lizard," the author wrote there, "and cut away the tail of it, and take that which cometh out, for it is like Quicksilver. After, take a wick and make it wet with oil, and put it in a new lamp and kindle it, and the house shall seem bright and white, or gilded with silver" (104).

Vermilion/cinnabar had been of interest to medieval alchemists such as Albertus because it was produced by the combination of what were believed to be the two principles of all metals, sulfur and mercury (Pamela Smith, "Vermilion" 39–40). The idea that sulfur and mercury were the two basic components of all metals derived from the enormously influential medieval alchemical text *Summa Perfectionis*, written by an author who called himself "Geber," which is the Latinized name for Jābir ibn Hayyān, the semi-fabulous eighth-century Arabic or Persian alchemist who is said to have written 3,000 books. As William Newman has shown, however, the *Summa Perfectionis* was not actually a translation from the

---

[22]   On dragon imagery in Western alchemy, see Abraham 59–60; for Hellenistic-Hermetic alchemy, see Hornung; the classic work, from the point of view of psychoanalysis, is Jung's *Alchemical Studies*.

Arabic (as it purported to be) but rather a text originally composed in Latin, and its real author was a thirteenth-century Christian—possibly the person who identified himself as "Paul of Taranto" in another work, who was evidently familiar with Arabic alchemy, and who is today known as "Pseudo-Geber." Although medieval alchemical texts such as the *Summa Perfectionis* were based, like the Scholastic sciences, on Aristotelian natural philosophy, they also elaborated a corpuscular theory of mixture, Newman shows, that was at odds with the Aristotelian theory of matter based on the concept of the four elements (water, fire, earth, and water) that was dominant in medieval matter theory. Thus, in this dominant strain of medieval or "Scholastic" Aristotelianism, substance was held to consist of prime matter and substantial form. In the event that various substances were compounded, it was believed that previous forms were destroyed and replaced by a new substantial form, without the possibility that the original components of a compound could be recovered. By contrast, alchemical matter theory, based on the more empiricist Aristotelian tradition of the *Meteorology* and the *De generatione et corruptione*, posited a corpuscular or atomistic conception of matter in which components of a compound retain their identity, as demonstrated experimentally by their recovery through alchemical procedures resulting in "reductions to the pristine state." For this reason, Newman argues, medieval alchemical texts such as the *Summa Perfectionis* must be seen as the true origins of the "Scientific Revolution," usually attributed to the works of such seventeenth-century English men of science as Boyle and Newton, many of whom had an active interest in alchemy (Newman, *Atoms* 24, 26–7).[23]

The fact that many of the seventeenth-century "fathers" of the Scientific Revolution, such as Boyle and Newton, had a patent interest in alchemy (and could thus be considered the early modern descendants of the medieval alchemist) was long considered a sort of *scandale* in the history of science, which traditionally considered alchemy as a medieval remnant that had inhibited the development of modern science until it was purged of its "religious" and "superstitious" aspects by the emergence of a secular and rationalist model science. More recently, however, historians of science such as Newman and Smith, as well as Mar Rey Bueno, William Eamon, and Charles Webster—building on the earlier insights of Walter Pagel and Allen G. Debus—have offered a thorough reevaluation of the role that alchemy played in the history of modern science epistemologically, socially, and culturally. Thus, Rey Bueno has studied the extensive diffusion of alchemical texts by medieval Spanish authors, such as Arnau de Vilanova, and sixteenth-century Italian and German authors, such as Girolamo Ruscelli and Paracelsus in sixteenth-century Spain, as well as the highly developed institutional infrastructure that alchemy had enjoyed there since the reign of Philip II, despite the fact that

---

[23]   See also Newman's *The Summa Perfectionis of Pseudo-Geber*. On Newton's alchemy, see Michael White, *Isaac Newton*; and Dobbs, *Foundations*. On Boyle's alchemy, see Lawrence M. Principe, *The Aspiring Adept*; also, Michael Hunter, "Robert Boyle and Secrecy."

alchemy was not taught (in fact, was despised) at the universities.[24] Pamela Smith, in her study of the German alchemist Johann Joachim Becher, has offered a sociopolitical model for understanding the resurgence of alchemy in the early modern period, arguing that, in the context of the increasing importance accorded to empirical knowledge, early modern alchemical philosophers such as Becher aimed to mediate between the immovable values of the landed nobility in the courts and the practices and movable values of the money economy of the commercial world. In effect, she argues, early modern alchemy framed the "commercial projects in the traditional idiom and gesture of noble court culture and translated the commercial values into [the] court (*Business* 5–6).[25]

Similarly, Eamon has drawn attention to the important cultural role that the medieval "books of secrets" generally, and the alchemical tradition particularly, played in the history of modern science. By fusing an interest in the material world with religious and spiritual concerns, the medieval tradition of alchemy offered legitimacy to materialist inquiry in the face of the Augustinian interdiction of *vana curiositas*, an interdiction especially with regard to occult phenomena that condemned curiosity for its own sake (or for the sake of self-glorification) but that licensed *iusta curiositas*—the kind of curiosity that is put into the service of the faith and especially the spreading thereof (Eamon, *Science* 59–66).[26] Naturalist inquiry thus became invested with a strongly spiritual, providentialist, and even apocalyptic-Christological dimension. As Eamon writes, the Latin Western books of secrets "understood the 'arcane wisdom' [contained in the Arabic books of alchemy] to be ancient in origin. They believed that all knowledge stemmed from a single divine revelation that was passed down from the Hebrew prophets to the ancient Chaldeans and Egyptians, then to the Greeks and Romans, to the Arabs, and finally to the Europeans, who were the 'sons and successors of the sacred writers and of the wise philosophers'" (Eamon, *Science* 39). Indeed, as Leah de Vun has shown, medieval alchemists such as Albertus, as well as Roger Bacon, Ramon Llull, John of Rupescissa, and Arnau de Vilanova, held a

---

[24] See Mar Rey Bueno's *Los señores del fuego*, "La Mayson pour Distiller des Eaües," "El informe Valles," "Juntas de herbolarios," and "Los paracelsistas españoles"; see also López Piñero, "*Paracelsus*"; Puerto Sarmiento, "La panacea áurea"; Puerto Sarmiento, Alegre Pérez, Rey Bueno, and López Pérez, *Los hijos de Hermes*; Javier Ruiz, "Los alquimistas"; Mar Rey Bueno and Alegre Pérez, "Los destiladores de su majestad"; López Pérez, *Asclepio renovado*; López Pérez, "Ciencia y pansamiento"; Goodman, *Power and Penury*; López-Terrada, "Medical Pluralism"; and Rodriguez-Guerrero, "La Primera Gran Red Comercial." On the special role of the Jesuits in alchemy, see Camenietzki Ziller and Martha Baldwin.

[25] See also Nummedal, *Alchemy and Authority*.

[26] On iusta curiositas in the Western theological tradition and Augustine, see Heiko Augustinus Oberman, "Contra vanam curiositatem." While Eamon still builds on Hans Blumenberg's classic account of the history of curiosity in the West (Blumenberg, *Legitimacy* 229–456), Oberman disputes the sharp contrast that Blumenberg saw between the Middle Ages and the "modern" age in this regard.

firm conviction in the providentialist significance of their "art," which would, they believed, play an "active role [...] in the apocalyptic drama" of Christian salvation history, especially in the conversion of Jews, Muslims, and pagans that would precede, according to Biblical prophecy, the coming of the Millennium (De Vun 6). In essence, thirteenth-century Christian alchemical philosophers had turned naturalist inquiry into a branch of theology, whereas the mainstream Scholastic establishment, especially in the universities, treated them as separate. As Stephen Gaukroger has significantly pointed out, it was this thirteenth-century *amalgamation*—rather than the separation—of natural inquiry with religion that set the stage for what he sees as the "anomalous" path that modern Western scientific culture has taken, as the methods of the empirical sciences were able to attain a historically unique cognitive hegemony at the expense of all other epistemologies (Gaukroger 18–19).[27]

These historical perspectives shed light on the rhetorical function that the language of alchemy plays in Monardes's natural history and in the early modern literature of the discovery of the New World more generally. The rich web of associations that alchemy afforded, at once scientific and salvific, allowed for the cultural appropriation and commodification—a sort of conquest[28]—of the New World's exotic and strange nature, the medicinal efficacy of which was known only from Native American (that is, pagan) medical knowledge.

The plausibility that Monardes's emblem of the dragon must be read in the context of alchemy and its medieval iconographic tradition finds support if we consider the changing physical presentation of his work as it went through its various editions.[29] Thus, the 1571 edition—where "El Dragon" first appeared— was dedicated to King Philip II, a well-known aficionado and patron of both alchemy and exotic medicine, the latter of which he championed by sending scientific expeditions to the New World and the former by establishing alchemical laboratories at his monastic refuge of El Escorial.[30] Also, whereas the early (i.e. 1565 and 1569) editions had been published without illustrations (by the Sevillian publishing houses of Sebastián Trujillo and Hernando Díaz, respectively), beginning with the 1571 edition, the volumes also included a number of woodcuts that embellished Monardes's descriptions and had probably been prepared (or commissioned) by a new printer, Alonso Escribano, who published both the 1571 and the 1574 editions. The 1574 edition combined the already-published first (1565/1569) and second (1571) parts of New World *materia medica*, such as the Flower of Michoacán, the copal, and the guayacán wood (the latter believed to be

---

[27]   For a critique of this development from the point of view of philosophy and the Humanities, see Gadamer.

[28]   On the notion of a "conquest" of nature, see Álvarez Peláez, *La conquista* 293–338.

[29]   Pardo-Tomás notes that Monardes did not share the general antipathy against alchemy prevailing at the universities (*Oviedo* 86).

[30]   On Philip's sponsorship of New World natural history and *materia medica*, see Varey, Chabrán, and Weiner's *Searching for the Secrets of Nature*.

a cure for the French pox).[31] Also, it included a new, third part with discussions of spices and plants found in the New World, such as cinnamon, rhubarb, and coca, as well as two tracts (already included in the 1565 and 1569 editions) of two marvelous antidotes, the bezoar stone (a calcinated concretion found in the stomach or intestines of certain Andean quadrupeds, including the llama, the alpaca, the vicuna, and the guanaco)[32] and the *escorzonera*, an Iberian herb introduced into medicine by the Catalan physician Pere Carnicer. Most curiously, however, it featured two tracts that seem unexpected in a volume ostensibly about New World *materia medica*. One of them, entitled "Libro que trata de la nieve," was a treatise on the medicinal uses of snow that had already been included in the 1571 edition. The other one was a new tract on alchemy and metallurgy entitled the *Diálogo del hierro y de sus grandezas*.[33] For the remainder of this essay, I would like to focus on the latter tract, in particular on the rhetorical purpose of its inclusion in Monardes's work about New World *materia medica*.

Alchemy and New World *Materia Medica*: Monardes's *Diálogo del hierro*

The *Diálogo del hierro* appeared with a frontispiece that aptly sets the stage for the presentation of its content: a female, witch-like figure with sagging breasts devouring two snakes that she appears to have stolen from Hermes's caduceus (see Figures 3.5 and 3.6). The image was the *impresa* (a signature "device") of Escribano's publishing house, which specialized in the printing of Spanish Renaissance literature of discovery, science, marvels, and secrets, such as Agustín Zárate's *Historia del descubrimiento y conquista de las provincias del Peru* (1577), Bernadino de Escalante's *Discurso de la navegación que los portugueses hazen à los reinos y provincias del Oriente* (1577), and Jerónimo de Chaves's *Chronographia; ó, reportorio de los tiempos* (1572), as well as humanist linguistic treatises and dictionaries such as Cristóbal de las Casas's *Vocabulario de las dos lenguas, Toscana y Castellana* (1570).[34] The image of the savage woman devouring Hermes's snakes allegorized the common humanist topos of the adulteration of ancient wisdom by modern-day degeneracy, especially the alleged perversion of classical knowledge of *materia medica* at the hands of the Arabs and their Medieval Latin translators.[35]

---

[31]   On the French pox (or *morbo gallico*), see also López-Terrada's chapter in this book.

[32]   As with the Old-World "Dragon Tree" and Monardes's New-World "Dragon's Blood," relatively familiar names, such as "rhubarb" and "cinnamon," were applied to plants from the East and West Indies alike; the "rhubarb of the Indies" was Michoacán root, for example. For a discussion of Monardes's treatment of the bezoar stone, see Stephenson.

[33]   On Monardes's *Diálogo del hierro*, see also López-Terrada in this volume.

[34]   On the role of the *impresa* or "device" during the sixteenth century, see Ashworth 140–42. On Escribano's *impresa* in particular, see Francisco Escudero y Perosso 28.

[35]   On the common humanist attack on Arabic medical writers, see Pardo-Tomás (*Oviedo* 92); also Stannard, "Dioscorides."

¹⁵⁷

DIALOGO DEL
HIERRO, Y DE SVS GRAN
DEZAS, Y COMO ES EL MAS
excelente metal de todos, y la cofa mas ne,
ceffaria para feruicio del hombre, y de
las grandes virtudes. medici,
nales que tiene.

HECHO POR EL DOCTOR
Monardes Medico de Seuilla.

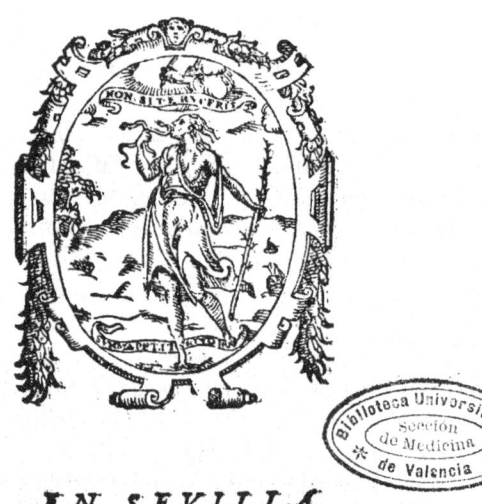

IN SEVILLA
En cafa de Alonfo Efcriuano.
1574.

Figure 3.5   Nicolás Monardes, Frontispiece to *Diálogo del hierro y sus grandezas*

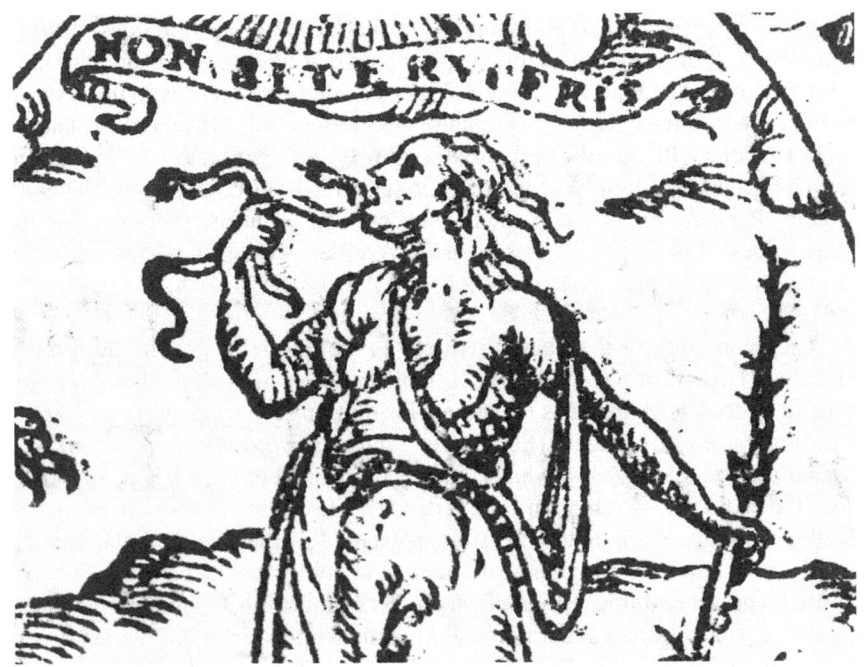

Figure 3.6   Nicolás Monardes, Frontispiece to *Diálogo del hierro y sus grandezas* (detail)

Overall, Escribano's *impresa* makes for an ambivalent fit with the content of Monardes's *Diálogo*. On the one hand, the humanist conception of history as a degeneration from a superior classical age—in particular the four-age theory based on Hesiod—constitutes the utopian intellectual background of Monardes's didactic proposal about the virtues of iron in the context of his discussion of New World *materia medica*: the adoration of gold and silver common in present-day Europe, which had resulted in the rape of the New World and the wreck of the Spanish economy, serves as a vivid reminder of life in the Iron Age, when iron is abundant and cheap, whereas gold is scarce and precious.[36] However, America, where gold is abundant and iron scarce, still exists in the Golden Age and has a moral lesson to teach Europe. Thus, the true riches of the New World, Monardes suggests, consist not in the gold and silver it provides for the royal coffers but rather in its therapeutic resources—its medicinal plants, stones, metals, and minerals—the raw materials that would be transformed by the Spanish artisan. On the other hand, however, Monardes's text does not seem to corroborate the negative opinion held by many Humanists of Arabic and medieval authorities on medicine. In fact, while the vast number of authorities cited in the *Diálogo*

---

[36]   On the debate on the effects that the influx of American gold had on the Spanish economy, see Vilches.

betrays a patent knowledge of metallurgy and alchemy on Monardes's part—so extensive that one modern historian speculated that he may have had "familiarity with the works of Paracelsus" (Stern 39)—we find no references to the sixteenth-century Swiss physician or the Renaissance Italian and German Neoplatonists, such as Ficino, Pico della Mirandola, Agrippa, etc.[37] Instead, we find citations from an expansive, inclusive, and eclectic selection of Greek, Roman, Hellenistic, Arabic, Persian, Jewish, and medieval Christian authorities—Plato, Aristotle, Dioscorides, Galen, Hermes Trismegistus, Averoes, Avicenna, Al-Rasi, (Pseudo-) Geber, Albertus Magnus, Ramon Llull, and Arnau de Vilanova, and many others (161r–171v).

The main body of the tract is written, as the title indicates, in the form of a dialogue. This form has, of course, a long tradition in Western literature going back to Plato, but Monardes's immediate inspiration seems to have been García de Orta's *materia medica* about (East) India—the *Colóquios dos simples e drogas he cousas medicinais da Índia*, which had been published in 1563 at Goa in India. As does the character of "Orta" in García de Orta's text, the "Doctor" in Monardes's *Diálogo* resembles the author himself, presented in the image of the Humanist scholar who combines an interest in theory and book knowledge with the practice of medicine. In addition, Monardes uses the dialog form to stage an intellectual exchange, not so much about colonial knowledge per se (as did García de Orta) but rather about epistemology. Thus, while the Doctor is on his way in the streets of Seville in order to see a patient, he meets one "Sr. Burgos," an apothecary, who is on his way to the Casa de Contratación (House of Trade) in order to view the gold, silver, and emeralds that have arrived with the latest fleet from the Indies. The Doctor decides to accompany him, but, upon arrival at the Casa, they find the doors still locked and begin a conversation about metals. The Doctor asks Burgos why he admires gold and silver—metals that are, in his opinion, much overrated. He announces that he will prove that iron is more excellent a metal than either gold or silver, because of both its medicinal properties and its usefulness to man in the making of tools. As though to dramatize Vives's call on scholars to "enter into shops and factories, and to ask questions from craftsmen, and to get to know about the details of their work" (Vives 209), the doctor therefore takes Burgos to the workshop of one Sr. Ortuño, a Basque miner and artisan who is an expert on iron mining and ironworking. At Ortuño's house, the three characters engage in a conversation in which each of the participants appears to personify one of the three branches in the Scholastic-Aristotelian division of knowledge between *episteme* (or *scientia*), *praxis*, and *techne*. Thus, the doctor personifies *episteme/ scientia*—theoretical knowledge based on the logical syllogism and geometrical demonstration; Burgos, whose name (which he shares with the historic Visigothic capital of Castile) associates him with the civic and political realm, while his

---

[37]   On the diffusion of Paralecelsianism in sixteenth-century Spain, see López Piñero's *El 'Dialogus'* and "*Paracelsus* and his Work"; also Rey Bueno, "Los paracelsistas" 41–56.

manifest interest in the treasure at the Casa associate him with commercial life,[38] personifies *praxis* ('things done')—the Aristotelian term for human knowledge, including such branches as history, politics, ethics, and economics. And the Basque artisan, Ortuño, personifies *techne* ("things made").[39]

In the Scholastic scheme of knowledge, there was not only a strict separation between the three realms but also a clear epistemological, ethical, and social hierarchy—*scientia* being regarded as the noblest, most certain knowledge, practiced by the social elite, and *techne* being regarded as the lowliest and least stable knowledge, practiced by the lower ranks of society, who had to work with their hands (H. J. Cook, "Medicine"). In the *Diálogo*, by contrast, Monardes underscores the equal "nobility" of artisanal work by giving his artisan character the name of "Ortuño"—an ancient Basque noble lineage whose name derives etymologically from the Latin roots fortuna (fortune) and hortus (garden), thus evoking the idea of empirical knowledge and the manipulation of nature by art and linking his art in alchemy to Monardes's own of botany or exotic horticulture.

Having underlined the equality of the three realms of knowledge, Monardes has his three characters engage in an egalitarian dialogue that is divided into two parts. The first part discusses the genesis of iron and steel, the methods of their production, and their technological uses; the second part treats their elemental properties and uses in medicine. The Doctor is the expert on the physical, (al-)chemical, and medicinal aspects of iron and steel; Ortuño is the expert on their technological production and uses; and Burgos is the expert on their pharmaceutical uses. However, whereas Burgos's theoretical learning seems somewhat limited (he only cites the Al-Andalusians Albucasis and Averroes on the preparation of medicines, and is otherwise mostly responsible for raising questions), the Doctor is the authority on the written record on iron and steel. Thus, he embarks on a highly learned disquisition on their origins and qualities. Iron and steel, he explains, are made "por via de Alchimia, y se haze dellos quinta essencia, como del Oro y Plata: dizen los Alquimistas que el metal mas aparejado para sus disignos y efectos es el Hierro" (by means of alchemy and from them quintessence, as gold and silver are made: the alchemists say that the metal most suited to their designs and effects is iron) (167 v). Citing a formidable, if eclectic, array of alchemical authorities, the Doctor argues not only that iron is created through the same means and of the same matter as gold and silver—"se haze y cría de los mismos principios y materia que se hazen el Oro y Plata"—but also that it is "más excelente" than gold and silver, "porque del tenemos más aprovechamientos y más necesidad que de todos los demás" (because it is more useful and necessary than all the other metals) (163v). Although all metals were equally engendered in the earth from substances placed there by God at the creation of the world, iron is singular in creation for its contrary qualities, being both hot and cold at the same time; this was an oxymoron

---

[38]   Burgos is derived from gothic baurgs, or walled villages.

[39]   On these Aristotelian categories and their Scholastic afterlife, see Long (*Openness* 16–45).

within strictly Aristotelian categories of mixture but a common idea within the alchemical philosophy, which understood all metals to be mixtures of "hot" sulfur (the "father") and "cold" mercury (the "mother") (Newman, *Atoms* 26).[40] Citing Avicenna, the Doctor explains that

> assi ha de tener la complexion y temperatura, que participe de entrambas calidades. Mediante el Azogue enfría, y por no tener humidad notable mezclada con estas calidades, es tan seco, y por esto duro y fuerte. Mediante el Sulfur calienta, consume, desseca, abre, conforta, provoca apetito, y haze las obras maravillosas que adelante diremos, que todas se hazen mediante el calor que tiene. (172v)

> (iron has a complexion and temperament that participates in both qualities. Through its mercury, it is cold and because it has no moistness mixed with these qualities and is so dry, it is hard and strong. Through its sulfur, it is warm; it consumes, dries, opens, and is comfortative, it stimulates the appetite and does marvelous things because of its warmth that we will explain.)

While he submits that some implements made of iron, such as the handgun, are surely inventions of the devil, more generally, iron and steel, not gold and silver, are the keys to power and dominion in the form of weapons. Indeed, it was Europeans' possession not of gold, but of alchemically produced iron, the Doctor argues, that allowed them to discover and conquer the New World. Not only did the iron needle in the compass assist their transoceanic navigations, but it also awed the Indians into submission: "Admirábanse los Indios al principio de su descubrimiento, quando veían a los Españoles coser con aguja, que les parecía cosa de milagro, y daban por una aguja mucho Oro" (When they were first discovered, the Indians marveled at the Spaniards, who sewed with a needle, which seemed something miraculous, and they traded a great deal of gold for one needle) (166v–r).

Significantly, Monardes dedicates the *Diálogo* to the second Duke of Alcalá de los Gazules, Fernando Enriquez de Ribera (1527–1594), who was not only one of the leading aristocrats of Andalusia but also the husband of Juana Cortés Ramírez de Arellano (?–1588), a daughter of the conqueror of Mexico, Hernando Cortés.[41] Monardes points out to the Duke that iron has great medicinal virtues—"grandes virtudes medicinales" (158v)—and also is an instrument by which "los valerosos ayan conseguido con el grandes titulos y fama" (the brave have won great titles and renown) (158v). The reference to titles and renown alludes to the role that the Duke's own ancestors, the "Admirals of Castile," had played in the *Reconquista* after Fernando III had created the title following his conquest of Seville in 1248. "[C]on sus vigorosos brazos, la lanza en el puño, la espada en la mano, venciendo batallas, ganando villas y lugares, el nombre y fama immortal, que hoy tienen

---

[40]   See also Debus, *The Chemical Philosophy*.

[41]   On the Duke's family history, see González Moreno. On the history of the title of the Admiral of Castile, see Ortega Gato.

consiguieron" (With powerful arms, gripping a lance, sword in hand, triumphing in battle, winning villages and towns, they won the name and immortal fame that they enjoy today) (158v). Moreover, through his marriage to Juana, the Duke had combined his illustrious lineage with that of Cortés, who, through "trabajos inmensos," conquered the New World and there won not only "lugares y villas" (villages and towns) but also "Reynos e Imperios" (kingdoms and empires) (158v). Surely, the Duke's own children will follow in the footsteps of these two great lines of ancestors and "imitarlos en las hazañas y hechos eroycos que hizieron: tomando por instrumento del Hierro, que a los tales, en exercicios militares les sera grande medio y ayuda" (emulate the feats and heroic deeds they did, taking for their instrument iron, which in such military endeavors will be a great and helpful tool) (158v). Thus, from the very outset, Monardes emphasizes the technological applications of the scientific interest in metals and the salvific consequences of these practical applications by effecting the triumph of Christianity and Spanish civility over infidels in Spain and pagans in America.

Conclusion

Synthesizing empirical discovery with textual tradition, as well as the scientific interest in the material world, with Christian militancy and messianic salvation, the language of alchemy lent a strongly transcendent, spiritual, and "magical" character to the early modern "hunt" for exotic spices and drugs in the early modern literature of the discovery of the New World. Unlike gold or Dragon's Blood, however, which was associated with a rich cultural web of associations and analogies in a long tradition of Old World alchemy and natural history, the majority of New World exotic plants, such as tobacco, entered the early modern literature of discovery "naked," decontextualized from their meaning in Native American cultures—as a sort of "secret" knowledge that early modern Europeans came to associate with idolatry and diabolism. Thus, the sixteenth-century literature of the discovery and conquest of the New World represents the first step in early modern natural philosophy that Francois Jacob has described as a "scraping clean" of living bodies: things "shook off their crust of analogies, resemblances and signs," he writes, "to appear in all the nakedness of their true outer shape [...] What was read or related no longer carried the weight of what was seen [...] What counted was not so much the code used by God for creating nature as that sought by man for understanding it" (Jacob 28). It is these dual processes that the anthropologist of modern science Bruno Latour has called "purification" and "hybridization," and that he sees as constitutive in the construction of the modern scientific "object" during the seventeenth-century Scientific Revolution in England (13–48).

It is at this juncture, then, that we can begin to see the significance of the European encounter with American nature to Stephen Gaukroger's question of why in the modern West the hermeneutic models of the natural sciences were able to establish cognitive hegemony—a hegemony that he deems to be "pathological" by comparative standards (Gaukroger 18). In medieval alchemy, the "hunt" for the secrets of nature between and beyond the categories of scientific reason had essentially been an esoteric tradition, limited in practice to private individuals, often operating in isolation and on the borders of religious orthodoxy. In the context of the European discovery and conquest of the New World, its rhetorical, hermeneutical, and epistemological models and methods became appropriated as instruments of the early modern and imperial state, such as the Spanish Casa de Contratación and Consejo de Indias (Council of the Indies). As historians of early modern Spanish science such as Antonio Barrera, Maria Portuondo, and others have argued, if the decisive factor in the emergence of modern science was the interaction between artisans and scholars, through which scholars began to hold artisans and their methods in higher esteem than in the past, this process "took place within the European imperial and commercial expansion of the sixteenth and seventeenth centuries. Merchants, royal officials, artisans, natural historians, pilots, and cosmographers came together in institutions such as courts and academies, where their economic and political interests overlapped" (Barrera-Osorio, *Experiencing* 8). It was this sixteenth-century synthesis of traditions, professions, and institutions in imperial Spain that would provide the model for Francis Bacon's "inquisitorial" model of science, especially his notion that "the nature of things betrays itself more readily under the vexations of art than in its natural freedom" (Pesic).[42] By "vexation" of nature, Bacon meant an "encounter between the scientist and nature in which both are tested and purified"—following the model of alchemy. Bacon's program of the "vexation of nature" became the model of science propagated by the Royal Society of London and informed the production of matters of "fact" in Boyle's airpump. Thus, Latour, in his brilliant reading of Stephen Shapin and Simon Schaffer's seminal *Leviathan and the Airpump*, may have intuitively put his finger on the colonial historical context from which the dual processes of purification and hybridization emerge. He writes that "Native Americans were not mistaken when they accused the Whites of having forked tongues. By separating the relations of political power from the relations of scientific reasoning, while continuing to shore up power with reason and reason with power, the moderns have always had two irons in the fire. They have become invincible" (Latour 38).

---

[42]   On the influence of sixteenth-century Spanish upon seventeenth-century English science, see Pimentel, "The Iberian Vision"; and Cañizares Esguerra, *Puritan*.

PART 2
Itineraries of Spanish Medicine

Chapter 4

"From Where They Are Now to Whence They Came From": News About Health and Disease in New Spain (1550–1615)[1]

Mauricio Sánchez-Menchero

There is so much distance by land, if only it were less, I myself would be the messenger.

—Juan López Talavera (personal letter, Mexico City, 1572)

Introduction

During the sixteenth century there were wide swaths of illiteracy among different cultural and socioeconomic groups, generations, and genders. In "towns and cities," however, "a greater number of tradesmen, shopkeepers, artisans and even journeymen could now read, put their signature to parish registers or notarial deeds, draw up a receipt, keep an accounts book or write a letter" (Chartier, Boureau, and Dauphin 1; also see Bannet 41). Letters and books with collections of models of letter-writing are invaluable to historians for, among other reasons, studying the lexical and syntactic change over time (Skaffarri et al.). But rather than considering linguistic issues, this chapter analyzes a corpus of transatlantic correspondence in order to explore first-person accounts of the medical cultures of Hispanic societies.

Indeed, as a Carmelite monk in Seville pointed out, "a letter is more persuasive than a very long book" because "in letters, more than in other longer pieces of writing [...] the writer selects *that which is liveliest and most passionate*" (Melchor de San Bartolomé, cited in Bouza 148; emphasis added).[2] In this chapter, I explore

[1] This chapter is the result of a research project sponsored by the UNAM (National Autonomous University of Mexico) through PAPIIT (Program to Support Research and Technological Innovation Projects) (IN 400911-3): *Geografías médicas. Discursos, prácticas y representaciones de la medicina en la Nueva España (siglos XVI–XVII)* and the *Cultura médica en la periferia colonial: Nueva España, 1520–1620* project, financed by the Spanish Ministry of Science and Innovation (HAR2009-11030-C02-01).
[2] On the effects of the manuscript referred to by the prelate, there is a very similar description in the booklet that Don Quixote and Sancho Panza found in that dusty suitcase where they discovered letters containing "complaints, laments, distrusts, flavors

early modern medical cultures through the letters of individuals, analyzing aspects linked to health that are poised at the intersection of the three areas discussed by David Gentilcore in the context of early modern Naples: family, religion, and "expertise" (*Healers* 2). The medical culture of New Spain was the result of a complex process of negotiation among medical cultures of very diverse origins and differing relationships to power, both factual and symbolic. It is important, therefore, to always keep in mind *who* was behind the different discourses, and *with what stated intention* those discourses were deployed (to the extent that intentionality is apparent in the letters). This can partly be inferred by format and genre (correspondence, reports, chronicles, legal testimonies in inquisitorial or other kinds of trials, responses to questionnaires) as well as the *intended audiences*; that is to say, *to whom* they were addressed and *where*, or to what setting their recipients belonged (Spanish cities, other towns in New Spain, or perhaps even, as in some cases, enemy European nations). These negotiations among indigenous and Western worlds impinge on the field of health during the phase of the Conquest and the early stages of colonization. There is no doubt that European university medicine, following the Hippocratic-Galenic tradition, arrived in Mesoamerica with the first physicians and surgeons. But these were so scarce that the medicine of physicians and surgeons was not the predominant discourse among the settlers, even after the medical culture they represented was implemented in institutions such as hospitals and universities. The variety of strategies Spanish settlers used for illness prevention and cure cannot be separated from the complex ethnic and cultural reality of New Spain, which included indigenous populations, Africans, mestizos, and mulattoes.

The immediate objects of my analysis—the letters themselves—are drawn from the collections of correspondence published by Enrique Otte, as well as research work by Concepción Company, Chantal Melis, and Agustín Rivero Franyutti. Although the corpus of letters I have used is primarily made up of correspondence between Spaniards settled in different Mexican towns and their relatives or acquaintances in Spain, it also includes letters sent by indigenous or African correspondents. Letters help us assess medical phenomena related to three concepts: distance, scale, and novelty.[3] In terms of distance, letters help us understand how being far from home became a medical issue: remoteness carried social costs and costs to health; descriptions of the danger of transatlantic passage itself reveal the physical and emotional costs of travel. Letters also tell us a great deal about the scale of particular medical phenomena. This sometimes implies horrifying frequency, as when one writer reacts to finding 30 neighbors dying every day for over a month during an epidemic. At other times, it is infrequency and

---

and troubles, favors and slights, some solemnly considered and others mourned over" (Cervantes 136).

    [3]   As David N. Livingstone says: "To understand the *history* of medicine [...] we must necessarily grasp the geography of medical, religious, and legal discourses [...] At every scale, knowledge, space, and power are tightly interwoven" (*Putting Science in Its Place* 11).

insufficiency that becomes a medical issue—the scarcity of medical practitioners and how this affected their fee structure. We know that the epidemics that ravaged New Spain during the sixteenth century were horrifying; letters give us a "bottom up" view of phenomena occurring on a hemispheric scale. In addition to distance and scale, letters, of course, can teach us about novelty—about the fears that new diseases caused and the worry about using unfamiliar medicines. Focusing on letters is in some ways opposed to large-scale, data-driven studies of demographic changes or statistical analyses. Letters tell us something that numbers cannot: how writers in New Spain might have rendered comprehensible the new world of medical cultures they encountered. In other words, it is as much the attempts to make the individual experience of a global monarchy legible as it is the events the letters describe that make this corpus of texts so valuable.

Letters are quite different from other documents considered in chapters dedicated to New Spain in this book. Transcripts of Inquisitorial trials are generated in a climate of antagonism and confrontation; the documents generated in any legal proceeding are the products of parties pitted against one another.[4] Requests for information from the monarch or from the state bureaucracy imply an imbalance of power; answers to surveys and questionnaires reflect this imbalance.[5] Letters may reveal the same level of animosity, jealousy, and rivalry that court proceedings do. And letters certainly encode relationships of power. But letters often construct the identity and authority of the correspondent through reference to the interior life of a particular person; this may be reflected in an attempt to produce a feeling of spontaneity, immediacy, or intimacy in the letter. Just as often, a letter may illuminate the life, the feelings, or the convictions of a letter-writer through careful craft and deliberation. As we shall see, a letter's immediacy does not indicate freedom from ideology; letters, like the other documents considered in this volume, can subtly and even conspicuously reveal power relations[6] (from family letters to commercial correspondence as well as other kind of letters: recommendations, condolences, those asking for mercy, etc.).[7] But there are also several models of letters in which we can observe various types of relationships in the form of the greeting in family spheres ("Sir and Father of Mine"; "My Highly Desired Lady Wife"; "My Son") or of subordination ("Most Magnificent Sir"). That is to say, the particular configuration of power relations, medicine, and personal appeal make letters a valuable source.

---

[4]   On Inquisitorial sources, see Morales's chapter in this volume.

[5]   In his chapter in this book, Pardo-Tomás examines responses to surveys and questionnaires—known as *Relaciones Geográficas*—and the scarcity of physicians.

[6]   As indicated by P. Bourdieu: "[...] one must not forget that the relations of communication *par excellence*—linguistic exchanges—are also relations of symbolic power in which the power relations between speakers or their respective groups are actualized" (37).

[7]   In 1617, Juan Vicente Peliger published a book with models for letters that readers could adapt to their needs. For example, to be granted permission to emigrate it was necessary to stress the hardships endured in the homeland, including illness (181–2).

Distance: Fear and the Crossing

Transatlantic migrants, before lighting out for the American paradise, had a great deal of mundane paperwork to do (such as obtaining a permit to cross the Atlantic).[8] Permits were often easier to come by than the courage it took to make the crossing. That is why letters from overseas, like a never-ending tide, exhorted those still in Spain to overcome their fear of the voyage. Juan de Mendoza, for example, wrote a letter from Zamora, Michoacán, in 1574, to his nephew Cristóbal de Ayala:

> Tell Alonso Díaz de Manzanilla for me that, since he has never made this voyage, despite having written to me that he would come, I believe he does not dare to come for *fear of the puddle*, and that he should not fear the voyage, that it is all in the starting-off, and that, if he wishes to come with the first armada, I have found him very good accommodations. (Otte 207)

Fear of the "puddle" (the Atlantic) was not unwarranted; many ships were lost to unpredictable seas. Urging a loved one to risk the voyage could lead to guilt. Juana Bautista did not know whether her sister had left Spain en route to the New World; hearing no news, Juana was assailed by guilt at having insisted that her sister make the trip, and filled with worry that because of "her sins" God might have allowed her sister to suffer "some mishap at sea" (Company 170–71). Luckily for Juana and her sister, nothing calamitous seems to have befallen either of them (at least up until 1572, when she described her concerns in a letter).

   Those who did plan to brave the crossing were offered abundant advice and warnings about the experience at sea and in America.[9] Hernán Sánchez wrote a letter in 1569 from Aranzueque to his brother Diego Ramos:

> I must warn you that it is a very laborious voyage, because you must negotiate the sea, and there is danger and risk in it although, the Lord be praised, it has been many days since one of the fleets has suffered an accident; because the route has been heavily traveled, and there are many skilled pilots. But you should still consider it, and write to me of your decision, and speak of it with my brothers […]. (Otte 219)

The call to adventure, as Joseph Campbell indicated, means abandoning the center of gravity anchored in social identity and venturing into an unknown beyond the self.[10] But which part of their world should travelers take with them to sea? Could one preserve familiar tastes and objects, or protect one's own welfare

---

   [8]   Part of the corpus is made up of letters from Spanish emigrants, presented by relatives at the *Casa de la Contratación* as part of their applications to go to the Indies.

   [9]   Margit Frenk, in her *Nueva lírica* book, includes the following humorous verse: "How will I cross, if I do not know how to swim? […] / Hey, sailor, would you help me?" (622).

   [10]   Campbell (54).

and health? Recommendations from those who had already gone through the experience of the crossing proved helpful.

Reading between the lines, one can ascertain the things they do not have and miss from their places of origin, as in this letter from Puebla, written by Sebastián Pliego to his wife, Mari Díaz, in 1581:

> For your time on the sea, they will give to each of you an *azumbre* of water, so bring twelve jugs of water, or if you want more, more. As for bread, for each of you bring one *quintal* of biscuits, and for everybody a *quintal* of raisins, three cured hams, almonds, sugar, an *arroba* of fish, another of *tollo* [a type of fish], especially a measure of garbanzos, hazelnuts. From home bring a good skillet and a grill, a rolling pin and a spoon. In Seville, buy a metal pot and plates and bowls, plus a kettle; of wine, two *arrobas* and of vinegar another two, and an *arroba* of oil, and whatever else you wish. Buy two chests to contain everything that you will eat, or they will steal it all from you [...] sleep on top of them, and do not sleep by yourself, but rather with my brothers [...]. (Otte 162–3)

References to the health and illnesses of travelers surfaced, above all, at two specific times: during the ocean crossing as they suffered from illnesses (such as scurvy, undoubtedly one of the most common on the journey),[11] and once they had docked at port,[12] when new and different ailments could attack the traveler during the land leg of the voyage that came next. Melchor Valdelomar, writing from Veracruz in 1574, warned his father-in-law, Lorenzo Martínez de Carvallar, about the "difficulty and danger still to come on the road":

> that is greater than one would believe, and [even after] leaving behind the dangers of the sea, [there are still] illnesses on land, that two-thirds of the people who came with us on the same fleet perished from, and this is regularly [...]. (Otte 85–6)

Indeed, after the hardships at sea, more were to come. In 1580, the physician Hernández Diosdado—"a man of considerable experience and practice in the things of this land"—recommended that travelers leave the port of Veracruz

---

[11]   The Italian sailor Pigafetta recounted in detail the troubles the crew was forced to face during the voyage led by Magellan in 1520–1521: "Our greatest misfortune was to be attacked by an illness in which our gums became swollen to such a degree that they made our teeth disappear, in both the upper jaw and the lower jaw and those who were attacked by it [scurvy] could not eat anything. Nineteen died [...] Besides those who died we had [...] sick sailors, who suffered pains in their arms, legs and other parts of their body, but they recovered. As to myself, I shall never be able to thank God enough because during all that time and in the midst of so many calamities I never had the slightest illness" (cited in Martínez 151).

[12]   Happiness and hope would spread out among the sailors when they caught sight of isome small bird [...] because it seemed like a sign of land, "together with a few clumps of grass [floating in] the water" (cited in Martínez 271).

"as soon as possible" (Acuña V: 301–8).[13] Diosdado explained that due to "the city's foul air, the water and the food had the distinction of making a significant number of travelers fall ill. It was not uncommon that the newly arrived were affected by strong fevers accompanied by chills and shaking, to such a degree that they could not stand up on their own feet [...]" (López de Mariscal 106).

There was no way around danger if one chose to travel. The price of the adventure was frequently illness, and sometimes death. Alonso de Alcocer told his brother, Juan de Colonia, that since arriving in Mexico, "I have not enjoyed a single day of health, because in this land all of those who come from Spain come down with a *chapetonada*, and it kills more than a third of the people who come here."[14] Once the first trials were overcome, the traveler had to adapt to new circumstances. Alcocer noted in 1577 that, if one were healthy, the rest was easy. Unlike in Spain, Alcocer noted—where "you will not be able to improve your fortune"—recent arrivals to the colonies found work quickly: "although they know nothing, they have no trouble finding work to earn their keep and one hundred pesos a year" (Otte 98–9). But there was a difference between finding work and adjusting to life on a different continent, as Alcocer's own life made clear.

In 1606 the astrologer Enrico Martínez, who had settled in the Americas, would write about the physical effects of moving to a new climate and changing his diet. Martínez's *Repertorio de los tiempos y historia natural de esta Nueva España* described, in Hippocratic-Galenic terms, the fate of Europeans who ate new foods that were "of less sustenance," and "easier to digest":

> those who come from Spain [...] to these parts, undergo certain changes according to their temperament and the celestial influence of these climes, and depending on the quality of the new foods they grow new blood, and the new blood produces new humor, and the new humor, new abilities and conditions [...] it is clear that the spirits of those who enjoy them are revived, and is evident from experience, in this kingdom the good skills of outsiders improve, and the skills that were not good are mended. (181)

The perception of the effects that the climate and foods of the Americas had on travelers is present in some letters. For example, Alonso Morales, who, in 1576, wrote to his cousin Juan Ramiro in Trujillo, describing his voyage to Puebla: "it cost us some effort to reach this city of Los Ángeles [Puebla], and when I arrived *the land hit me* and I fell gravely ill, but Our Lord saw fit to restore me to health" (Otte 159; emphasis added). María Díaz describes to her daughter a harrowing crossing during which the ship was dismasted in 1577; once in Mexico City,

---

[13]   About the contents of the account by Hernández Diosdado, see the chapter by Pardo-Tomás in this volume.

[14]   A *chapetonada* was an illness that affected travelers from Europe. According to Corominas, this term comes from *chapetón*, referring to the "European who has recently arrived to Spanish America and, therefore, is untried, a greenhorn, in the country's difficulties, [around] 1555."

"God saw fit to afflict your father with diarrhea and fever." Suspecting that the illness was caused by the local climate, Díaz and her husband depart Mexico City, with "the hope of some improvement." Díaz continues:

> fifteen days later he relapsed into the same illness, in which God saw fit to take him. And I assure you that I would have been much happier to have also been buried with him that day, rather than to be widowed and defenseless so far away from my own country. (Otte 97)

Scale: The Scarcity of Physicians

In the letters studied, a few references are made to the professions of physician, surgeon, and apothecary. A lack of competition could sometimes be advantageous for the physicians who were in New Spain, as we see in the letter of Hernán García. García's brother-in-law, Andrés Toribio, "was very well versed in his trade" as an alchemist. So in 1583 García wrote to Catalina Núñez, his sister and Toribio's wife, to convince them both to travel to Mexico. García promised Toribio that "in three years [he would be earning] eight thousand pesos" (Otte 166). Miguel Hidalgo in 1587 wrote a letter from Cartagena to his father-in-law, Juan Martínez, promising similar riches: "the two or three surgeons or apothecaries who are here earn thousands since there are no physicians available here in the three months it takes the fleet to make the journey" (Otte 301).

There are not many descriptions of therapeutic procedures or healing practices coming directly from European healers settled in the Indies in the sources I analyzed; when descriptions do appear, they surface obliquely and apparently betray relations of mistrust between patient and physician. A good example is that offered by the case of Melchor Valdelomar, whom we have already seen writing from Veracruz about the dangers of the ocean crossing. He told his father-in-law how his wife, Inés, had miraculously recovered from a fever, even though the doctors had ruled her condition a hopeless one:

> [...] all the physicians of Mexico had said her case was hopeless, and it was God who chose to give her health. She is now fine and very lovely and fat and having just given birth to a daughter, the loveliest born in this kingdom [...]. (Otte 85–6)

If one could afford it, it was perfectly possible to receive medical care from several physicians at the same time in Mexico City in 1584. Hernán Ruiz told his wife, Mariana de Montedoca, in Seville about such a case:

> Since I departed that land I have not had a single day in which I was healthy, and all of July and August I spent in bed, having been told that I would die and *the doctors wanted to open me up*, they were saying that my illness was *poctema* [sic] [an abscess] in the liver. *I never gave my consent* [...]. (Otte 108)

Without a doubt, Hernán Ruiz's doctors were simply following Galen's instructions concerning the treatment of abscesses when they advised that he be "opened up" (Galenus 308). But as Ruiz adds in his letter (and this makes it even more interesting), he did not agree to be operated on "because he suspected that his illness was because of food or because of spells." Although he does not clarify, the spells may have been cast after he arrived in the colonies.[15] Ruiz was sick a long time, and weak with fever. After recovering, he wrote in a letter dated 1584 that the physicians may not have approached his cure properly. Ruiz wondered, "if they made their best efforts, or if they [the first physicians] gave me the wrong cure at the start of the illness." Here, he alludes to the fact that after he dismissed his first physicians, Ruiz was treated by three new doctors. The team of new doctors finally cured him, after "twenty-two" bloodlettings "from the main vein in my right arm," in addition to the inevitable purges administered "four times [at] the start of the illness" (Otte 108).

Yet another bit of correspondence is intriguing for its portrayal of the economic hardships caused by disease and discomfort. In Mexico City in October 1573, Bartolomé de Morales was suffering from a headache that he thought would drive him mad; a cup was applied to his head to draw out the pain, but this left him "stiffer than a rod." After having spent "over three hundred pesos" on "medicines," the "doctor and everything else," Morales still found no relief. Eventually, his pain abated, but once his headache resolved, Bartolomé de Morales suffered a grave accident. He was riding at night on a street and collided with a "wooden stake driven into the ground." The blow caused his left leg to be wedged between the pole and the horse, "leaving it so twisted, that the kneecap was pushed into the back of his knee." But what is really remarkable is how Bartolomé de Morales gave thanks to God because instead of calling a physician to care for him, "a native Indian" who knew how to return his leg "to its proper shape" was called in, and he thus avoided having to "walk with crutches," which is what he had feared when he saw how badly his knee had been injured (Otte 72–3).[16]

---

[15]   On food poisoning it should be noted that it is a kind of spell in which "[...] the harm is linked to a specific individual because of the ill will of she who prepared the food. In other words, the bite of food, the drink, constitute the embodiment of evil [...]" (Bernard 126). Bernardino de Sahagún, in *Discurso sobre cosas y policía exterior, del padre al hijo*, revealed the importance that indigenous people gave to meals, "since there are many enemies who despise a person secretly; take care that no one give you food or drink that could be something poisonous; mostly, you should be careful about this with people who wish you ill [...]" (Sahagún, *General History* 361–2).

[16]   In the *Relaciones Geográficas* corresponding to Malinaltepec and Atlatlauca (Oaxaca), reference is made to "The many medicinal herbs used by these Indians, and the ones they know how to describe what their uses are include: For a broken or twisted arm or leg they take the bark of a tree that they call Yandandaqueno in their own language and Cacalosuhil in Mexican. If placed on a broken bone, and by applying heat and bandaging, they say it helps to cement bones [...]" (Acuña, II: 47–59).

It should be stressed that this type of information pulled from private letters tells us a lot, frequently in a way that is completely normal and natural. Letters provide information about therapeutic procedures that were oftentimes totally unlike those of academic medicine. They also tell us a great deal about the relationships between Spaniards and Indians in the field of healing. These relationships are characterized quite differently in letters than they are in trial documents and judicial proceedings. In judicial documents, an air of tension or hostility often pervades portrayals of relationships among different ethnic groups; logically enough, there are many accusations of criminality. But letters are quite different in this respect and, to a greater extent, represent an atmosphere of more amicable relationships. Judicial texts are of great interest, however, in those cases in which Spanish or creole witnesses explain or justify Indian curing methods suspected of being linked to sorcery or idolatry. Witnesses presented arguments that give us clues about medical practices, but in a context that necessarily suggests a power relationship.[17] Accounts in letters, on the other hand, although often less rich in detail, are far more spontaneous. Even when their letters may, in fact, have been carefully composed, letter-writers often seek to convey a sense of immediacy and spontaneity.

Letters also reveal the different range of reactions to illness and healing strategies used by immigrants from the Old World. For example, when Spaniards in New Spain fell ill they turned to the Galenic or Hippocratic medicine taught in European universities. That did not mean patients declined to complain about the fees they had to pay physicians. Neither did it mean that patients were hesitant to lament their doctors' ineptitude. In 1561 Antonio Mateos told his wife about having fallen into a river with his horse and how "cold entered his gut," making him so ill and so weak "that he could barely bring a jug of water to his lips." So Antonio Mateos attempted one cure and during the "month of August" he "spent nine days sweating." There was no improvement. He had to spend "money first with foolish physicians and then God had the grace to send me a physician who cured me in twenty days" (Otte 145).

The ineffectiveness of doctors and physicians in the colonies is illustrated in the following quotation from Juan de Brihuega, in which he tells his brother about the poor medical care his wife received in 1572: "My wife has been very ill with

---

[17] An example of these kinds of documents was written in Michoacán in 1618 and refers to a healing through a superstitious curing ceremony carried out in 1608. The account says that an Indian called Alonso had cured an 11-month-old infant. Among the interesting elements in this account are the description of the healer as an "old man, aged about fifty years," who entered the living room of the house and began curing the baby, "whose soft spot on top of his head had dropped." To conduct the healing, the document notes, the Indian asked for "clay bowl with embers, copal and cotton." It should be noted that in this case the child's health was achieved through the desperation and audacity of his parents in calling an Indian healer, but also, and above all, because of the way Alonso, the doctor, acted—because even though he used techniques and elements linked to indigenous culture, such as copal and clay bowls, he had the sense to mix them with Christian elements to be able to act and not be labeled an indigenous sorcerer by Spanish authorities (Company 241–3).

a pain in her side and her condition was very risky because she was seven months pregnant and *they did six bloodlettings* and it is because of this that her situation became so grave" (Otte 154). Sometimes there was nothing left to do except pray. For a patient whose home and family were far away, who had no money and no hope of assistance, God was the last resort.[18] Francisco Ramírez provides a good example of how illness often drove patients into such precarious situations that turning to prayer or divine intervention was sometimes the only option available. He speaks of it in this letter from 1582:

> My health is not good and I recently recovered from a long and dangerous illness. It has been God's grace to give me health and this year I have suffered four illnesses, all of them strong and that put at risk my life, that I offer to God to serve Him with it. (Otte 193)[19]

The use of relics also appears alongside prayer. In 1575, Gregorio de Quintana described the holy relics he utilized as amulets when facing a long and difficult illness. Quintana tells his brother:

> [I]t has been more than two years that I have been very ill, for more than a year my hands and feet were paralyzed and to go out I needed to take two Negroes and go on horseback, and it was the Lord's will to give me health, *but I still have some relics* [...]. (Otte 213–14)

Novelty: New World Medicines

Correspondence also gives us information about settlers of Spanish origin who gathered information from Indians; the Spanish were attempting to find plants and remedies native to New Spain that they could use as substitutes for European plants that were either difficult or impossible to acquire. One example is found in the medicinal use of cocoa. Cocoa was already widely consumed as "chocolate," and people frequently justified their consumption by referring to cocoa's therapeutic uses. Thus, Ana de Herrera, a mulatto woman, wrote a letter to her mother from the secret dungeons of the Inquisition with an urgent request:

---

[18]   In this regard Antono Torrijano told his wife about how he had "such a hard time until he was able to enter" New Spain, "I spent all that time ill and now I am penniless. But it pleased God that I should come out of it alive and I give thanks to Him" (Otte 163–4).

[19]   The same feeling of impotence when coping with illness could be felt by a patient, not in New Spain but in the metropolis: "From your [letter]," dated 1577, "I found out that your worship was ill from fevers (malaria), and because of that chose to spend the winter at home. I was saddened that your worship was afflicted with such a disease because, even though it is not dangerous it is very sad and vexing. I do sincerely want to know how the illness left you and please let me know everything about it. Your worship must care for his health since it is very important and it is a shame to see how all of us are slowly beginning to fail" (Otte 184–5).

To please do me the favor of sending me a bit of ground chocolate made into tablets, because Mrs. Francisca has given it to me to drink, because Luisa ground it for her a few times and she has found that it has sat well with her for a stomach pain that she has [...]."[20]

Despite the success in choosing to use some plants native to the Americas, Spaniards continued to insist that they be sent medicines made in the metropolis. They were hesitant to employ herbs or other remedies that were different from those to which they had always been accustomed. Furthermore, in order to avoid the risks of using local remedies, many Spaniards preferred those that were prepared under the supervision of apothecaries.[21]

A good example of the hesitancy of Spaniards to use American medicinal plants and substances is Miguel Navarro's letter of 1564 to the king. Navarro was a Franciscan friar and he wrote to request that the monarch send more friars because "many of those who are here on this apostolic mission have died recently." To justify his request Navarro explained that due to the "intolerable hardships" that the monks endured, they frequently fell ill. It was difficult to find the "remedies and medicines to cure them," even though there were "two infirmaries, one here in Mexico and another in the city of los Ángeles [Puebla]." Navarro went on to say that, since the friars were "poor and [had] no money," they lacked funds to buy the materials and medicines from Spain "from whence they must come." Thus, the monks ended their letter with the following request:

That we receive sufficient alms so that father Joan de Mansilla, who is the person that this province sends to the general chapter on business that it might have, may buy with the alms in that kingdom, while he is over there, the necessary drugs and medicines for both infirmaries, and that he bring them himself when it is time for him to return. (Company 150–51)

Scale: Epidemics, Propaganda, and Numbers

References to epidemics abounded in the letters of the period. One typical example is the letter that, in 1576, Juan López de Soria sent to the Countess Ribadivia; in it, he related the grave labor problems he faced at his Tlaxcala estate due to

a pestilence among the people of the area [... of whom] it is said more than 80,000 have died, and on our property more than 200 have succumbed, and

---

[20]   AGN/Inquisition/vol. 207/f. 1 [Letter from 1594]. Another therapeutic use of chocolate ìdiluted in hot waterî was to use it for the bloody flux (dysentery), as mentioned in the *Relación Geográfica* de San Andrés, Guatemala (Acuña I: 130).

[21]   Luis de Oviedo, an apothecary in Madrid, said that it was not enough to just "grind the substance of the medications we grind very well since if you take a rose, that contains the same substance for different medicines, it needs to be ground differently according to the different parts on to which it is to be applied [...]" (*Methodo* 139).

among them some Negroes, so now the estate is at a standstill and we [...] are giving the order to find people, but it cannot be done [...] God in his mercy *protect the Spanish people*, who as yet have hardly been touched, but who remain in great fear. (Otte 96–7; emphasis added)

Spaniards had taken note of how their arrival—and the subsequent herding of native Indians into villages,[22] and compelling the reorganization of the indigenous population—caused ecological changes and epidemic outbreaks. The fact is that while the Spanish population remained largely immune to the epidemics, disease stalked the native Indians. The challenge to explain or at least question the causes of all this misery surfaced many times in letters. A few friars pointed out, in a letter to the king dated 1569, that:

The natives of this land [...] have decreased in large numbers and are much fewer. The cause, only God knows, because it would be reckless judgment for us to venture an answer.[23]

Although these religious men refused to seek out and explain the causes of the pandemic, they noted social changes carefully. What they saw and wrote about was a "new model of monetary tribute" applied to the indigenous population on "isolated lands, where there is no employment and where the native Indians have nothing more than a small amount of maize, chili and beans that they cook." The friars knew this arrangement aggravated the situation of the indigenous population. They demanded that the king[24] do something to halt it to prevent further errors, because:

---

[22]   Fernández Christlieb and García Zambrano point out that while the housing and buildings of the pre-Hispanic *Altepetl* (political unit) were usually scattered across remote hillsides or located on agricultural land and perfectly integrated into the environment, the communities that the Spaniards set up for the Indians, and that they called "towns," were built on flat land, away from rural areas, nature and the mountains and were densely populated places crammed with buildings (13–14).

[23]   With the refrain "only God knows," the Spaniards absolved themselves of any blame. The notion appeared in the *Relación Geográfica* de Teozapotlán, Oaxaca, where it was noted that in earlier days "the number of people and great personages in the town where the court was established was far greater; but today, there are far fewer people and almost no one of importance. What are the causes of all this death and destruction, *only God knows*" (Acuña II: 159; emphasis added). Attempts to explain divine will in relation to events such as death also appeared in popular songs: "Forget not that God watches you / Forget not that he is watching / Remember that you will die / Bear in mind that you do not know when" (Frenk 927).

[24]   In 1550, almost 20 years before the case of these friars, the priest Toribio Benavente "Motolinía" wrote to the king detailing, among other complaints, the ill treatment meted out to the Indians through the system of tributes in kind that, on occasion, had no value whatsoever for the Spaniards: "They also give honey and fish, frogs and a lot of other *sacalinjas*, bad and causing great trouble to Indians and of no great interest to Spaniards" (Company 127–32).

in this land money has been dwindling significantly, and furthermore, the little that there is, is not enough for these isolated peoples [...] for them to maintain themselves and their children and that there be any left over to give in monetary tribute in reales each year. (Company 161–5).[25]

Although the epidemics primarily affected the indigenous population, those of European and African origins did not always remain unscathed. Estate owner Diego Ruiz de Andrada, in a 1565 letter, wrote that his wife was on the point of death, quite possibly from an outbreak of smallpox.[26] Faced with the poor health of his wife, whom he gave no thought to leaving until he saw "what our Lord has in store for her," he had been forced to sell 1,500 bullocks and 100 cows. The cattle had to be driven from Oaxaca to Tuxtla with the help of those who had survived "very great pestilence." Andrada claimed that "for more than a month has each day seen no fewer than twenty, and 25 and 35 dead. Likewise in Xalapa it has left me with almost no one who did not fall ill. And so a Negro and two mulattoes, a female Negro and a child, her daughter, have died. It is God's will" (Melis and Rivero Franyutti 99–100).

In addition to epidemics, the livestock business also had an impact on the natural balance of the ecology of these lands. One example is a description from Pedro de Solórzano to his brother in 1582 of the trade of Guatemalan cocoa beans in Mexico City, which enable Pedro to acquire an estate "of several houses that have cost me more than four thousand ducats and a farm of *cows and mares that will be one thousand heads*" (Otte 104–5; emphasis added). A second example shows that the consequences of the Spanish livestock operations were already beginning to be felt by other hacienda owners in the Puebla region; Alonso de Viñuelas described these repercussions in his letter, sent in 1583. In this area of central Mexico the farms established were of small livestock—pigs, sheep, goats—that needed pastureland, which meant that cultivated fields were reduced to fallow land. So it is quite understandable that Viñuelas described the land as "so ravaged and exhausted, that some suffer more need here than there [in Spain], although there is always work for those who want it, and they earn enough to eat because as there is so much land, there is never a shortage" (Otte 104–5).

In the *Relación Geográfica* de Tenango one can read a description similar to Viñuelas's, although the text adds commentary about the climate:

---

[25]   The authors of the *Relación Geográfica* de Poncitlán, Nueva Galicia showed their objection to the tributes imposed on the native peoples that were an added burden to the disease and death that stalked their communities. It was a situation far different from what has been considered the idyllic, though illusory pre-Hispanic past: "They were healthier when they were pagans, because bouts of illness had been far more spread out over the years and hit every once in a while. And the cause of it they said is because they had not been worked, nor knew what work was, as they do now, and all they did was act freely and work when and how they wanted to, because the tribute that each gave to his lord was practically voluntary" (Acuña X: 196).

[26]   In 1565 in Zinacantán, Chiapas—near Tuxtla—a smallpox epidemic struck that killed half the population (García Acosta, et al. 115).

> The borders [of the town] abound with pastureland, they wither and become dry since this is a very cold land. The natives reap plentiful maize and raise chickens and some pigs, and, in the mountains, there are mountains of oaks and pines [...]
> It is not a land where you would find fruit nor orchards because it is a very cold land [...]. (Acuña V: 278)

However, the majority of letters contain a different opinion: the 1594 correspondence of one settler, Juan Cabeza de Vaca, conveyed an image of the richness of the land and of the lavish living conditions of the Spanish. In the Valley of Mexico, he declared, there were harvests of

> wheat and maize twice a year, and every fruit in Castille and many more of this land can be had, [...] and so poor people are better off here than they are in Spain because here they give orders all the time, they do not have to work themselves and they always ride on horses [...]. (Otte 130)

The tendency to embellish the living conditions of the Spanish in New Spain, including those of the poor, functioned in general terms as a "recruitment mechanism" for the readers of the letters on the other side of the Atlantic. It was pro-emigration information, designed to encourage friends, relatives, or compatriots to undertake the journey to Spanish American soil. This insistence was probably the result of the conquerors' anxiety about being overmatched. Despite the demographic catastrophes visited upon the natives, the indigenous population was still far larger than that of Spanish settlers.

One example will suffice to indicate the extent to which this feeling is transmitted in the letters written from New Spain. In a letter dated 1572 and directed to the King of Spain, Diego de Santillán wrote of the need to repopulate the land of Yucatán. Ill health and the approaching death of the conquistadors had only served to highlight the considerable imbalance between the populations of the vanquishers and the vanquished:

> the conquistadors are all now very old and ill. And so this land is in danger, not only from corsairs, but also from the natives because for the two hundred and fifty, at the most three hundred, Spaniards who might be here, there are more than eighty thousand native Indians [...]. (Melis and Rivero Franyutti 110–12)

Conclusion

In all of the examples cited in this study, one finds that the information contained in letters is important because epistolary discourse—within its stylistic and generic limits—can contribute significantly to efforts to reconstruct the medical cultures that were forged in New Spain. The communicative function of a private letter was only fulfilled when the person to whom it was addressed had received it, read it, and understood the message within, such as excuses for failure to send money due to illness or medical expenses. However, this information contributes valuable data to our understanding of the ways in which unfamiliar diseases and therapies were perceived; correspondents' reactions to the health risks involved in the transatlantic passage; the scarcity of medical practitioners; the social costs of being far from home; and how letters might be used to encourage reluctant emigrants.

One of the reasons that letters are so revealing is that they deal with intimate family matters; we find correspondents linked by various ties of kinship, and acting as they did for quite varied reasons, from promoting spousal reunion to demanding the arrival of relatives willing to work (Gálvez Ruiz 87–8). And let us not forget the interracial and religious contacts that would shape the lineage of the caste family groups with all the cultural exchanges of discourse, practice, and forms of medicine (Bel Bravo 28).

As we have seen, the analysis of private correspondence helps elucidate the medical strategies that were devised in American lands (Kuklick and Kohler, 1). Of course, the same context of distance, scale, and novelty can be observed in another type of letters, namely those exchanged between authorities and scientists sent to carry out research in the new colonial possessions. For example, the first physician (*protomédico*) Francisco Hernández, in his first letter to Philip II, justified the lack of information he was sending the king by stating that he had an illness, probably a kidney or urinary disorder (Hernández 51). Before resuming his work, he first had to get well:

> September 22, 1572.
> [...] I think this care and pain have been part of a long and serious illness, from which the Lord at present, as by a miracle, had spared me, because my works remain to be finished, and Your Majesty to be served, and I am at present convalescing. Because of the extremely weak state in which I find myself, I cannot give Your Majesty a more detailed account of the whole [...]. (Hernández 51)

It remains, then, to examine the epistolary exchanges between scientists and authorities, in addition to the letters written in the monasteries and convents of New Spain. These tasks will be undertaken in future research.

As we have seen, letters are a marvelous source for the reconstruction of the experience of health and sickness during the sixteenth century. Lestringant wrote that "to observe the XVI century through the mirror of letters and correspondence is not to look through the wrong end of the telescope, and much less spy through a keyhole in a lock, a loathsome practice rightfully denounced by Rabelais." It is, instead, "to penetrate into" the heart of the century "by the surest and least illicit of means" (Lestringant qtd. in Carrera de la Red 639). If we are to see clearly into its heart, a great deal more work must be done. Scholars need to carry out new studies of similar kinds of letters, preserved in convents and monasteries. Ultimately, this research will help us document negotiations regarding the processes of legitimization, institutionalization, and commercialization of materials, practices, and medical knowledge exchanged through the main terrestrial and oceanic routes around the world.

Chapter 5
Literary Anthropologies and Pedro González, the "Wild Man" of Tenerife[1]

M. A. Katritzky

Introduction

This chapter presents two previously unconsidered German print culture documents relating to Pedro González, born in the 1530s on Tenerife in the Spanish Canary Islands, who passed the medical condition hypertrichosis on to several children and grandchildren. The defining physical symptom of hypertrichosis is permanently or temporarily growing long hair over most of the face and body. Despite its numerous cultural representations in mythology, folklore, and literature, hypertrichosis occurs in human physiology only as a permanent, inherited trait, as in the case of the Gonzalez family, or as a temporary pathological symptom. HLA (hypertrichosis lanuginosa acquisita), a form of non-congenital hypertrichosis, is a significant indicative symptom for certain medical conditions, notably some cancers, and for severe malnutrition, starvation, or anorexia. Extensively recorded in this latter context by physicians (Strumia) and historians of disasters such as the nineteenth-century Irish Potato Famine, but previously overlooked in connection with the medieval Wild Man tradition, HLA may underlie the Wild Man's acquisition, during the famine-ridden twelfth century, of his defining hirsuteness.

The two documents under consideration here are an account occurring in writings attributed to Philip Melanchthon (1497–1560) first published in 1563, and an image in a work by Eberhard Werner Happel (1647–1690) published in 1685

[1] Earlier versions of this paper were presented at two workshops, and I thank their organizers and delegates (John Slater, Maríaluz López-Terrada and José Pardo-Tomás: *Medical cultures of early modern Spain*, Valencia, October 2011; Jacques Lezra, Michael Armstrong-Roche, and my friends and colleagues in Theater Without Borders: *Mobility, Hybridity and Reciprocal Exchange in the Theatres of Early Modern Europe*, NYU-Madrid, May 2011). For supporting this research, my thanks also to The Open University Arts Faculty Research Committee and Caitlin Adams and the OU REST team, to The Wellcome Trust, and to the Herzog August Bibliothek and its staff and Fellows (most especially Jill Bepler, Asaph Ben-Tov, Judit Ecsedy, Christine Johnson, Bob Kolb, Hiram Kümper, Cornelia Niekus Moore, and Charlotte Colding Smith).

(Figure 5.1, p. 126).[2] As well as expanding our knowledge of the González family, these two documents raise wider implications for the early modern classification, representation and reception of hypertrichosis sufferers. Melanchthon's text illuminates connections between hypertrichosis and the demonic, and Happel's image situates the González family within the medical context of similar cases. Both Melanchthon and Happel make strong connections between hypertrichosis and hairy-bodied peoples and creatures of classical mythology and fable, the medieval traditions of the hairy anchorite and the Wild Man, and non-European indigenous peoples. Conceptually, the González family stands at the intersection of mythological, folkloric, religious, anthropological, and medical discourses; their story suggests ways in which classification systems, theology, and medical cultures engaged these seemingly disparate fields. As monstrous humans, they fell within the legal category "persona miserabilis." Developed by medieval legislation to address certain female, old, disabled, or otherwise politically disadvantaged Old World groups, this was extended in the mid-sixteenth century to entire indigenous New World populations of the expanding Spanish empire.[3] Contextualized within the known historical record, the newly identified documents of the Wild Man of Tenerife presented here illuminate early modern ideas about definitions and borders of the human—with respect to the supernatural, the zoological natural world, and indigenous peoples brought within the jurisdiction of Spain's civil and canon law by the long reach of its cultural and military influence.

Happel's extraordinary composite image of 1685 occurs in *Relationes Curiosae*. This five-volume publication is stylistically derivative of popularizers of sensational fact and fiction, such as Erasmus Francisci (from whose substantial volumes Happel sometimes pirated whole pages almost verbatim), but journalistically innovative in gathering together material first published in a pioneering, weekly German-language periodical over the decade 1681–1691. This journal established Happel as one of central Europe's most widely read seventeenth-century authors. Figure 5.1 portrays Pedro González with three of his own hairy offspring and three other "shaggy-haired humans," all seven images based on previous iconographic sources.[4] Roundels featuring portrait heads of

---

[2]   Melanchthon's account is previously uncited in this (or, as far as I know, any) context (Manlius sig.D7). Bondeson (13) notes in passing, and without a reproduction or volume or page reference, the version of this illustration in the 1729 edition of Happel's five-volume *Relationes curiosae*; on Happel, see also Schock.

[3]   Duve, 43–6. On infantilizing evaluations of New Spanish *indios* by the Old Spanish, and on monsters and monstrous births, see the chapters by José Pardo-Tomás and Enrique García Santo Tomás in this volume.

[4]   Engraving: Happel, *Relationes curiosae* II, 1685: plate opposite p. 312. For images A–D, see Aldrovandi (16 [D & E], 17 [B], 18 [C], 21 [A]); for F, see Isaac Brunn, *Barbara Urslerin ward geboren ihm Iar 1633 den 18 February in Augsburg* (1653), single-leaf publicity broadsheet (reproduced in Holländer 153); for G, see de Bondt (84–5, Lib. V, "Historia Animalium," Capvt XXXII: *Ourang Outang sive "Homo silvestris"*).

Pedro González and his son Arrigo are suspended from a broad "family" tree growing from the top of a rustic slope overlooking a wooded, hilly landscape whose European vegetation is exoticized with palm trees, perhaps with reference to Tenerife. Below them in the middle distance, two González daughters stand to the left. To the right, behind her harpsichord, stands Barbara Urslerin, the only adult hypertrichosis case known to have been born in the seventeenth century. All three women are fully dressed in early modern European clothes. The naked, hairy-bodied male crawling in the lower left foreground depicts a classical forerunner of the medieval hairy anchorite and Wild Man, a member of the Himantopodes, an example of the "marvellous races" addressed in the following section. At the exact center of the image stands a second completely naked figure, a hairy-bodied female, according to the accompanying text intended to depict a Javanese *Ourang Outang* or Wild Wooddweller. I would argue that this central portrait also draws iconographically on a much-circulated representation of the fourteenth-century Italian hairy girl discussed below (Figure 5.2).

In combining seven derivative portraits into one original new composite, Happel's image contextualizes the González family within early modern understanding of their medical condition and validates their continuing journalistic interest well into the late seventeenth century. Melanchthon's text offers significant new insights into the family's early history. Commenting on the Catholic court of the Spanish Habsburgs, it occurs in a section on "evil spirits and devils" in Johannes Manlius's published collection of the sayings of the resolutely Protestant Melanchthon. It adds considerable weight to scant hints by writers such as Giulio Cesare Scaligero suggesting that González may have spent a significant period in Madrid between being taken from Tenerife and being presented to the French king in Paris:

> I would never have believed that the four-footed forest creatures with human form called satyrs could be found, if experience had not made me a believer. When Sulla returned to Rome again from the Mithridatic war caused by Marius, who murdered the best and most excellent statesmen of Rome, such a satyr was brought to him during his journey. He was like and similar to humans in many ways. When commanded to talk, he just muttered to himself in ways that no human could understand.[5] I am entirely of the opinion that this spirit was the devil, and that he was demonstrating what type of citizens Sulla would find in Rome. Thus, it is said, King Philip of Spain, the son of Emperor Charles V, led two such satyrs around with him a few years ago. They were two hairy little mannikins,[6] or at least of quite similar face and figure to humans, but as for the rest irresponsible and bestial like other animals. They too made some

---

[5]   According to a seventeenth-century English translation of Melanchthon's source text (Plutarch's 'Life of Sulla'), "he was ask'd by several Interpreters who he was, when with much ado he sent forth a harsh unintelligible Noise, like the Neighing of a Horse, and crying of a Goat, in mixt Consort: *Sylla* dismay'd at it, turned aside in detestation" (Plutarch 255).

[6]   "menschle" (Latin edition: "homunculus").

secret murmurings such that nobody could understand. Without a doubt, they were demonstrating some future event. In his *Life*, St. Ambrose records that such satyrs appeared to him and met with him. I am of the opinion that they were devils. (Manlius sig.D7)[7]

Melanchthon here repeatedly refers to the reason why early modern congenitally physically exceptional humans and animals were termed monsters, namely their perceived "demonstrative" role as supernatural omen-bringing messengers, warning the vigilant of significant future events. Because of their social and religious significance, every such birth that came to public attention was recorded as a matter of course. The development of printing provided a cheap, portable, and profitable way of spreading news of their births and activities through broadsheets, prodigy books, and other publications. Rulers aspired to indicate their magnanimity and power by taking unusual human monsters under their personal protection, making them valuable "tokens" in the aristocratic gifts-for-patronage exchange economy. As well as being subjected to considerable medical scrutiny, some monsters earned their keep traveling the fairground circuits as independent live performers or being exhibited or shown by itinerant promoters. Dead or alive, monsters were highly prized as collectibles for the curiosity cabinets or service of medical and noble collectors and patrons. This collectibility shaped the lives of Pedro González and his family. My suggestion here is that there are many advantages to considering documentation relating to them, whether texts such as Melanchthon's or images such as Happel's (Figure 5.1), within the context of what, I further suggest, may usefully be described as literary anthropologies.

Literary Anthropologies and the "Marvellous Races"

The term "literary anthropologies" is here used to refer to anthropological categories drawing on pathology and cultural fantasy, based on accounts in which, as for many reports of unfamiliar humans or other primates documented by early modern New World explorers and other travelers, any degree of eye-witness authenticity or empirical scientific authority is obscured with heavy layers of expectation and influence generated by literature, folklore, and mythology. The most decisive influence on European literary anthropologies is the "marvellous races of the East".[8] Classical anthropologists such as Pliny or Alexander defined this heterogeneous assortment of humans, hybrids, and animals by distinctive physical or cultural characteristics. Sometimes, as with the Astomi (Apple-Smellers), Gorgades,

---

[7]   The first edition of Manlius's work was published in Latin in 1563; the present author's translation is from Johann Huldreich Ragor's 1566 German translation.

[8]   See Friedman (*The Monstrous Races*, 11–16, 164, 200) for its excellent treatment of classical and early modern conceptualizations of monstrous or Plinian races.

Gorillae, and Himantopodes, these include all-over hairiness.[9] Despite isolated expressions of skepticism by theologians and naturalists such as St. Augustine or Albertus Magnus, the existence of the "marvellous races" was overwhelmingly accepted by medieval thinkers from Isidore of Seville onwards, and further promoted by the garbled deceptions of Sir John Mandeville, lesser armchair travelers, commercially minded writers such as Happel, and their credulous book illustrators. Depictions of them became a familiar feature of medieval bestiaries, renaissance world maps, even of authoritative early modern natural histories and cosmographies such as Konrad von Megenberg's *Buch der Natur* (Augsburg 1475) or Hartmann Schedel's *Nuremberg chronicle* of 1493, Conrad Gesner's four-volume *Historia Animalium* of the 1550s and Ulisse Aldrovandi's *Monstrorum historia* of 1642. By the early modern period, the profoundest cartographic and ethnographical influence of the stereotypes and vocabulary of "marvellous races" had shifted from the Old World to the New. Fully expecting to encounter members of the "marvellous races" of the East, explorers such as Columbus or Vespucci reported on New World cannibals and female warriors, and, as Braham puts it, "whole regions of Latin America—Amazonia, Patagonia, the Caribbean— are named for the monstrous races of women warriors, big-footed giants, and consumers of human flesh" (17–24).

Deep-seated anxieties about defining the borders of the human, of the type expressed in the tradition of the "marvellous races," are discernible in human records since earliest antiquity. The pre-Enlightenment concept of the human as a zoological phenomenon was not well defined. Early modern classification systems blur the boundaries between human and non-human in unpredictable ways, with their generous inclusivity of a wide range of hybrids, such as mermaids or centaurs, and almost total unfamiliarity with the great apes.[10] In Europe, anatomical identification and investigation of great apes with rigorous reference to actual live or dead specimens was systematically pursued only from the seventeenth century. Preceded by millennia of literary anthropologies, this work represents a fundamental contribution towards clearing the scientific path, from hierarchical classification theories primarily based on Aristotle's "Great Chain of Being" or the biblical Creation Story to the new vistas opened up by Darwinian evolutionary theory. Galen, said to have dissected apes as well as humans, was one of many medical forerunners who heralded the new scientific approaches. However, perspectives based on literary anthropologies, rather than driving out these newly invigorated anatomical investigations, persisted alongside them. Legends of inter-species births, some already recorded by medieval historical authorities, were endlessly recycled by early modern writers whose debates on bestiality habitually invoked the possible generation of monsters and monstrous races, and demonic involvement. Popular examples, usually involving the type

---

[9]   Similarly, traditional Far Eastern literary anthropologies feature "the country of fur-covered people" (Sato 375, 378).

[10]   See, for example, Knowles 138–9.

of familiar animal species favored by traveling showmen, include the hairy-bodied Swedish boy born after his mother was raped by a bear; the sons born to a Portuguese woman raped by an ape on the Indian island to which she was banished; or the Frenchwoman condemned to the stake with her Maltese lapdog, allegedly the father of her daughter.[11] On August 24, 1661, Samuel Pepys viewed "the strange creature that Captain Holmes hath brought with him from Guiny; it is a great baboon, but so much like a man in most things, that though they say there is a species of them, yet I cannot believe but that it is a monster got of a man and she-baboon" (no page no.). Even in his weighty mid-seventeenth-century *History of Scotland*, William Drummond of Hawthornden felt it appropriate to refer to a "Taile told of a poor miserable Fellow accused of Bestiality; [who ...] at his *Arraignment* confessed, That it was not out of any evil intention he had done it, but onely to procreat a Monster, with which (having nothing to sustain his life) he might win his bread going about the Countrey" (256).

Prior to the refinement of concepts such as species and sub-species extinction, inter-species or hybrid infertility, dominant and recessive inheritable traits, and mutant genes, disagreement and confusion impeded understanding of the causes of "monstrous" congenital nonconformities and the principles underlying the inheritance of physical characteristics. Central to the early modern debate was the challenging nature of resolving differences in cultural and scientific anthropological approaches, complicated by anxieties concerning the permeability of borders between humans and animals, and the challenges of differentiating between exceptional congenital physical characteristics ("monstrous" traits), those recurring as standard physical traits of particular human gene pools, and temporary pathological symptoms (such as HLA). Such anxieties inform Happel's image (Figure 5.1) and texts influenced by the literary traditions of satyrs, anchorites, and Wild Men.

Satyrs, Anchorites, and Wild Men

The physical symptoms of hypertrichosis shared by some members of the González family closely correspond to two exceptionally popular and widespread medieval types, the linked Wild Man and hairy anchorite traditions obliquely acknowledged in the central and lowest portraits of Happel's image (Figure 5.1). Unlike the physically varied "marvellous races," who also demonstrably influenced the expectations of Spanish New World explorers, the European Wild Man or *Homo sylvestris* was consistently characterized in medieval art and literature by his shaggy-haired body, inarticulateness, and liminal humanity. According to Richard Bernheimer, the defining characteristic of this "hairy man curiously compounded of human and animal traits," generally understood to be incapable of human speech, is all-over shaggy hirsuteness: "a growth of fur, leaving bare only its face, feet and

---

[11]   Guazzo 29 (Book I, Chapter X); Torquemada 31–3; Happel, *Relationes curiosae*, I: 15–16, III: 399. See also Janson 275–6.

hands, at times its knees and elbows, or the breasts of the female of the species" (1). In a posthumously published Lenten sermon, the Swiss preacher Johannes Geiler von Kaysersberg (1445–1510) identifies five categories of Wild Man (sigs. xxxix^v–xxxxi^R). One of them, the hermit ("solitari"), acknowledges the tradition's debt towards "the legend of the hairy anchorite," concerning certain holy Christians whose bodies were said to have been covered all over by long hair. The legend's traces are rooted in accounts of hairy-bodied, desert-inhabiting Semitic demons, such as the Assyrian Enkidu and Gilgamesh, and Old Testament Hebrew characters such as Samson, Nebuchadnezzar, Ishmael, and Esau (Williams; Mobley).

For some Christians, such as St. Onofrius or St. Paul of Thebes, the condition was said to have become a permanent physical manifestation of divine grace; for others, such as Mary Magdalene, St. James, or St. John Chrysostom, a temporary penance for sinfulness. These latter inspired a flourishing European literary tradition, which left its mark on the *Amadis*, Juan de Flores's fifteenth-century fictional narrative *Grimalte y gradissa*, and the persistent Catalan hagiography of Juan Garín.[12] The Basle physician Thomas Platter the Younger, one of the earliest foreign visitors to the Monastery of Montserrat to record the Garín legend told there, illustrated his substantial account of February 1599 with one of his rare sketches, depicting Juan Garín as a hairy anchorite or Wild Man (T. Platter 359–63). Drawing on local oral sources and the much-reprinted *Historia* of Montserrat compiled by a former abbot, Pedro de Burgos (1460–1536), and perhaps also on *El Monserrato*, the epic poem of 1587 by Valencian Cristóbal de Virués, Platter relates that Juan Garín gave his name to a hermit's cell at Montserrat, uninhabited since his own time there during the late ninth-century reign of the first Duke of Barcelona, Guifré el Pilós (Wilfred the Hairy). Two devils had tricked Garín into exorcising, then raping, murdering, and burying the Duke's daughter. He fled to Rome to confess his crimes and absolved them by crawling back on all fours to Montserrat, withdrawing into the forest, discarding his clothes, and (much like Happel's Himantapodes in Figure 5.1), growing furry hair all over his body. Seven years later, Garín was caught by the Duke's hunting dogs. Unrecognized, he was kept at the ducal court in Barcelona like an exotic household animal. The Duke's infant son, seeing him eat like a dog, cried out to him: "Levántate, fray Juan Garín, levántate, ponte derecho, y mira al cielo, que tú has cumplido la penitencia" (Rise, brother Juan Garín, rise, stand up and look at the sky, because you have completed your penance) (T. Platter 362). Having stood upright again at last and confessed his crimes to the Duke, Garín helped the Duke seek the body of his wronged daughter, only to discover her alive and wishing to found a convent.

Although HLA-related symptoms provide a plausible explanation for the hirsuteness of early Christian fasters such as Juan Garín, the link is previously unnoted in this context. Exceptionally, an account of St. Wilgefortis identifies secondary growth of lanugo hair as a medical symptom of her fasting, without, however, referring to the hairy anchorite or Wild Man traditions as a whole (Lacey).

---

[12]   As late as 1892, it inspired Tomas Breton y Hernandez's opera *Juan Garín*.

Neither is the nuanced awareness of malnutrition-induced temporary hirsuteness reflected by Geiler von Kaysersberg's Wild Man classifications noted in modern scholarship. His survey of the wide range of influences on the medieval Wild Man tradition is also relevant to connections made by Melanchthon and Happel between hypertrichosis sufferers and some persistent categories underlying literary anthropologies. He identifies four further categories of Wild Man in addition to anchorites: satyrs ("sachanni"), Pygmies ("pigineni"), "diaboli," and "Hyspani." Pygmies, still classified as Wild Men by writers such as Francisci or Happel, were a major sub-category of the classical "marvellous races."[13] The term "Hyspani" specifically refers to a feral couple captured in medieval Spain, as documented by Albertus Magnus and others. However, it may also incorporate the Reform humanist's references to indigenous peoples of the Spanish empire and his thinly disguised sectarian slur on Europe's then most powerful Catholic nation. Catholics returned the compliment in kind, as when Aldrovandi alleges the existence of "infinite numbers of Wild Men with no desire for any kind of interaction with the coastal inhabitants in Ireland, an island subject to the English king" (16). "Diaboli" and "sachanni" acknowledge the Wild Man's affinity with Semitic devils and classical satyrs.

Greek, Roman, and biblical accounts of satyrs (e.g. Isaiah 34.14) were extremely influential on the medieval Wild Man tradition. Long before their Renaissance reintroduction into art by Dürer (Kaufmann 35, 41), or onto the stage in the satyr-plays or pastorals of Italian dramatists such as Giovanni Battista Giraldi Cinthio (Henke 111), satyrs exerted a palpable iconographic influence on the linked traditions of the hairy anchorite, early Christian devil, and Wild Man.[14] Classical sources uniformly describe satyrs as human-faced, tailed, and horned *animals* with hairy goat legs, as opposed to *humans* with characteristic bestial physical traits, but obscured their attitudes to the physical boundaries of the human with generously vague elasticity. Roman ethnographers strongly contrast their views on the "marvellous races," whom they regarded as distinct mixed-gender, self-reproducing groups, with their descriptions of the inter-species mating habits of the male-only satyrs. However, they are not forthcoming on mundane details such as whether satyrs' matings with nymphs, who looked like normal human females, resulted in offspring whose physical traits were hybrid or pure, randomly distributed or gender-specific. As libidinous abductors of human females, classical satyrs were consigned to the pagan pantheon demonized by Christian theologians, who followed the lead of St. Jerome in regarding them as hairy *incubi* or devils (van der Lugt 180). Significant aspects of their layered profane, diabolical, and sexual

---

[13] Francisci 351; Happel, *Relationes curiosae* IV: 242. According to Colin Turnbull, who studied and lived with the indigenous Pygmies of the Democratic Republic of Congo's Ituri Forest for three years in the 1950s, their "head hair grows in peppercorn tufts, and the body hair varies from one extreme to the other; some Pygmies are covered thickly from head to foot" (24).

[14] On the forest as a transgressive, even supernatural, literary space, see Sanders, *Cultural Geography* 65–100.

dimensions were inherited by the Wild Man and, as explicated by Melanchthon and other renowned Reformation theologians and evident from popularizers such as Happel, informed attitudes towards hypertrichosis cases.

As indicated by writers such as Thomas D'Urfey, popular perceptions of the González family as a discrete hairy tribe of the type of the "marvellous races" (despite its numerous non-hairy members), even as Wild Men, persisted throughout the seventeenth century. D'Urfey refers to Pedro González and his daughter Antoinetta in 1690 in the context of Isabella Pallavicina, Marchesa di Soragna, who adopted the eight-year-old Antoinetta. Perhaps through being an acquaintance of the Marchesa, the Bolognese physician Ulysses Aldrovandi was able to medically examine Antoinetta and other González family members. The detailed colored drawings of them commissioned by Aldrovandi formed the basis for their portrait woodcuts in *Monstrorum historia*,[15] his posthumously published treatise of human and zoological physical abnormalities of 1642, copied in later publications such as Happel's (Figure 5.1):

> *Pliny* and *Solinus* make mention of diverse Hairy Nations; and *Lycosthenes* Writes of a certain Island, the Inhabitants whereof have all their Parts, except their Faces and Palms of their hands, cover'd over with long Hair; part of the Hide of such a Savage, a certain Sarmatian sent unto *Ulisses Aldrovandus*, and is kept in the *Musæum* of the Bononian Senate: These kind of Wild Men were first seen at *Bononia*, when the beautiful Marchioness of *Soranium* coming thither, was nobly receiv'd by the *Illustrissimo Marcus Casalius*, who brought with her a Hairy Girl of eight Years of Age, being the Daughter of a Wild Man born in the *Canaries*, whose Effigies [*marginalium: Aldrovand. in Monst.Hist.*] *Aldrovandus* expos'd to the view of all his Friends as a great Rarity; there are, as *Eusebius* also writes, in the East and West *Indies*, Wild Men who are born smooth like our Infants, but as they grow up have Hair covering their whole Bodies. (D'Urfey 201–2)

As Spain's first non-European colony, mainly known for exporting excellent sugar[16] and for providing a stopover off the coast of North Africa for explorers en route to the New World, Tenerife, the birthplace of Pedro González, was associated in the minds of most sixteenth-century Europeans less with their own continent than with Africa or the New World.[17] Humanist ethnographical investigations prompted by enquiries into the historical *ur*-German, following the Renaissance rediscovery of Tacitus's *Germania* of 98 AD (Leitch 37), and above all by the discovery and exploration of Old and New World territories and peoples, gave Wild Men (and hypertrichosis sufferers) renewed relevance in early modern

---

[15]   These woodcuts are on pages 16–18. On the González family, see also 473, 580ff.

[16]   Guarinonius comments that "every country traditionally offers its own special fruits and gifts, thus the best sugar is from the Canary Islands: (49); he writes of "the best Canarian sugar" (1161).

[17]   For insightful discussions of the status of the Canary Islands—between the Old World and the New—see Abulafia; and Wiesner-Hanks (49–64).

medical, cultural, and popular circles. One indication of this is the keen interest they attract from Thomas Platter the Younger. As well as the legend of Juan Garín, his travel journal singles out two depictions of Wild Men he saw in England in 1599. In Greenwich, the physician admired a richly jeweled salt cellar shaped like a Wild Man clad in feathers; at Hampton Court, Cornelius Ketel's now lost portrait painting of the native American couple brought live to England from the New World by Sir Martin Frobisher in the 1580s, described by Platter as a "lively and natural portrait of the Wild Man and Wild Woman [...] they both looked like Wild People, they wore furs and the woman carried a child" (T. Platter 863–4, 834–5).

The central female in Figure 5.1 is intended to depict the hairy-bodied bipedal creature known on the Indonesian island of Borneo as the *Ourang Outan*, or "Wild Man of the woods."[18] Similar hirsute forest dwellers, such as the Sumatran *orang pendek*,[19] still flourish on the anthropological fringes and occasionally trespass into serious academic studies.[20] Indonesian usage of the term "orangutan" to describe the ape *Pongo pygmaeus* is a twentieth-century development reflecting Western influence. During the seventeenth century, when the term first entered European languages, its literal Malay definition was human "forest person." Early modern European usages, reflecting total unfamiliarity with such forest people and their zoological status, indiscriminately apply the term to Asian Bushmen or alleged Eastern equivalents of the European Wild Man; Asian or African apes such as the orangutan (*Pongo pygmaeus*), siamang, baboon, or chimpanzee; or occasionally even forest gods (Mahdi 170–80, 291).

Happel's central female is not derived from Nicolaes Tulp's groundbreaking illustrated anatomical researches, first published in 1641, identifying as a great ape the creature described in his Latin text as an "Indian satyr [...] called

---

[18]   Happel, *Relationes curiosae* II: 316 (the first of two pages numbered 316, as 313–16 are repeated).

[19]   A "cryptid or cryptozoological [...] ground-dwelling, bipedal primate that is covered in short fur and stands between 80 and 150cm [...] tall" (Wikipedia, accessed September 5, 2012).

[20]   In the 1970s, Russian anthropologists led by B.F. Porshnev proposed a reclassification of Neanderthal man from extinct human to extant animal, identified by them as the "hairy, mute, non-sapient" bipeds variously referred to in earlier times as satyrs or Wild Men, and in their own time as the Yeti, Sasquatch, etc. (Porshnev, Bayanov, and Bourtsev; Bayanov and Bourtsev). Illuminating in this context is Judith C. Berman's identification of the medieval Wild Man as "the ur-image of the hairy Cave Man [...] the 'truth' of the Cave Man image is derived from his Wild Man forebear and not from the archaeological record" (293, 297). Although they refer neither to Wild Men nor to satyrs (or their highly distinctive inter-species mating pattern), the theory of Paul H. Mason and Roger V. Short is also potentially relevant to their interpretation. According to these two Australian anthropologists, evidence from DNA analysis of Neanderthal fossils indicates that until some 250,000 years ago, "male Neanderthals were able to reproduce with female humans but that the reciprocal cross was absent, rare or sterile" (2).

by the Indians orang-autang or Wild Man [*homo sylvestris*]" (284).[21] Instead, it draws on the literary anthropology of another Dutch physician, Jakob de Bondt, based in Java from 1625 to his death in 1631 (or his posthumous editor, Willem Piso).[22] Whether or not he ever saw a great ape himself, de Bondt's posthumous illustrated account of the *Ourang-outan* in 1658 follows a persistent iconographic tradition, apparently initiated by an incunabula of 1486, whose impressive plates were based on the drawings of Erhard Reuwich, a professional artist hired to accompany Bernhard von Breydenbach to Jerusalem to record his pilgrimage. Its final plate, bearing the title "These animals are truthfully depicted just as we saw them in the Holy Land," features eight real and imaginary animals labeled by name, including a giraffe, a crocodile, a unicorn, and a camel, this last led by a tailed, naked, hairy-bodied female biped labeled only as "Name unknown."[23]

Happel's engraving reflects some of the major concerns of the seventeenth-century European medical establishment. Was the hairy-bodied Indonesian *Ourang-Outan* human, ape, or hybrid? Were individuals with the medical condition of hypertrichosis born with it or temporarily afflicted? If congenital, were they exceptional monsters born to normal humans, members of a discrete, self-generating species or sub-species of human, liminal Wild Man or animal, or supernatural beings fathered by demons? By the nineteenth century, medical specialists such as the Berlin physician Dr. Max Bartels were vocal in identifying certain types of unusual human hirsuteness as "atavistic throwbacks to the animal kingdom."[24] Similar ethnographic issues are currently being revisited by contemporary anthropologists and medical experts in the context of the discovery of 13,000-year-old human bones on the Indonesian island of Flores in 2004. They disagree as to whether the Flores bones are evidence of "the remarkable discovery of a new species of the genus *Homo*, a new kind of human dubbed *Homo floresiensis*" that flourished alongside *Homo sapiens* on the island some 18 to 13 millennia ago, and "may even still be living on Flores" (Forth 13–14), or simply microcephalic dwarf specimens of *Homo sapiens*, physically deformed by the exceptional congenital condition ME: "myxoedematous endemic (ME) cretins, part of an inland population of (mostly unaffected) Homo sapiens."[25]

---

[21]   Tulp's pre-dissection depiction of this ape (plate XIIII), identified by modern specialists as a chimpanzee, not an orangutan, led to numerous derivative images. Some, with Bondt's "Ourang-Outang" and Francisci's copies after Tulp and Bondt, are reproduced and discussed by Mahdi (Fig. 29). Mahdi's comprehensive treatment of early modern Germanic usage of the term "orangutan" translates *Homo sylvestris* as "forest man," and discusses glosses of the term "orangutan" as human forest man or bushman, but not as subhuman European Wild Man (173–4).

[22]   Mahdi 174–6. Again, Happel's copy is mediated by Francisci (374 & Plate XI.11).

[23]   "Non constat de nomine." See also Janson 270, 333.

[24]   Bartels, "Ueber abnorme Behaarung beim Menschen I" 118. See also I: 127; II: 150, 163, 167, 183–5.

[25]   Obendorf, Oxnard, and Kefford 1294; these authors also note "striking parallels" between *ebu gogo* and ME cretinism, including "the retention of lanugo hair in sporadic cretins."

Anthropologists are taking into account reports by the current inhabitants of Western Flores concerning the *ebu gogo*, said to have been a discrete tribe of dwarf-like, possibly non-human, hairy cave-dwellers approximating the possible appearance of *Homo floresiensis*, allegedly exterminated by the ancestors of the current Nage tribe "between 1750 and 1820" in retribution for stealing their harvests and abducting their children (Forth 14–15). Similarly, local tales and myths collected from Indonesians in Makea by seventeenth-century European travelers about the antisocial behavior of the *Ourang-outan* informed early modern scientific debate and filtered down into popular media representations, such as Happel's central female (Figure 5.1). This follows de Bondt's *Ourang Outang* in downplaying scientific anatomical analysis conclusively identifying the creature as an ape, foregrounding its liminal, hybrid qualities at the very borders of the human even further by drawing on a much-copied and widely circulated fanciful representation of a hairy girl born in Tuscany in 1355 (Figure 5.2, p. 127).[26]

The Tuscan Hairy Girl, 1355

Modern historical surveys of hypertrichosis were inaugurated in the 1870s by Max Bartels's monograph-length, rambling, three-part article considering diverse cases of abnormal human hair distribution over a three-century period, with the emphasis on contemporary case studies. Following the lead of Bartels, many medical historians still present Pedro González and his family as the earliest historically documented cases of hypertrichosis. Bartels excludes from his chronological tables of hypertrichosis cases numerous sparsely documented pre-sixteenth-century cases, such as the Wild Couple captured in thirteenth-century Saxony noted by Albertus Magnus; the hirsute boy born in 1282 to a woman who had looked at pictures of bears during her pregnancy (Lykosthenes 445); or a fourteenth-century case briefly noted by Aldrovandi (580–81).[27] This last, which Bartels alludes to in passing via Aldrovandi, provides a precedent for imperial sponsorship of a child afflicted with hypertrichosis. It involved Anna von Schweidnitz (1339–1362), distantly related to the Spanish Habsburgs through her maternal great-grandmother Klementia of Habsburg. In 1354, the year after Anna became the third of the four wives of Emperor Charles IV (1316–1378), the couple traveled from Prague to Rome, where Charles was crowned Holy Roman Emperor

---

Loren Eiseley cites the Geneva scholar Carl Vogt's 1864 diagnosis of the Neander skull as "that of an idiot or microcephalus," and similar, now discredited reactions to Eugene Dubois's 1891 discovery of *Pithecanthropus erectus* ("the Java ape man"), as symptoms of what she identifies as a "slow shift from a belief in living *normal* links passing slowly to a notion of living Microcephalic *abnormals* as in some manner *representing past normals no longer existent in the living world*" (459–63, Eiseley's emphasis).

26   Woodcut: Aldrovandi, 579 (Caput VII, Icone I).

27   See also Bartels II: 169; for the tables, see I: 124 and II: 182.

in April 1355. According to the Florentine chronicle of Mattea Villani, shortly thereafter, during the return journey,

> when the emperor was at Pietrasanta, as a great wonder, and a new and strange thing, he was presented with a hairy little girl aged seven years old, woolly all over like a sheep, with badly coloured red wool, and she was covered with this wool all over her body, right up to her lips and her eyes. The empress, completely amazed to see a human body covered by nature in such an extremely marvellous way, commanded her ladies in waiting to feed and care for her, and took her to her court. (III: 77)[28]

That 15-year-old Anna was indeed so fascinated by this little girl that she took her back to the imperial court in 1355 is confirmed by the Bishop of Bisignano, Giovanni de'Marignolli (1290–1357). Engaged by Emperor Charles IV in 1355 to work on the *Annals of Bohemia*, this former delegate to the Emperor of China from Pope Benedict XI's papal court at Avignon, interpolated his contributions with Far Eastern reminiscences. His brief note of the Italian hairy girl—incidentally confirming that she was a redhead—is closely followed by a passage that has been identified as the earliest European eyewitness account of the indigenous Veddar tribe of Sri Lanka (Kennedy 76), where de'Marignolli had been marooned for several months of 1349:

> So the most noble Emperor Charles IV brought from Tuscany a girl whose face, as well as her whole body, was covered with hair, so that she looked like the daughter of a fox! Yet is there no such race of hairy folk in Tuscany: nor was her own mother even, nor her mother's other children so, but like the rest of us. [...] We do not suppose that such creatures exist as a species, but regard them as natural monstrosities. [...] The truth is that no such people *do* exist as nations, though there may be an individual monster here and there. [...] There are also wild men, naked and hairy, who have wives and children, but abide in the woods. They do not show themselves among men, and I was seldom able to catch sight of one; for they hide themselves in the forest when they perceive any one coming. Yet they do a great deal of work, sowing and reaping corn and other things; and when traders go to them, as I have myself witnessed, they put out what they have to sell in the middle of the path, and run and hide. Then the purchasers go forward and deposit the price, and take what has been set down. (Yule 379–83, in translation)

The case attracted Europe-wide attention. Antonio de Torquemada summarizes it in his *Jardín de flores curiosas*, published in Madrid in 1570 and translated into English in 1600. He furthermore adds a case of a boy with hypertrichosis shown around Spain for money by his father, linking this latter case directly to the diabolical by following it with the tale of a monstrous child, born to a German actor who refused to remove his devil costume before sleeping with his wife:

---

[28]   Libro Quinto, cap. 53, "D'una fanciulla pilosa presentata all'imperadore"; present author's translation from the original Italian.

I haue heard of a woman deliuered of a child all couered ouer with rough haire, the reason wherof was, that she had in her chamber the picture of Saint Iohn Baptist clothed in hairy skinns, on which the woman vsing with deuotion to contemplate, her chyld was borne both in roughnes & figure like vnto the same. [...] Marcus Damascenus [...] said [...] that it hapned [...] neere the Citty of Pysa. [*marginalium*: "the place is called *Petra Sancta*"] It is not long since that there went through Spayne a man gathering money, with the sight of a son of his couered with hayre, in such quantity so long & thicke, that in his whole face there was nothing els to be seen but his mouth and eyes: Withall, the haire was so curled, that it crimpled round like Ringes, and truely the wilde Sauages which they paynt, were nothing so deformed, and ouer their whole body so hairie as was thys boy. [... *marginalium*: "A wonderfull monster borne in Germany"] I will neyther wonder at this, nor at any such like, seeing that in this our time it is known & affirmed for a matter most true, that certaine Players shewing of a Comedy in Germany, one of them which played the deuill, hauing put on a kinde of attyre most grisly and feareful, whe[n] the Play was ended went home to his own house, where taking a toy in the head, he would needs vfe the company of his wife without changing the deformed habite hee had on, who hauing her imagination fearefully fixed on the ouglie shape of that attire with which her husband was the[n] clothed, conceaued childe, and came to be deliuered of a creature [*marginalium*: "A wonderful monster"] representing the very likenes of the deuill, in forme so horrible, that no deuil of hell could bee figured more lothsome or abhominable. (Torquemada sig. 10)

Jody Enders's insightful discussion of a French version of this legend lacking the dimension of a monstrous birth, located in Bar-le-Duc in 1485, refers neither to this German case nor to one documented in a luridly illustrated German broadsheet of 1569, of a Jesuit dressed as the Devil, who was stabbed to death for attempting to frighten a Protestant maiden into relinquishing her faith.[29] Wild Man and devil costumes were extremely popular at masquerades and carnivals. Accidents in connection with them were widely interpreted as divine punishment, as with the Bal des Ardents of 1392, when four masqueraders in Wild Man costumes were burned to death and King Charles VI of France seriously injured,[30] and two German carnival conflagrations. One at Waldenburg Castle in Württemberg, Germany, on February 7, 1570, fatally injured several masqueraders, including the host, Duke Eberhard

---

[29] *Newe zeytung / Unnd warhaffter Bericht eines Jesuiters /welcher inn Teüffels gestalt sich angethan / in welcher gestalt / er ein Euangelische Magd / von ihrem Glauben abzüschrecken vermeint / und darob erstochen ward.* Single leaf broadsheet, Augsburg 1569 (reproduced in Strauss 1335).

[30] Froissart sigs.CCXLIII–CCXLIIII: "Of the aduenture of a daunce that was made at Parys in lykenesse of wodehowses / wherin the Frenche Kynge was in parell of dethe." The original illustration of this episode is in London: Froissart, *Chroniques* IV, part 2, illuminated manuscript, Bruges c.1470. British Library, Harley 4380, f.1ʀ. It was considered newsworthy as late as 1707 (Happel, *Continuation* I: 427–8, illustrated).

von Hohenlohe (1635–1670), when their devil costumes caught fire.[31] In the other, at Georg von Schleinitz's court near Meissen in Saxony, a group of noblemen, including the host, burned to death when their shaggy bear costumes caught fire during his wedding festivities (Grundmann 191–3; Wesenigk 81–3; Gräße 58–9).

Despite serving at the French court, the surgeon Ambroise Paré does not appear to have known of the González family, absent from the chapter on monsters in his monumental medical treatise, first published in Paris in 1570. In it he presents the fourteenth-century Tuscan case, commonly diagnosed as a case of maternal influence:

> *Damascene* reports that he saw a maide hairy like a Beare, which had that deformity by no other cause or occasion than that her mother earnestly beheld, in the very instant of receiving and conceiving the seed, the image of St. *John* covered with a camells skinne, hanging upon the poasts of the bed. (Paré 978)

Paré's plate is iconographically closely related to Aldrovandi's (Figure 5.2), and to another in the anonymous *Aristotle's masterpiece*, of which successive editions were in print from 1684 to the 1930s, most also illustrating a short-lived hirsute boy said to have been born in 1579 or 1597 (Katritzky, "Images"). As the most widely read medical guide published in pre-modern England, this popular vernacular publication ensured that Paré's fanciful metamorphosis of the woolly-haired Tuscan child into a naked, hirsute adult woman became the most widely circulated book illustration of a hypertrichosis case.[32]

The González Family

The much more diverse visual and textual records of the González family contribute rich insights into their appearance and travels. Pedro González, the son of physically normal, Spanish-speaking parents,[33] was taken as a boy to the French court, where he received a classical education. In adulthood, González served as a French court servant from 1556 to at least 1560. With his wife, Catherine (d.1623), and their growing family of children, at least four of whom were to take after him and at least three of whom inherited her normal hair distribution (Zapperi 46–7, 81–2, 115, 215),[34] he was moved as a living Wild Man from the royal court of

---

[31]   *Ein ser erschröckliche doch warhafftige Geschicht / so sich begeben hat in dem landt zü Wirdenberg / auff dem schloß Waldenberg genand.* Single leaf broadsheet, Nuremberg 1570 (reproduced in Strauss 1337).

[32]   This case is also noted by Montaigne: "There was also presented vnto *Charles* king of *Bohemia*, an Emperour, a young girle, borne about *Pisa*, all shagd and hairy over and over" (45); *pace* my incorrect identification in *Healing, Performance and Ceremony* 205.

[33]   As indicated in the correspondence of Duke Wilhelm of Bavaria (April 3, 1583, quoted below).

[34]   The date of birth of the oldest son, Paolo (non-hairy), is unknown. Zapperi suggests birth dates for Madeleine/Maddalena (c.1575, hairy), Henri/Arrigo (c.1580–1656, hairy),

Paris, via Flanders and the alpine regions, to the ducal court of Parma, and finally to the Farnese country villa at Capodimonte. He is first noted in a dispatch of April 18, 1547, to Ercole II d'Este from his envoy to the French court, Giulio Alvarotto. It documents the presentation as a gift to Henri II and Catharina de'Medici on March 31, 1547, of a boy aged about 10 years old, hairy all over "just like Wild Men of the woods are painted," speaking Spanish, and dressed in European manner, but allegedly found in "the Indies."[35] A comment in the physician Realdus Columbus of Cremona's consideration of excessive human hair, first published in 1559, is probably registering an early sighting of Pedro González: "Nevertheless I saw a Spaniard of this type, with hair growing from every part of his body except his face and parts of his hands" (470). A Latin treatise of 1557 by another Italian physician, Giulio Cesare Scaligero, contains a definite reference, noting a hairy Spanish boy referred to in France by the nickname "Barbet" (a colloquial term for the shaggy Flemish hunting dog, the "Watterhund"): "brought from the Indies, or, as some think, born in Spain to parents from the Indies" (sig.177ᵛ).[36]

In one of his medical case studies, the Basle physician Felix Platter (older half-brother of Thomas) notes that the González family left the French court to enter the service of the Farnese family, noted collectors of monstrous humans:

> *Some Men are very Hairy.* It is vulgarly supposed that there are Wild Men that have Hair all over their bodies, except the tip of their Nose before, on the Knees, the Buttocks, and Palms of the Hands, and Soles of the Feet, as they are painted. But this is false, for none of the Cosmographers have mentioned any such, though they left not out the most brutish, as the Amazons, Canibals, and Americans, and others that go naked, and yet are not Hairy, but pul out Hairs where they grow. But this is true, that there are many of both Sex, especially men, more hairy then others, on their Thighs, Arms, Belly, Breast and Face, such I have seen. There was one at *Paris* very Gracious with King *Henry* the second, that lived at his Court, who had very long hair all over, except a little under his Eyes, his Eyebrows, and Hair in his Forehead were so long, that he was forced to tye them Back from hindering of his sight. He married a smooth Woman like others, and had by her Hairy Children, which were sent into *Flanders* to the Duke of *Parma*, I saw them in *Basil, An.* 1583. and got their Pictures, when they were to go into *Italy* with their Mother, a Son of nine years old, and a Daughter of ten:[37]

Francesca (c.1582) and Antonietta/Tognina (c.1588, hairy); the youngest sons were born in Parma in 1592 (Orazio, hairy) and 1595 (Ercole).

[35]   Alvarotto's dispatch is in the Archivio di Stato di Modena (Zapperi 189).

[36]   "Hispano puero: quem ex India aduectum, alij parentibus Indicis in Hispania natum putant."

[37]   This incorrect translation of Felix Platter's original wording of 1614 ("masculum 9. & fœminam 7. Annorum") demonstrates the ease with which such inaccuracies are introduced. If Platter intended to record the boy's age not as nine years but as nine months, then the two hairy children accompanying Catherine can be identified as Madeleine, aged around seven years in 1583, and her then possibly nine-month-old brother Henri. On my reasoning for accepting that, as recorded in his publication of 1614, Platter examined

the Male was more hairy in the Face then the Female, but all her Backbone was full of long bristles. But since (as we showed in Anatomy), there are Hairs in all the Pores of the body, it is no wonder that there are more in some then others, as the Nailes. But this is a greater wonder, that in some places they should grow so orderly, as in the Eyebrows, and in others scarce to be seen. There are Hairs in the Palms of every ones hands as appears by Children, but they are smal and continually worn away, which makes the Hand appear smooth.[38]

Possibly, they were presented to the Farnese family because of the family connections of Margareta of Parma, illegitimate daughter of Emperor Charles V,[39] and thus half-sister to King Philip II. Margareta's first husband, Alessandro d'Medici, who died when she was 14, had been an illegitimate brother of Henri II's wife, Catherina de'Medici. A former Regent of the Netherlands herself, Margareta of Parma returned from Flanders to Italy for the last time in 1583, after supporting her son Alessandro Farnese for several years in this post (Hertel 174; Zapperi 200–202). However, "Don Pietro González Selvaggio"[40] and his family arrived at the Farnese court in Parma only in May 1591 (Zapperi 93, 214). During the 1580s, the Bavarian and central European Habsburg courts exhibited an extraordinary flurry of interest in the González family. This generated correspondence and major portrait paintings of the family by several renowned artists based at these courts, some of which are still on display at the former seat of Archduke Karl's brother, Ferdinand of the Tirol, Ambras Castle, near Innsbruck.[41]

The Flemish artist Joris Hoefnagel, active in Spain during the 1560s, was based in Munich during the period from 1578 to 1590, when he completed commissions for the Bavarian ducal family as well as their neighboring Habsburg relatives. Duke Wilhelm V of Bavaria's attempts to acquire a living Wild Man date back to at least 1571, when Duke Philipp zu Hanau responded to his enquiries with assurances that there were none in his forests.[42] A brief Latin biography of "Petrus Gonsalus" inscribed on the back of Hoefnagel's double portrait of González and his wife, Catherine, concludes with the sentence, "He appeared in Munich, Bavaria, in the year 1582" (Zapperi 195–6).[43] On April 3, 1583, Wilhelm drafted a letter to be sent from Munich to Archduke Karl's wife, his sister Maria, in Vienna:

Catherine González in 1583 with a "boy of 9 [months?] and a girl of seven years," and not, as suggested by Zapperi (88–93, 214), eight years later, in early 1591, with her 11-year-old son Henri and 8- or 9-year-old daughter Françoise, see also Katritzky, *Healing, Performance and Ceremony* 205–7.

[38]   F. Platter, Culpeper, and Cole 365–6; based on Platter's original German-language edition of 1614. See also Wiesner-Hanks 183–4.

[39]   An uncle of Wilhelm V of Bavaria's mother, Anna of Habsburg.

[40]   Selvaggio is the Italian term for Wild Man.

[41]   For texts and images, see Zapperi 194–7; for a discussion of the portraits, see also Hertel 169–76.

[42]   Munich Bayerisches Hauptstaatsarchiv (BHStA), Fürstensachen 426/I: March 10, 1571; Baader 74.

[43]   "Conparuit Monachij boiorum a[nn]o 1582."

Concerning my Wild People, I want to have them portrayed full-length to send to you. I've also written to France to enquire everything about his origins, comings and goings. But he himself will know little, as he left when he was very young, and was presented to the king. Apart from that they aren't wild, as they are called. The man is a very refined, modest and polite person, apart from being so shaggy. The little girl is also very refined and well mannered; if she didn't have the hair in her face, she'd be a pretty little girl. The boy can't speak, he is very foolish and diverting. The old father and mother are not hairy, but like other people, and if I understood correctly, they were Spaniards. I also want to send you a full-length portrait of the old man, I have it life-size, he is not a tall person.[44]

In a letter he sent a month later, on May 10, 1583, Wilhelm specifies "his Wild People" themselves, as well as their painted portrait, among various commodities he shortly intends to have sent to Maria in Vienna: "I want to send you and your husband the Wild People and the painting at the earliest opportunity. I will send the stove to Vienna, to your house."[45] These letters were sent in response to correspondence of 11 March 1583, in which Archduke Karl warmly thanks Wilhelm for

the little panel portraying the hairy man together with his wife and children, which y[our] e[steemed self] sent me via my chamberlain, von Herberstain. This is certainly a thing that is well worth seeing. I would ask y[our] e[xcellency], insofar as it is possible, that y. e. would send me full-length portraits of the two children, and have the little boy depicted naked, while he is still so young.[46]

This final phrase suggests that Karl knew that the growing infant himself was present in person at the Bavarian court, and strengthens the possibility that Pedro and Catherine González and their two hairy children were associated with the entourage of Margareta of Parma, journeying from the Netherlands to Italy during late 1582 and early 1583, and that they passed through Basle and spent time in person at various courts of her Munich and Habsburg relatives.

Melanchthon's account contributes important new information to this already detailed narrative. As well as referring to Pedro González's demonstrative role and substantiating his early childhood links with Madrid, Melanchthon uniquely documents the existence of a second "manikin" of similar size and appearance, almost certainly another young male hypertrichosis sufferer. The condition's distribution appears to be consistent with control by a dominant gene. These only exceptionally skip a generation, suggesting that hypertrichosis can be passed on only by direct inheritance from a parent manifesting it or through spontaneous

---

[44]   Munich BHStA Geheimes Haus Archiv (GHA), Korr.Akt 606 V, f.212ᵛ (file draft of letter sent); Zapperi 194–5.

[45]   Munich BHStA.GHA, Korr.Akt 606 V, f.214ᴿ (a draft of the letter sent, as recorded on the verso in a scribal hand of similar date also providing a list of subjects covered in the letter, whose item "Rauchen leüt und tafln" ("hairy people and pictures") distinguishes between the people and their portraits.

[46]   Munich BHStA.GHA, Korr.Akt 609 III/3, f.61.

mutation in a reproductive cell prior to conception. As neither of Pedro González's parents exhibited the physical symptoms of hypertrichosis, and the condition is extremely rare, if Pedro's companion was human, he can only have been his identical twin brother.

By 1592, the González family had settled at the court in Parma, and around 1608, its surviving members were retired to the Farneses' rural seat at Capodimonte. No such noble protection was afforded to Barbara Urslerin, the only sufferer of hypertrichosis born in the seventeenth century known to have survived into adulthood. She competed with other physically exceptional humans trying to make a living touring European fairgrounds. Several documents have escaped previous attention in this context. I here suggest that an illustrated broadsheet records Urslerin's birth in the village of Mursellers near Kempten, Bavaria, on February 16, 1629 (Figure 5.3, p. 128),[47] and that the report of an unnamed, bearded, three-year-old girl with all-over body hair, in the medical case studies of the Jewish physician Zacutus Lusitanus (1575–1642), is an eyewitness commentary on Barbara Urslerin confirming that her parents showed her around Europe for money as early as 1632.[48]

Linking his account of Pedro González to Plutarch's account of the Roman general Sulla's meeting in Dyrrachium (now Durres, Albania) in 86 AD with a satyr captured nearby enabled Melanchthon to connect hypertrichosis cases of his own time with the classical satyr and the Christian devil. If the young González could evoke comparison with demons, Barbara Urslerin was systematically compared to a dog. For some of her spectators, the multilinguality and harpsichord-playing she demonstrated during her shows were appreciated more as proof of her humanity than as skills in their own right. Like Urslerin, the González family attracted the close interest of a wide range of medical professionals. Unlike her, they also attracted the patronage of European royalty and nobility, including King Philip II and his Habsburg relatives. Their interest ensured that the impact made by Pedro González and his family was confined neither to Spain nor to their own lifetimes. Early modern understanding of the "marvellous races" and of satyrs, devils, hairy anchorites, and above all, the Wild Man, are fundamental to the period's multilayered medical and cultural reception of congenital and temporary hypertrichosis. Viewed within the context of literary anthropologies based on the traditions of classical myths, legends, and fables, documents such as Melanchthon's account or Happel's image confirm that through their persistent afterlife in European print culture, the González family exercised a lasting impact on medical culture far beyond Spain itself.

---

[47]   Nuremberg, Germanisches Nationalmuseum (Holländer 277; Alexander & Strauss 338).

[48]   Lusitanus, *Praxis medica admiranda* 504: "*De Monstris. Puella barbata.* Pvellam vidi ætatis trium annorum, formosam, & pulchram cum barba magna, cui totum corpus nimis hirsutum erat, & ex eius auribus, pili crassi, hirti, numerosi prodibant, ita oblongi, vt palmum & dimidium æquarent. Hoc monstrum circulatores lucrandi causâ publicè ostentabant."

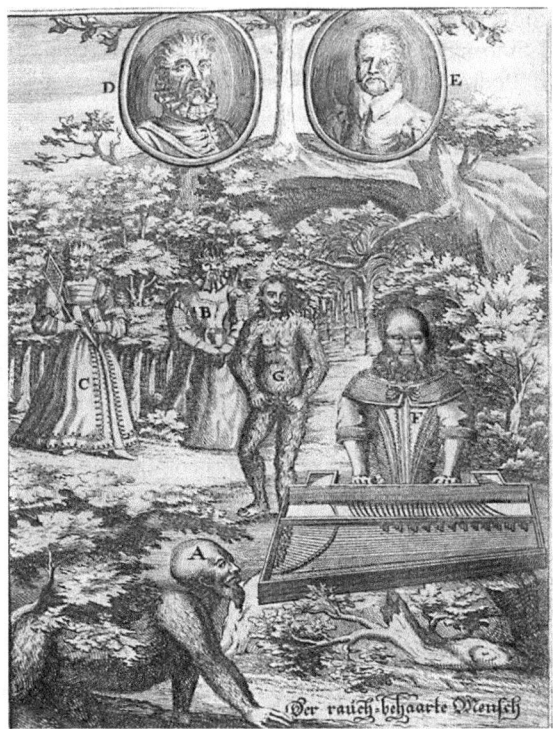

Figure 5.1   Eberhard Werner Happel, *Shaggy-haired humans* (Der rauch-
              behaarte Mensch), engraving, *Relationes curiosae* II, 1685: plate
              opposite p. 312. Depicting A: classical "Himantapodes"; B, C, D,
              E: "The hairy-bodied Canary Islander" (Pedro González with a son
              and two daughters c.1600); F: "The hairy woman of Augsburg"
              (Barbara Urslerin c.1655); G: Javanese *Ourang Outang* or Wild
              Wooddweller

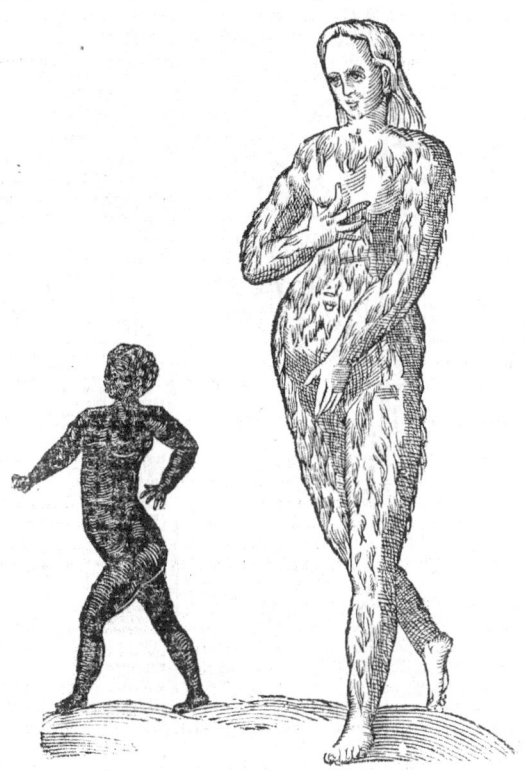

Figure 5.2   Ulysses Aldrovandi, *Infans Aethiops, & Virgo villosa* (A black
infant and a hairy maid), woodcut

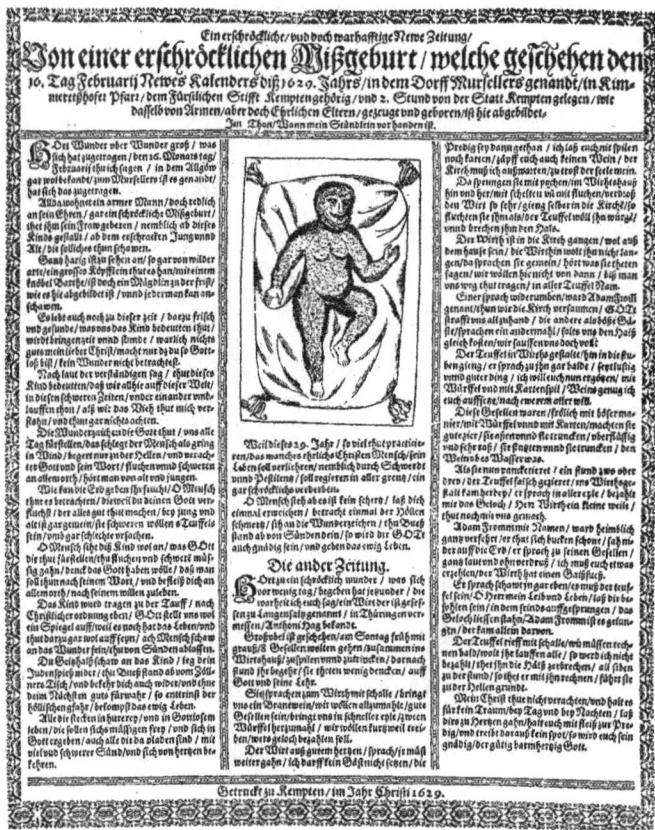

Figure 5.3   Christoph Kraus, *Of a frightful misbirth (Von einer erschröcklichen Mißgeburt)*, printed single-leaf broadsheet published in Kempten, 1629. (This previously unidentified newborn is here identified as Barbara Urslerin.)

Chapter 6

The Medical Cultures of "the Spaniards of Italy": Scientific Communication, Learned Practices, and Medicine in the Correspondence of Juan Páez de Castro (1545–1552)[1]

Elisa Andretta

Introduction

During the middle decades of the sixteenth century, Trent and Rome were not only centers of the Roman Catholic world, but also significant points at which Spanish cultural and political influence was clearly felt in Italy. Rome, the seat of pontifical power, was in the process of redefining its role as the world's capital. Trent, as seat of the eponymous Council, was temporarily invested with near-absolute centrality; it was there that a plan was elaborated that would guide much of Europe's cultural and spiritual life over the next century and beyond. Spain would take a significant interest in the developments in these two cities. The correspondence between two emblematic imperial subjects, Juan Páez de Castro (c.1510–1570) and Jerónimo Zurita (1512–1580), illustrates both the intensity of the Spanish concern for Italy and the ways in which this concern shaped intellectual life on the Iberian peninsula. Both men were historians and witness to important ecclesiastical developments of the time. Páez de Castro was to become imperial historiographer.[2] Zurita was Secretary of the Inquisition and went on to be one of the most important historians in Aragon.[3] Páez de Castro's letters to Zurita were written between 1545 and 1552, first in Trent, and later in Rome,

---

[1] My thanks to José Pardo-Tomás for his comments at various stages in the preparation of this chapter. This research was supported by Fonds National Suisse "Ambizione grant" PZ00P1_137043 / 1.

[2] On Juan Páez de Castro, see Domingo Malvadi, *Bibliofilia humanista*, and Martín Martín, *Vida y obra*.

[3] The letters are published partly in Uztarroz and Dormer's *Progresos de la historia in Aragon* I: 525–61 (which will hereafter be referred to as *Progresos*), and partly in Andrés, "31 cartas."

where he moved in 1547.[4] In the letters, Páez de Castro provides his friend Zurita with detailed information about his stay in Italy and first-hand testimonies on the important cultural and political-religious transformations taking place. In addition to informing Zurita carefully on the Council's workings, he wrote of exciting, even transformative intellectual experiences.

The two men shared philological passions, and Páez de Castro could be confident of Zurita's interest in the humanist milieus of Rome and Trent.[5] Páez de Castro describes public and private libraries and who visited them; enumerates the activities of some Italian printing offices; and names the works—ancient and modern—recently published or still in progress in Italian literary-scientific circles. Conversations with learned men and descriptions of their scientific endeavors have an important place in his correspondence. Clearly, these letters were designed to feed Zurita's curiosity about the world of letters abroad. Through his letters to Zurita, however, Páez de Castro also tries to keep alive his connection to Spanish cultural and political life. The letters are an important means to communicate, almost in real time, the experience of Italy to the Spanish world. In this way, Páez de Castro justifies his presence in Italy and prepares his return home.

The correspondence between Páez de Castro and Zurita provides modern readers with a privileged insight on the cultural trajectories of a Spanish intellectual in mid-sixteenth-century Italy. Páez de Castro belongs to the Castilian cultural élite and thus considers Italy the ideal place to enrich his knowledge of the classical world and to refine his cultural profile. For figures such as Páez de Castro, the intensifying political relationships between the two peninsulas—Iberia and Italy—made possible new forms of cultural exchange. The official responsibilities of Spanish ambassadors, viceroys, cardinals, and the members of their circles may have obliged them to spend periods in Italy, but these stays also created opportunities to develop private collections and libraries, as well as build personal relationships within Italian intellectual circles. Páez de Castro's letters to Zurita are particularly valuable because they shed light on the workings of a scientific culture, on the one hand, and exchange between Spain and Italy, on the other. Although neither a physician nor a man of science, Páez de Castro zealously cultivated scientific and, in particular, medical interests. Among his interlocutors were many Spanish and Italian physicians. Especially significant is his attention to anatomical and naturalistic studies. On several occasions, he played a crucial mediating role in the production of medical knowledge itself, passing from witness to actor.

Examining the Italian experiences recounted by a Spanish humanist within the context of other journeys that men of science and letters from Spain undertook in

---

[4]   On Zurita, see *Jerónimo Zurita: su época y su escuela*; Iso; and Domingo Malvadi, *Disponiendo anaqueles*.

[5]   Zurita, like Páez de Castro, was educated in Alcalá under the guidance of *Comendador griego*, the famous Hernán Núñez de Guzmán (1475–1553) (Domingo Malvadi, *Disponiendo* 11–12).

Italy elucidates the cultural and scientific exchanges between the two peninsulas. Furthermore, it permits a clearer understanding of the forms that scientific knowledge took, the channels by which this knowledge circulated between Spain and Italy, and the consequences of this circulation at a moment in European history when the interactions among medical cultures, other forms of cultural production, and politics were particularly important.

In recent years, numerous studies have focused on aspects of the relationship—political, religious, and cultural—between Spain and Italy in the early modern age, and in particular on the Spanish presence in Italy.[6] Rarely, however, have these studies explored the medical and scientific exchanges that tied the two areas, despite the fact that, as James Amelang noted, "there were few physicians in 16th century Spain who did not look eastward to Italy as the main locus of medical authority," while "a different sort of medical practitioner headed in the opposite direction" (443).[7]

Medicine and Natural History in Trent at the Time of the Council: The Aristotelian Academy

Juan Páez de Castro was born around 1510 in Quer (Guadalajara) and was trained at the universities of Alcalá and Salamanca, where he not only studied law but also devoted himself to mathematics, history, philosophy, and ancient languages.[8] When he reached Trent he was already a renowned humanist.[9] He arrived in the alpine town following Francisco de Vargas y Mesía (d.1566), who was "Fiscal del Consejo de Castilla" (the imperial lawyer appointed to the Council by Charles V).[10] Through the intercession of another humanist, Gonzalo Pérez (1500–1567),[11] Páez de Castro entered the circle of the imperial ambassador, Diego Hurtado de Mendoza (1503–1575). Mendoza employed him as a "literary agent" and perhaps even gave him a few informal diplomatic missions (Martín Martín 17).

Páez de Castro's stay in Trent was the fulfillment of a long-standing desire to go to Italy. His expectations were high, both for the intellectual exchange and for

---

[6]   See Cantù and Visceglia; Dandelet and Marino; Hernando Sánchez; and Visceglia.

[7]   Some interesting lines of research in this area can also be found in Carlino, "Tre piste."

[8]   See Páez de Castro's own "Método para escribir la historia," dedicated to Charles V (published in Eustasio). On his education and relationship with the universities of Alcalá and Salamanca, see Domingo Malvadi, *Bibliofilia humanista* 17.

[9]   In a sixteenth-century list of the Spaniards present in Trent, he is described as "immensa eruditioni seu sacrae sive profanae vir" (Gutiérrez 662).

[10]   "Yo vine por inducción del secretario Zurita y por la voluntad que yo me tenía de antes, de ver Italia; y lo principal fue ofrecerse esta jornada del Concilio, para lo cual fue llamado el Sr. Licenciado Vargas, fiscal de su Majestad y de su Consejo, que es la más honrada y docta persona que he visto en mi vida y víneme en su compañía y así me estoy ahora," Letter to Augustín Cazalla (06-07-1645), ctd. in Andrés 519.

[11]   See González Palencia.

the possibility of entering into contact with the ancient cultural heritage coming to light thanks to the work of renowned humanists, copyists, and printers. He was not disappointed.[12] Thanks to the Council, Trent had become a cultural center. Among the cardinals, political representatives, and their staffs (including important physicians),[13] there were famous humanists and bibliophiles (Jedin 539–46). Some brought their private libraries with them, adding to the city's preexisting collections, and Trent temporarily acquired unique library resources (Jedin 547).

Mendoza was a towering figure in Spain's humanist culture and his library was among the most important of the itinerant collections temporarily housed in Trent.[14] Mendoza moved his rich collection of printed books and manuscripts from Venice to Trent, and did not hesitate to make it available to scholars gathered there, even to those belonging to opposing political parties.[15] The ambassador soon became an important figure for Páez de Castro (Hobson 81). As he described in detail to Zurita, Páez de Castro began assiduously to visit Mendoza's library, which included texts on theology, philosophy, medicine, music, and astrology.[16] But in addition to the library, Páez de Castro seems to have been greatly impressed by Mendoza's own scholarship, finding it "muy varia, y estraña" (highly varied and remarkable).[17] The two men shared a great interest in Aristotle, which they read entirely in Greek. The slow pace of the Council may have caused Mendoza some impatience, but it gave him time to work on his translation and commentary of the *Mechanica*; Páez de Castro followed this undertaking with great interest. Mendoza was quick to share his progress and even commissioned Páez de Castro to purchase new works that would expand the ambassador's collections (Martín

---

    12   The first letters to Zurita (e.g. Trent, 10-08-1545) exude high expectations. He excitedly describes the first meetings of scholars—"congresos de Letrados de muchas naciones"—and provides brief portraits of the learned men already in the city and those who are expected to arrive (*Progresos* 529).
    13   Besides the Council's physician, Girolamo Fracastoro, the personal doctors of various cardinals and diplomats were in the city. Among these was Balduino Balduini, Cardinal Del Monte's doctor, whose activity in Trent is well documented (Merkle 224–5, 228, 790, 831, 841, 843).
    14   On Mendoza, an extraordinary political and cultural figure, see González Palencia and Mele; and Spivakovsky. On his stay in Italy, see Stefania Pastore, "Una Spagna antipapale?"
    15   "La biblioteca di Mendoza supplì a quella del concilio, che non si era riusciti ad apprestare, ma essa divenne anche strumento di lavoro e punto di attrazione per gli umanisti presenti a Trento" (Jedin 322). About Mendoza's library see in particular Hobson. About the liberality with which he offered to loan his books, see González Palencia and Mele 259–60.
    16   "Los libros que aquí ha traído son muchos, y son en tres maneras, unos de mano Griegos en gran copia, otros impressos en todas facultades, otros de los Luteranos, y todos estos están públicos para quien los pide, si no son los Luteranos que no se dan sino a los hombres que tienen necessidad de los ver para el Concilio" (*Progresos* 530; Trent, 10-08-1545).
    17   "Es gran Aristotlélico, y Mathemático; Latino, y Griego que no hay quien se le pare; al fin él es un hombre muy absoluto" (*Progresos* 530; Trent, 10-08-1545).

Martín 17). These missions led to stimulating visits and meetings in Padua, for example, where Páez de Castro entertained Lazzaro Buonamici (1479–1552) and visited the home of Pietro Bembo (1470–1547). He was greatly taken with Bembo's library, collections of art and antiques, and the botanical garden "con muchas herbas, y arboles exquisitos" (with many herbs and exquisite trees) (*Progresos* 539–40; Trent, 08-06-1546).

Thanks to Mendoza's patronage, Juan Páez de Castro could largely devote himself to the philosophical *otium*. His erudition was appreciated to such a degree that in December 1545 he was chosen to write the history of the Council (*Progresos* 534–35; Trent, 14-12-1545). He took up the study of Plato, but more importantly, thanks to Mendoza's copies, he amended several of Aristotle's works, focusing mainly on *De animalibus*[18] and the *Physica* (*Progresos* 535; Trent, 14-12-1545). Around the same time, his interest in Aristotelian natural philosophy led him to study medicine. He read Hippocrates and Galen and bought their works in Greek in Venice, intending to assemble a small Greek library.[19] This interest in medicine developed rapidly during his time in Trent.

Páez de Castro's studies in Trent were not lonely at all. He had a confidant in Mendoza, with whom he could share his passions and doubts, and he came into contact with other learned men in the city. It was in this context that, in August 1545, he conceived of the ida of creating a "great academy of erudite men dedicated to understanding in Aristotle."[20] The initiative was intimately linked to the studies conducted by Mendoza, but Páez de Castro was probably the driving force. The first meetings were scheduled for that winter. Scant information about the Academy remains. What little we have comes from Páez de Castro's letters, and these letters, as H. Jedin noted of the artistic and cultural exchanges at Trent, leave many questions unanswered.[21] We do not know, for example, how often the Academy met or how the meetings were structured. We do know that the Academy met in parallel with the first sessions of the Council, where the doctors gathered imposed a ban on the free interpretation of scripture. And Páez de Castro indicates that natural philosophy and the study of the human body, including the

---

[18] "Mi estudio principal es Aristóteles, y procurar emendar mi libro con los exemplares del señor Don Diego, donde hallo cosas maravillosas, que hay tantos monstruos vencidos, tantas cosas añadidas, tantas quitadas, que no se puede creer, principalmente en los libros *de animalibus*, y los que van debaxo deste nombre" (*Progresos* 533; Trent, 14-12-1545). A few months later Páez de Castro is quick to say that this study was "el mayor trabajo que tuve en mi vida en cosa de estudio" (*Progresos* 536; Trent, 24-03-1546).

[19] "Estoy determinado de hacer librería Griega; he comprado mas de cinquenta ducados de libros, y entre ellos a Galeno, y Hipócrates" (*Progresos* 534; Trent, 14-12-1545). The two posthumous inventories of Páez de Castro's library ordered by Philip II (Martín Martín 39, 41–4) show how this idea soon became reality.

[20] "[…] gran academia de hombres muy eruditos, que se dedican todos a entender en Aristóteles, *dum sub nivibus stupet alma tellus*" (*Progresos* 532; Trent, 09-08-1545).

[21] "[…] uno sprazzo di luce, […] sufficiente per illuminare un lato della storia del Concilio, del quale noi non sappiamo quasi niente" (Jedin 546).

body's functioning and the curative properties of plants and minerals, were the Academy's main topics of study.

Páez de Castro names three physicians who participated in the meetings: "Fracastorio," "Iulio," and a "Medico" and "gran Herbolario" who remains unidentified (*Progresos* 538; Trent, 25-03-1546). "Fracastorio," or Girolamo Fracastoro (1478–P1553), was appointed physician of the Council in 1545. Páez de Castro's letters mention Fracastoro often, calling him "a great friend of mine, and a learned man who makes no great show of his learning."[22] Páez de Castro also informs Zurita of the debate caused by *De contagione*, a synthesis of Fracastoro's natural philosophy that had just been published in Venice, saying that "some like it and others do not" (*Progresos* 539; Trent, 08-06-1546). "Iulio" refers to Giulio Alessandrini (1506–1590) from Trent. Alessandrini was nearly three decades younger than Fracastoro and had studied medicine and philosophy at the University of Padua. Alessandrini was eventually appointed physician to Emperor Ferdinand I, later to Maximilian II, and finally to Rudolf II (who had been educated at the court of Philip II of Spain). Alessandrini was a fine Hellenist and Latinist, as well as a great connoisseur of Galen, a number of whose works he wrote commentary on and translated. Over the years, Alessandrini prepared the *Galeni enenatiomaton aliquot liber*, dedicated to Madruzzo, Cardinal of Trent; the book was published in Venice in 1548, just a few years after Páez de Castro established the Academy.

Textual and philological concerns were clearly a central preoccupation of the Academy. Immediately following his decision to convoke the Academy, Páez de Castro went to work finding the Aldine edition of the *opera omnia* of Aristotle (Venice, 1495–1498) and a few Greek and Latin commentaries on the Stagirite— probably made available by Mendoza—along with other books and codices.[23] The study of texts, however, was accompanied by direct observation of nature and the human body. On March 25, 1546, Páez de Castro reports that the Academy had performed an anatomical dissection in its first winter. This was "the best in the world," attended by only a few and conducted with diligent reference to Galen and Vesalius (whose groundbreaking *Fabrica* had been published shortly before).[24] Páez de Castro had previously expressed interest in anatomical studies and his desire to go to Padua to attend dissection (*Progresos* 533; 14-12-1545). But the report of March 25, 1546 is particularly noteworthy for two reasons.

---

[22]   "[…] gran amigo mio, y hombre muy docto, mas poco aparente" (*Progresos* 539; Trent, 08-06-1546). On Fracastoro, see Pastore and Peruzzi's *Girolamo Fracastoro*, as well as Pennuto. On his appointment in Trent, see Alessandro Pastore.

[23]   "Lo principal que tengo de traer es, Aristóteles de impresión de Aldo, y todos los comentarios Griegos que hallare, y algunos Latinos, que serán Averrois, y S. Thomas" (*Progresos* 531–2; Trent, 09-08-1545).

[24]   "este ibierno [invierno] una anotomía la mejor del Mundo, y con muy pocos, y mui doctos […] he pasado todo lo que haze a este menester diligentemente, confiriendo a Galeno, y a Vesalio" (*Progresos* 538; Trent, 25-03-1546).

First, it indicates that philology was, from the Academy's beginnings, paired with anatomical study. Conceptually, this was the coupling of the systematic, textual study of Aristotle with Paduan Aristotelianism, which conceived of anatomy as a "natural philosophical enterprise" (Klestinec 51), a conception later widely developed in Padua, first by Jerome Capodivacca and then by Jerome Fabricius d'Acquapendente.[25] In more personal terms, the presence of Fracastoro and Alessandrini, both significantly influenced by their time in Padua (Ongaro) alongside Páez de Castro, an early follower of Mendoza's humanism, further suggests ties, at least virtual, between the Aristotelian Academy of Trent and the University of Padua.

The second reason Páez de Castro's letter of March 25, 1546, is significant is related to the conditions under which the anatomical dissection was performed. We cannot be sure of the method used for the demonstration, nor do we know who was in charge of the material dissection. We do know, however, that not many people were present. In this privileged context, which ensured a good view for the lucky few, the study of the body was carried out by meticulously comparing Galenic doctrine to Vesalius's recent contributions to anatomy. Vesalius had been a lecturer in the study of anatomy at Padua between 1537 and 1542. Again, we find constant dialogue between textual authority and the direct observation that was contributing to a new conception of the human body. Páez de Castro maintained that he valued the knowledge gained from anatomical dissection over everything else he had learned.[26]

While dedicating the long winter of 1545–1546 to anatomy, Academy members planned to develop a second front for their research, also located at the intersection of the ancients and *observatio*. During the following summer, they wanted to investigate herbs and metals, because, as Páez de Castro explained, there were "great mines" in the region, "principally silver and iron mines." In conjunction with their investigations of *materia medica* they planned to return to their studies of Galen.[27] In May of 1547, Páez de Castro reports that the preceding year's expeditions to the countryside had been fruitful. He tells Zurita, "I spent part of the past summer studying herbs and plants and had the Ruel's herbal as my companion," and goes on to say that alongside Giulio Alessandrini he investigated "silver and copper and the many other metals we have nearby."[28]

---

[25]   See Cunningham's "Fabricius" and *The Anatomical Renaissance* 167–90; French, *William Harvey's Natural Philosophy* 3–17; and Klestinec 51–2.

[26]   "[…] que precio más que este estudio que quanto sabía" (*Progresos* 538; Trent, 25-03-1546).

[27]   "[…] tener Academia de yervas, y de metales que hay aquí muy grandes minas, principalmente de plata, y hierro, y passaré otro pedazo de Galeno" (*Progresos* 538; Trent, 25-03-1546).

[28]   "me ocupé este verano passado algun tiempo en yervas, y plantas, tuve por familiar a Ruelio, autor herbario […] unos minerales de plata, y cobre, y otros mil metales que tenemos aqui junto, y esto hago en compañía de Iulio Alexandrino, Médico muy excelente" (*Progresos* 546; Trent, 25-03-1546).

These medical studies of plants and minerals led to broader considerations of natural history. Natural historical research was already in full swing on both the Iberian and Italian peninsulas and was related to Páez de Castro's interests.[29] He collected numerous works on natural history by classical and modern authors.[30] In one letter written at Trent, he expressed the desire to get the *De metallis* of the "germanicus" Agricola.[31] Páez de Castro's curiosity was not limited to texts; he demonstrated interest in the collection of *specimina* and was favorably impressed by the Venetian Senate's plan to establish a Garden of Simples (medicinal plants) in Padua (*Progresos* 539; Trent, 08-06-1546). He told Zurita that he was looking forward to the time when the two of them could examine his modest collection of specimens together.[32] Páez de Castro even hoped to travel to the New World to see *naturalia*.[33]

Páez de Castro's letters portray Trent in the early years of the Council as not only the "crossroads of European politics," but also an important center for the development and dissemination of philological, medical, and scientific cultures between Spain and Italy (Jedin and Prodi). As we have seen, the correspondence with Zurita tells—if only in the most general terms—of an academy of Spanish design where Spanish humanists and Aristotelians of the Paduan school combined textual study and first-hand observation of nature, all while enjoying access to an extraordinary trove of books and codices brought to Trent during the Council.

Scientific Knowledge, Humanistic Culture, and Politics in Spanish Rome

Two years after the founding of the Academy, in February 1547, Juan Páez de Castro was able to summarize his intellectual sojourn in Trent in bold terms. He tells Zurita:

> I am altogether absorbed in my work on Aristotle and better prepared than any Christian who has ever undertaken the task, equipped with my personal faculties and with books; I have sufficient linguistic facility and I know more than enough mathematics for Aristotle; I have come by a great knowledge of anatomy, which has cost me a good deal of trouble; I understand the law, which is extremely necessary; and as far as poetics and rhetoric [are concerned], I don't find myself lacking. I have done extensive examination of the very fine minerals we have

---

[29]   On the renewal of naturalistic studies, see among others Jardine, Secord, and E. C. Spary; Ogilvie; and Egmond, Hoftijzer, and Visser. On the Italian context, see Olmi; and Findlen, *Possessing Nature*. On Spain and its American colonies, see Pardo-Tomás, *Oviedo*.

[30]   On the "naturalistic library" of Páez de Castro see Domingo Malvadi, *Bibliofilia humanista* 132–5.

[31]   Letter to A. Casalla (Trent, 19-03-1546), Andrés 520–21.

[32]   "[...] quando nos veamos placiendo a Dios, que cierto en este Lugar hay aparejo para saber dos cosas, yervas, y minerales" (*Progresos* 546; Trent, 31-05-1547).

[33]   "Podrá v.m. creer que tengo deseo de ver aquel mundo, y que no pierdo esperança de lo ver" (*Progresos* 543; Trent, 26-10-1546).

here in Trent. As far as books, I have the best-corrected texts of Aristotle that anyone has had in eight-hundred years. I have all of the Greek commentaries published and have looked at others at Leoncio's shop in Padua. Among those authors who came after the Greeks, I have the finest texts in the world, what there is of Averroes, Saint Thomas, and Latins, such as Boethius, although these are worth little in comparison to the Greeks. I compare everything that Galen refutes, or that Aristotle declares with the texts we have that contend the opposite. In addition, I put Plato and Aristotle side by side and compare them, and all of this while enjoying the greatest ease, in the finest place in the world, with health and energy, for which I thank God. So, this is my study, which will go on as long as the Council lasts, probably two years or a little more.[34]

Beginning in December of 1545, however, Páez de Castro's productive *otium* in Trent was "disturbed" by repeated invitations to move to Rome. Urging him were prominent figures of the Spanish community in the Eternal City, including the doctor Juan Aguilera (d.1560) and the humanist and antiquarian Antonio Agustín (1516–1586). The prime mover of these invitations was, however, Cardinal Francisco de Mendoza y Bobadilla (1508–1566), whom Marcel Bataillon called a political mainstay of Charles V's in Italy and a shining example of a Castilian aristocracy immersed in humanism.[35] Mendoza y Bobadilla's motivations for inviting Páez de Castro to Rome are not entirely clear, but it is conceivable that they were of a dual nature. On the one hand, Cardinal Mendoza was a great bibliophile, and probably saw in Páez de Castro the ideal figure to build and oversee his library collections (Graux 43–6, 61–78; Bataillon, "Benedetto Varchi" 6–12). On the other, the arrival of a humanist like Páez de Castro would swell the

---

[34] "Yo estoy todo metido en Aristóteles con el mayor aparejo que jamás creo que Christiano lo emprendió, assi por las artes que tengo en mi persona, como por los libros, porque de mi parte tengo pericia de la lengua bastantemente, y tengo cognición de lo que toca a Mathemáticas más de lo necessario para Aristóteles; entro con gran conocimiento de anatomia, que me ha costado mucho fastidio; tengo para lo moral la facultad de Leyes, que es asaz necessaria; y para la Poesia, y Retórica, creo que no me falta; he hecho gran inquisición de minerales, que los tenemos aqui en Trento muy buenos. De parte de libros tengo los textos de Aristóteles más correctos que los ha tenído hombre de ochocientos años a esta parte. Tengo todo quanto se ha impresso Graece de comentarios, y cotejados algunos con la Libreria de Leoncio en Padua. Tengo textos de la traslación vieja los mejores del mundo, y lo que hay de Averroes, y S. Thomás, y algunos otros Latinos, come es a Boecio en toda la Dialéctica, aunque todos valen poco en comparación de los Griegos. Saco todos los lugares que Galeno reprehende, o declara a Aristóteles, y confiero los textos que alega con los que tenemos. Allende desto voy juntando a Aristóteles con Platón, y los Platón sobre Aristóteles, y todo esto con el mayor ocio, y mejor aposento del mundo, y con gran salud, y fuerza, gracias a Dios por todo. Assi que señor mio este es el estudio, el qual concluiría en dos años que durasse el Concilio, o en poco más" (*Progresos* 544; Trent, 17-02-1547).
[35] "l'un des piliers de la politique de Charles Quint en Italie et une des gloires de l'aristocratie castillane éprise d'humanisme" (Bataillon, "Benedetto Varchi" 3).

ranks of those who supported Spain's imperial ambitions at a time of great tension between the Papacy and Charles V.[36]

Páez de Castro reacted with some irritation to the invitations of the "Spanish Romans."[37] He was simply not convinced that Rome could offer him anything Trent did not have in a greater degree.[38] On several occasions he confided to Zurita that his greatest desire was to enjoy life in the Alpine town a bit longer, to go on consulting Diego Hurtado de Mendoza's library, and to continue following the slow progress of the Council. He managed to stall for several months, but when it was announced in May of 1546 that Mendoza would take the place of Juan de Vega as ambassador to Rome, Páez de Castro was convinced the fates were conspiring to bring him to the papal city. This belief, however unwelcome, intensified his interest in Roman affairs.[39] In February 1547, he made his first short stay in Rome and immediately entered into contact with the most important cultural figures of Spanish Rome.[40] He also began to appreciate the city's library resources. He identified the Vatican Library as particularly promising for his studies, but he also put great hopes in private libraries, such as those of cardinals.[41]

Once back in Trent, Páez de Castro began to plan for his future in Rome. At first he aspired to the post of secretary at the embassy. He quickly gleaned, however, that it was not to be. Undaunted, he entered the service of Cardinal Mendoza y Bobadilla, who had promised him substantial benefits through his doctor, Juan Aguilera.[42] At the same time, Páez de Castro began to explore how the city might

---

[36]   Concerning the complex balance between the two powers during the first period of the Council, see Bataillon, "Benedetto Varchi" 10–12; Signorotto I: 259–80; Firpo 245–61; Stefania Pastore; and Levin.

[37]   "Aguilera y el Cardenal de Coria me fatigan" (Andrés 521; Trent, 7-07-1546).

[38]   "Porque a la verdad en toda Italia no hay mejor conversación que aquí, donde está gran parte de España, y lo mejor de Italia" (*Progresos* 539; Trent, 08-06-1546).

[39]   He even began to intervene in the affairs of Rome, advising Ambassador Mendoza to appoint Juan Aguilera as family doctor, despite (or perhaps because of) the fact that Aguilera dwelt at the Apostolic Palace (*Progresos* 544; Trent, 17-02-1547).

[40]   Among these was Antonio Agustín, with whom he claims to be familiar: "Al señor Antonio Agustín tengo muy familiar, es gran amigo de v. m. no vi en mi vida hombre más curioso, ni más honrado, tiene muy buenos libros, principalmente en su professión" (*Progresos* 545; Trent, 31-05-1547). About "Spanish Rome" see Dandelet's much discussed *Spanish Rome*, as well as Hernando Sánchez; and Visceglia. On Spanish intellectual sociability in Rome, see Amelang, "Exchanges."

[41]   "Yo ando rebuelto en la Biblioteca Vaticana, y creo que sacaré buenas cosas, y lo mismo haré en librerías particulares que las hay buenas" (*Progresos* 545; Rome, 27-02-1547).

[42]   The letters document in detail the uncertainty of Paéz de Castro and the negotiations; see in particular Andrés 524–5, 528, 533–6. It was Bataillon who put emphasis on the "material" dimension of the humanist's Italian stay: "on nous excusera d'avoir cherché à voir de quoi *vivait*—ou, comme il dit, mangeait—le plus savant des compagnons du Cardinal de Burgos" (Bataillon, "Benedetto Varchi" 19).

further the studies he had begun in Trent. Rome had its own books, plants, trees, and minerals.[43]

Páez de Castro moved to Rome permanently in October 1547, only months after his first visit.[44] He lived there until 1550 under the protection of Cardinal Mendoza y Bobadilla (Martín Martín 18). Despite the fact that Páez de Castro was not officially in the service of Hurtado de Mendoza, who was now the Roman ambassador, the two men did not break ties. Hurtado de Mendoza continued to rely on Páez de Castro's services.[45] As a "servant of two masters"—Cardinal Mendoza y Bobadilla and Ambassador Hurtado de Mendoza—Páez de Castro entered into Roman intellectual life with the best credentials.[46] He came into contact with the world of copyists and printers working for the cardinal, augmenting his own library of Greek texts and perhaps working as the cardinal's librarian (Graux 44). At the same time he met men of science and letters within the Spanish community and beyond, becoming a regular visitor to the Pope's own library and the libraries of various cardinals (*Progresos* 547; Rome, 17-06-1548). This made it possible to continue the work he began in Trent and to explore new fields. Páez de Castro did not give up his commentary on Aristotle's texts, although he showed a growing impatience with this research and a renewed interest in Platonic and skeptical philosophy.[47] When the weather improved, he hoped then to devote himself to the topography of the city and to antiquarian studies.[48] But he was increasingly

---

[43]   "Creo que allende del interés, me holgaré mucho en aquella ciudad por los grandes aparejos que hay en todas disciplinas; desde allí yo escribiré muy largo todo lo que sucediere. Aquí entendido en hierbas y árboles y minerales con gran suceso, todos mis estudios terminan en Roma" (Andrés 535–6; Trent, 22-08-1547).

[44]   The first letter written after his transfer is dated October 20, 1547 (Andrés 537–8).

[45]   "El Sr. D. Diego de Mendoza me ha hecho grandes favores porque ha dicho al Cardenal tanto bien de mí, que el Cardenal fue forzado a le decir que si su Santidad se quería servir de mí que él holgaría de ello; y D. Diego asióse de aquella palabra y dijo que le besaba las manos; el Cardenal quedó harto congojado y al fin la cosa se resolvió con decir que las casas de entrambos eran una misma cosa; que yo me estuviese hasta que se ofreciese en que D. Diego se pudiese servir de mí" (Andrés 537; Rome, 20-10-1547). This quote also provides proof of a certain agreement between the two Mendozas, which was not destined to last. On the complex relations between the two Mendozas in the Roman years see Bataillon, "Benedetto Varchi" 19–39.

[46]   On Roman scientific culture in the early modern period and the city's cultural infrastructure, see A. Romano, *Rome et la science* and "Rome, un chantier pour les savoirs"; and Donato and J. Kraye.

[47]   "Agora entiendo en hazer en Latino a Sexto Empyrico Cheroneo, que sono dos libros de Philosophia de los Pyrrhonios, haré una prefación en que porné grandes cosas de lo que toca para nuestra Religión, *et effugiam vitiligatores*; v.m. advierta lo que en esta parte tiene notado" (*Progresos* 550; Rome, 01-09-1549). Some attention to sceptical philosophy is clear in the letter to Zurita on August 10, 1545 (*Progresos* 530). On Páez de Castro and the manuscript "Sexti Cheronei[s] libri tres de Sceptica disciplina et charactere," see Floridi 70–71.

[48]   In August of the same year he plans to devote himself to "antiguallas, y ver estas ruinas muchas vezes" (*Progresos* 548; Rome, 01-08-1548).

interested in mathematics and started new, ambitious projects in natural history.[49] Rome seemed to suit Páez de Castro just as well as Trent had. According to the correspondence with Zurita, mathematics and natural history consumed Páez de Castro during his Roman years.

It was on these fronts that he entered into close relations with two of the central figures in the circle of scholars who gathered around powerful Spanish cardinals. The first of these was Juan Aguilera, personal physician to Juan Álvarez de Toledo (1488–1557).[50] The second was Andrés Laguna (1499–1559), Mendoza y Bobadilla's personal doctor.[51] The cardinals had recruited Aguilera and Laguna for personal and political reasons. Renowned physicians provided the cardinals' familiae with skilled medical attention. And Laguna, in particular, had already proved his absolute loyalty to the emperor. The confluence of personal and political motivations was not uncommon; at the time, the appointment of a personal physician was dictated by complex reasons, public and private.[52] Juan Aguilera was a physician and astrologer trained in Salamanca, where he held the chair of astronomy until being called to Rome.[53] Andrés Laguna was invited to Rome at the end of 1545 from Metz, where he found himself after a long sojourn through Europe.[54] For both physicians, working for an eminent cardinal guaranteed protection and the possibility of entering into a circle of learned humanists.[55] In addition, Aguilera's and Laguna's privileged positions made them sought after

---

49   "Por otra parte leo a Theophrasto, confiriéndole con la translación de Theodoro Gaza, y con Plinio: hallo muchos descuidos del Intérprete, y muchos de Plinio, y por otra parte gran ayuda en Plinio, y en el Intérprete. Pero como agora en nuestro tiempo la historia de plantas se ha llegado muy al cabo, todavía hay buenas cosas" (*Progresos* 548; Rome, 01-08-1548). On the philological activity of Páez de Castro see Domingo Malvadi, *Bibliofilia humanista* 133–4.

50   On Juan Aguilera see Navarro Brotons, "La actividad astronómica" 185–216 and "Aguilera, Juan." Information about Juan Aguilera's stay in Rome can be found in Marini 369–71.

51   On Laguna, see Hernando y Ortega; Dubler's edition of Dioscorides, *La materia médica de Dioscórides*; Bataillon, *Le docteur Laguna, Lección Marañon*, and *Erasmo y el erasmismo* 286–326; González Manjarrés; García Hourcade and Moreno Yuste; and Pardo-Tomás, "Andrés Laguna." Detailed information concerning Laguna's life and work are in the "estudios introductorios" to Laín Entralgo (ed.), *Pedacio Dioscórides Anazarbeo, acerca de la materia medicinal* XIII–CLV.

52   On the role of doctors as political mediators, see A. Carlino, "Medicina e politica."

53   Laguna recalls the circumstances of Aguilera's arrival in Rome in the dedication addressed to Aguilera in April 1548 (*Epitomes* 4r–5v).

54   As stated by the doctor himself: "Quam sane tibi insitam, cognitamque in studiosos omneis benignitatem, abunde etiam sum ipse expertus: quippe quum me anno quadragesimo sexto supra millesimum, ex Germania redente, ubi primum attigi Romam, quam munificentissime exceperis, exceptumque praefeceris curae valetudinis tuae, ac postea in dies magis summa liberalitate locupletaveris" (Laguna, *Epitomes* 6v).

55   On the scientific and medical patronage of Cardinal Juan de Toledo see Carlino, "Tre piste."

by other members of the Curia, such as Paul III and his successor, Julius III. This proved lucrative, and the fact that they were esteemed within papal circles probably made them exceptional go-betweens among the Spanish community and the various factions of the Curia.[56]

Despite busily practicing medicine, both Aguilera and Laguna wrote books of ambitious scope during their Roman years. Aguilera devoted himself to the creation of an astronomical instrument and the preparation of his *Canones Astrolabii Universalis*, published in Salamanca in 1554. Laguna worked on his well-known Spanish translation of Dioscorides's *Materia Medica*.[57] Moving in many of the same circles, Páez de Castro was well aware of the scholarly efforts of the two physicians. Humanist correspondence attests to the relationship between Páez de Castro and Aguilera, and Laguna expressly acknowledges his great intellectual debt to Páez de Castro in the dedication to his translation of Dioscorides.

As we have seen, Aguilera began his correspondence with Páez de Castro when the latter was still in Trent. We might even consider Aguilera the architect of Páez de Castro's move to Rome. Their early correspondence is dedicated to the material considerations related to the humanist's move to the papal city. Once ensconced there, however, the two men started an intense intellectual exchange. "During stolen moments," Páez de Castro writes, "doctor Aguilera and I discuss mathematics."[58] Mathematics was of consuming interest to Aguilera, who was at work on his astronomical instrument, a "Quadrante universal" or "universal quadrant." Páez de Castro describes it as "something that no one has invented until now," specifying that it is a series of tables of "all the heavenly movements, very easy to use and very precise."[59] Drawing on the work he had done on Aristotle's *Mechanica* in Trent, and confident in his knowledge of mathematics, the humanist claims to have helped Aguilera complete the extraordinary quadrant (*Progresos* 548; Rome, 01-08-1548).

While Páez de Castro maintained ongoing conversations about mathematics with Aguilera, he discussed natural history and *materia medica* with Laguna. We saw previously that while in Trent, Páez de Castro acquired classical texts on natural history, studied Aristotle's *De historia animalium*, and went afield

---

[56]   At the Archivio Segreto Vaticano there are several works related to the benefits conferred to Juan Aguilera by the popes: Archivio Segreto Vaticano, Reg. Paul. III, t. 154, p. 29; t. 182, p. 225; t. 188, p. 2; t. 201, p. 316; t. 225, p. 159; Julii III, t. 224, p. 181; t. 38, p. 30. Concerning the benefits obtained by Andrés Laguna in exchange for his services at the Apostolic Palace, see Nelson (whom I thank for providing me with a draft of the article).

[57]   "Por donde al Illustríssimo y reverendíssimo Cardinal de Mendoça (debaxo de cuya sombra y amparo se fabrican estos nuestros trabajos) [...]" (Dioscorides, *Acerca* [ed. 1555] 84).

[58]   "el Doct. Aguilera, y yo a ratos hurtados entendemos en Mathemáticas" (*Progresos* 547; Rome, 17-01-1548).

[59]   "[...] cosa que nadie hasta agora lo ha inventado [...] unas Tablas de todos movimientos, de operación muy fácil, y muy ciertas, y otras cosas bien apacibles" (*Progresos* 547; Rome, 17-01-1548).

to collect plant specimens in the mountains. Rome had established itself as an important center for naturalism almost a century before. Thanks to the support of popes beginning in the mid-fifteenth century, Rome became noted for, on the one hand, the recovery, edition, and publication of ancient works and, on the other, its excellent gardens (Siraisi, "Life Sciences"). Systematic instruction in the use of medicinal plants began at the Roman university in 1513. The Vatican's garden, the Hortus Vaticanus, was expanded during the pontificate of Paul III; other botanical gardens in Rome, often guarded by the court physicians, adorned the residences of many cardinals and noblemen.[60] The city seemed to Páez de Castro a particularly suitable place to develop his study of natural history. He spent his first "Roman summer" immersed in the study of Theophrastus's *Historia plantarum*, comparing a manuscript to which he had access to Theodore Gaza's edition and to Pliny's *Naturalis Historia*. He planned to work next on Theophrastus's *De plantarum causis*.[61] Páez de Castro acquainted Zurita with these efforts, asking Zurita, in turn, to send him the commentary that Zurita was writing on Pliny (*Progresos* 549; Rome, 15-09-1548).

Naturalism took up all of the following year: in January 1549 Páez de Castro informs Zurita of his scholarship, in which he compares Theophrastus's text not only with Gaza's edition and Pliny, but also with Dioscorides.[62] After the completion of this work he intends to do the same type of comparison with Aristotle's texts.[63] In September 1549 he announces the conclusion of his work on Theophrastus. Noting the numerous shortcomings of Gaza and especially those of Pliny, he proposed an entirely new edition of the *Naturalis Historia*. This work, together with the other translations of classical natural history, including Zurita's commentary, would have rendered "a vastly corrected Pliny," in which the errors of Hernán Núñez de Guzmán (1475–1553), who had been Páez de Castro and Zurita's teacher, would be avoided.[64] At the same time, Páez de Castro tells Zurita

---

[60]   On the historical-naturalistic practices in early modern Rome, see Andretta and Brevaglieri.

[61]   "Estos meses de calor entendí en leer a Theophrasto de *historia plantarum*, tengo notados grandes lugares contra Plinio, y contra Theodoro Gaza; otra temporada conferiré lo de *causis*, y después lo que Gaza trasladó de Aristóteles, y creo se juntará buena cosa; tengo un exemplar de Theophrasto de mano, que no es poco hallarlo, aunque es muy incorrecto, pero ayuda quando menos pensamos" (*Progresos* 549; Rome, 15-09-1548).

[62]   "Estos días he entendido en Teofrasto que tengo un ejemplar de mano razonable y voy cotejando a Gaza y a Plinio y a Dioscórides; hallo cosas muy buenas y lapsos graciosos de Plinio y Gaza y lugares que están corruptos en Plinio" (Andrés 541; Rome, 22-01-1549).

[63]   "Acabado esto tengo intención de hacer otro tanto en Aristóteles con las traducciones de Gaza y Plionio y con mis textos que creo son los mejores que ahora hay en el mundo" (Andrés 541; Rome, 22-01-1549).

[64]   "Yo creo que escriví a v.m. como entendía en Theophrasto, téngolo concluido, en que hay grandes lapsos de Gaza, y grandes de Plinio, en algunos cayó el Comendador, pero restan muchos; estoy determinado de le trasladar de nuevo, en teniendo oportunidad juntamente con todos los otros opúsculos que están por trasladar: assí que con esta

that he wants to get in touch with Spanish naturalists, such as Miguel Monterde (c.1505–1571).[65]

While Páez de Castro was strengthening ties between the Italian and Spanish traditions of natural history, he came into contact with Laguna in Rome. The profiles of the two learned men have many similarities and their paths often traced the same itineraries through Italy. Both men spent time in Rome and Trent, although not always at the same time, and Laguna had collected herbs in the Dolomites. Both men were friends with Francisco Vargas and both were related to the circles of Mendoza y Bobadilla and Hurtado de Mendoza; they served Cardinal Mendoza y Bobadilla during the same year.[66] Despite all of these coincidences, evidence of the relationship between Páez de Castro and Laguna is scarce. One significant mention, however, indicates the crucial role played by Páez de Castro in assisting Laguna in his translation of Dioscorides. Laguna writes:

> Juan Páez de Castro, a man of rare learning and a highly respected imperial historian, assisted me in this enterprise by sharing with me an extremely old Greek codex and a manuscript of Dioscorides thanks to which I was able to correct seven-hundred places in the text that until now have tripped up Dioscorides' other commentators, whether in Latin or vernacular languages; it is for this reason that all of Spain can justly celebrate the completion of a faithful translation, something that Spanish can claim but Latin cannot; this success may be judged by any who wish to compare my translation with any other.[67]

Laguna had begun to copy and collect manuscripts useful for his work on Dioscorides years before in Paris, and continued to do so all through his European *peregrinationes*. It was, however, upon meeting Páez de Castro in Italy, in the

---

diligencia, y con lo que el Comendador ayuda, y con lo que v.m. por su parte traerá notado, creo haremos un códice de Plinio muy emendado, por esso v.m. tenga atención a juntar todo lo que tiene en Plinio, porque acá lo comuniquemos" (*Progresos* 550; Rome, 01-09-1549).

[65]   "Del Doctor Lucena tengo entendido como el señor Monterde es aficionado a secretos naturales, y conocimiento de yervas, y plantas [...] v.m. le diga, que le beso mil vezes las manos, y deseo que nos comuniquemos, porque me avisasse de algunas cosas que por fueza ternán notadas en Theophrasto, en quien como digo yo hize harta diligencia" (*Progresos* 550–51; Rome, 01-09-1549).

[66]   Both were part of the circle in the wake of "[...] Illustrísimo y Reverendísimo Cardenal de Mendoza, cuando, desde Roma, fue a recibir al Serenísimo Príncipe Don Filipo, Rey Católico de Inglaterra, la primera vez que pasó in Italia" (Dioscorides, *Acerca de la material medicinal* [1555] 17–18). About this journey, see also *Progresos* 549.

[67]   "Assí mesmo el Doctor Juan Páez de Castro, Varón de rara doctrina, y Digníssimo Coronista Cesáreo, me ayudó para la mesma empresa, con un antiquíssimo códice Griego, y manuscripto, del mesmo Dioscórides, por medio del qual restituy más de 700 lugares en los quales hasta agora tropeçaron todos los intérpretes de aquel author, ansí Latinos, como vulgares; por donde se puede justamente alabar toda España que le tiene ya transferido y más fielmente, en su lengua española, que jamás se vio en Latina, lo qual podrán fácilmente juzgar aquellos, que quisieren conferir mi translatión con todas las otras" (Dioscorides, *Acerca* [1555] "Epistola Nuncupatoria"). See also Laguna, *Annotationes* 3r.

shadow of Cardinal Mendoza, that Laguna came to a turning point in his careful philological work; it was thanks to this meeting that his Spanish edition was, at least according to Laguna, superior to all previous editions.[68] Laguna's expression of gratitude to Páez de Castro may be gracious and self-congratulating at the same time, but it also tells an important story. It shows that Páez de Castro was willing to share his treasured manuscripts and findings, not only with old friends, such as Zurita, but with new colleagues, such as Laguna. In Rome, as in Trent, and throughout his correspondence with Zurita, we find Páez de Castro building important relationships based on the exchange of knowledge and shared access to valuable works of scholarship. As Laguna attests, Páez de Castro's generosity led directly to the success of one of the most famous works of natural history to be published in Spain during the sixteenth century.

Conclusion

Juan Paez de Castro, Juan Aguilera, and Andrés Laguna were all marked by their stays in Italy, stages in much longer journeys that ended in all three cases with a return home. Juan Páez de Castro was appointed chaplain and royal historiographer in 1550. His history was never published, but the manuscript was consulted on several occasions by Philip II as he was establishing the library of the Escorial.[69] Páez de Castro's private library became part of the royal collections. Juan Aguilera returned to Salamanca to teach, where he was one of those who contributed to the renewal of the university curriculum and the introduction of Copernicanism into the program of study.[70] Andrés Laguna's annotated translation of Dioscorides was reprinted several times in the course of the sixteenth and seventeenth centuries and constituted an important contribution to the development of Spanish naturalism. Through the translation of Dioscorides's *Materia Medica*, Laguna contributed, on the one hand, to the systematization of the knowledge of the ancients on the basis of comparison with direct observation, and on the other, to the establishment of specialized and precise botanical terminology. From the seventeenth century onward, the text became an obligatory point of reference for Spanish apothecaries.

The generation of Spanish men of science and letters who lived in Italy during the troubled years of the end of Charles V's reign and worked in the service of cardinals and ambassadors assisted in the formation of a renewed Spanish medical culture that found refuge and assistance in the courts of nobles and clergymen. Of course, this medical culture had many points of reference beyond Italy and

---

[68]   The codex probably entered the collections of the Escorial together with the other volumes of Paéz de Castro's library, later destroyed by fire in 1671. On the history of this manuscript see Graux 97–9; Guzmán Guerra; Miguel Alonso XCI–XCII.

[69]   See in particular the "Memorial del Dr. Paéz de Castro sobre la importancia de establecer librerías reales en el reino," published in Martín Martín 77–83.

[70]   See Bustos Tovar; and Navarro Brotóns, "The Reception."

Spain, notably the Low Countries and the New World. It was not at any moment, however, a unidirectional transfer from one region to another; there was always exchange.[71] Significantly, exchange among medical cultures was made possible by networks of communication that often tracked contemporaneous religious and political channels. Juan Páez de Castro's itinerary, his experiences in Italy, and the way in which he brought those experiences to bear on his subsequent work in Spain show how elite medical cultures were constructed across professional and political boundaries.

---

[71]   An example is the influence of Laguna's *Dioscorides* on the Italian naturalists; another is the fact that the Italian translation of Juan Valverde's *Historia del cuerpo humano* (Rome, 1559) was the one of the first discussions of the *nova anatomia* in Italian.

PART 3
Textual Cultures in Conflict, Competition, and Circulation

Chapter 7
"Offspring of the Mind": Childbirth and Its Perils in Early Modern Spanish Literature

Enrique García Santo-Tomás

La carne muerta luego cría gusanos
(Dead flesh soon breeds worms)
—Francisco Santos, *Día y noche de Madrid*

Bodies in Crisis

The intersection of medicine and literature is one of the fields that offer the richest potential for any Golden Age specialist, especially now that critics are embracing a much-needed interdisciplinary perspective. The figure of the surgeon, to cite a typical case, continues to be one of the most fruitful archetypes of seventeenth-century fiction, whether through the portrayal of the *matasanos* (quack) in texts of a satirical and burlesque nature or that of the *galeno* (learned doctor), in whom sincere hopes of recovery are vested. Medicine is openly depicted in a wide range of genres and modes, from the *comedia* to the *baile*, from the picaresque to the courtly novel, from the sonnet to the ballad. Wherever the symptoms of courtly love appear, for example, so too does the doctor. Like astrologers or cobblers, physicians are remarkably versatile creations, in that they are often veiled in an aura of mystery. Half mystical, half heretical, they derive this aura from their secret knowledge, their personal art of achieving the improbable. From the very beginnings of Petrarchist poetry in the Iberian Peninsula, writers adopted models inherited from the Middle Ages when speaking of the process of seduction or the humoral balance of the body in love. And yet we do not need to cite specific allusions in order to detect the traces of medical practice, which so intrigued people during the Baroque. After all, there has always been medicine without doctors and pharmacopoeias. The popular beliefs, superstitions, and home remedies we so often find in literature have always existed: processes like bloodletting, purgatives, and eating clay are poised between high and low, ceremonial and improvised, abject and sublime. It is therefore safe to say that the cultural output of this period, from the *Quixote* to the most ephemeral Baroque dramatic texts, is incomprehensible unless one takes into account the medicine of the time.

Although the image of the doctor in early modern fiction has been studied in some detail,[1] the field is far from exhausted. Pioneering studies by historians of science in Spain, from José María López Piñero onwards, have shown us that medical texts constituted a publication phenomenon of extraordinary dimensions; as a result, medicine, in its various facets, has been the object of intense scholarly attention. There is a great deal of ground to cover, because the scope of the material is vast. My concern, therefore, is not to focus on the representation of a particular practitioner or symptom in the fiction of the time, but rather to explore how received knowledge of specific medical practices influenced the praxis of writing, not only in terms of lexical and metaphorical usage but also in the formulation of content: how, in other words, what was published in one field reverberated in the other. What I want to consider here is what we would now call obstetrics, perhaps the most *literary* or aesthetic discipline of all, given the visual and poetic seductiveness of its raw impact. I shall leave aside the traditional figure of the *galeno* or academic doctor and concentrate instead on one of the least explored figures of the period, the midwife or birth attendant, with the aim not so much of looking at the mechanisms involved in representing them, but rather of connecting them with a whole symbolic view of Baroque decline. This view is expressed—more fully, perhaps, than by any other writer—in the work of the moralist Francisco Santos (Madrid, 1623–Madrid, 1698), the last of the great Baroque novelists, in whose writings the narrative trends of the seventeenth century converge.

Offspring of the Mind

The Baroque exhibited a taste for representing bodies "in transition," whether in the process of maturation, reproduction, evacuation, or putrefaction. Painters like Holbein and Bruegel the Elder offer us copious oneiric, allegorical, and phantasmagorical visions of mutilated, mixed, or dismembered beings, not to mention all the body parts that take on lives of their own. The influence of Bosch's fantastic, abject creatures can be measured by the frequency with which his name is mentioned in Golden Age fiction.[2] Bosch and the authors who invoked his name deployed a particular conception of the human body; as Mikhail Bakhtin pointed out, the phenomenon of the Carnival and its inverted view of life plays a predominant role. It is a world of uninhibited behavior and tasteless jokes, where the "opened" or severed body, along with all its functions, is exploited and exhibited.[3] In this worldview it was the metropolitan landscape, more than

---

[1]   See, for example, Simón Palmer, "Hipócrates y Galeno"; David-Peyre.

[2]   The influence of Bosch on Spanish literature has been studied by Levisi; Iffland I: 128–30, II: 43–9; on Bosch's presence in the poetry of Lope de Vega, see Sánchez Jiménez 347–74.

[3]   The idea of the opened, dissected, or mutilated body has been the object of renewed attention in recent years; see Sawday 213–29 and Hillman and Mazzio's anthology.

any other, that became the backdrop of choice for artists and authors, as cities like Seville and Madrid gradually established their calendar of festive celebrations during the sixteenth century.

Childbirth is therefore located at the very center of the festivity, subverting an entire medical tradition that, from an academic perspective, investigated every phase and element of the process.[4] Birth attendants were controversial figures in pre-modern Europe: frequently older and already with children of their own, they had been trained by their own mothers, aunts, or grandmothers. Gail Kern Paster explains that because "women in early modern Europe ordinarily gave birth under conditions monitored only by other women, childbirth in the period has been interpreted as an inversion of customary gender hierarchies—one of those instances of temporary but genuine female empowerment" (165), an example of what Natalie Davies nearly 30 years ago called "women on top" (124–51). In Hapsburg Spain, women sought the care of midwives or *madrinas* ("matrons"), who may have been known to them through family connections but were generally well regarded in their communities. Midwives even acted as witnesses in cases of rape or examinations of virginity, as López Terrada reminds us ("Medical Pluralism" 11). Although in general terms it is true that before "childbirth belonged to medicine, it belonged to women," in early modern Spain it is generally difficult to pinpoint a before and after: midwifery was often in flux (Wilson 70). Between 1477 and 1523 a decree required the *Protomédicos*—that is, the royal first physicians, head of the tribunal of the *protomedicato*—to examine any woman who wished to practice this profession before issuing an official permit.[5]

An excellent theoretical consideration of the lacerated body is offered in Connor. On the relationship between pain and language—which I shall not address here—I refer readers to Scarry's classic study. For an interesting range of theoretical readings of the phenomenon of childbirth, see Adams.

[4] On the evolution of the role of the mother in sixteenth- and seventeenth-century Spain, see Nadeau, "Authorizing"; Moncó Rebollo; Morant. For a recent general survey on medical practices by women in Europe, see the monographic issue of the journal *Dynamis* 19 (1999) entitled "Mujeres y salud: prácticas y saberes" ("Women and health: practices and knowledge").

[5] With regard to the *protomedicato*, López Terrada has written that "The powers of this court were delimited in accordance with its purpose and those over whom it held jurisdiction (i.e. health workers); it was not subordinate to the Consejo Real. The functions of the tribunal were twofold. First, it examined and granted licenses to physicians, surgeons, and apothecaries, as well as to *especieros* (spice sellers), herbalists, *ensalmadores* (bonesetters), and midwives. Second, it controlled the exercise of the various medical professions. In this capacity, the *protomedicato* had both civil and criminal jurisdiction; practitioners were subject to both economic and corporal sanction. It prosecuted and punished unauthorized medical practice, especially when the magic arts (*artes mágicas*) were involved, but also in cases of unlicensed exercise of 'empirical' and scientific medicine" ("Medical Pluralism" 10). This gives us an idea of the precarious position of many midwives in the period, subject to constant changes of opinion according to the success of their efforts. For the European context, see Whaley 91–130.

After 1523, however, the *protomedicato*'s licenses were only issued for professions such as surgeon, barber, or what we would now call an apothecary. This left the way clear for any woman who wished to assist a family member, neighbor, or friend in childbirth, although in some cities, such as Zaragoza, the College of Physicians trained midwives. As Teresa Ortiz has pointed out, a very influential part in the development and transmission of midwifery was played by the studies of Damián Carbón, *Libro del arte de las comadres y del regimiento de las preñadas y paridas de los niños* (*Book of the Art of Midwives and the Management of Women Pregnant with and Newly Delivered of Children*) (Mallorca, 1541); Francisco Núñez, *Libro del parto humano en el cual se contienen remedios muy sutiles y usuales para el parto dificultoso de las mujeres* (*Book of Human Parturition Containing Very Subtle and Useful Remedies for Difficult Childbirth in Women*) (Alcalá, 1580); and Juan Alonso de los Ruyzes de Fontecha, *Diez privilegios para mujeres preñadas* (*Ten Privileges for Pregnant Women*) (Alcalá, 1606). In such works one detects a very obvious tension in assigning a specific role to "external" agents such as midwives. On the one hand, midwives were at the very center of the authors' theoretical and practical speculations; on the other, midwives were excluded from the possible readership, given that they most of them were illiterate and these manuals were peppered with quotations in Latin.[6] It was not until the beginning of the eighteenth century that childbirth came under the control of surgeons and priests (except in cities like Málaga, which had a large Moorish population devoted to this occupation); it was finally regulated in 1750 by a royal decree from Ferdinand VI, giving full power back to the *protomedicato* and granting direct licenses to women interested in practicing this profession.

Within this catalogue of horrors and curiosities, a large number of Golden Age texts include the image of childbirth as an expression of the laborious effort by which good literature is created.[7] One often encounters the expression "partos del ingenio" (offspring of the mind), for example, in authors like Alonso Jerónimo de Salas Barbadillo,[8] who complained of the constant demand for new titles in the

---

[6]   This was a constant theme outside Spain, as Mazzoni points out: "While the knowledge embraced by medicine was and is a written discourse, a discourse assuming that all knowledge must be propositional and subject to theorization, midwives' knowledge, on the other hand, was orally transmitted and eminently pragmatic. Significantly, this experiential type of knowing is closely related to the knowing of the pregnant woman herself: midwives relied heavily on their personal experience of childbirth for their ability to empathize and care. It is therefore not surprising that, along with the invalidation of midwives' knowledge, the pregnant and birthing woman's own knowledge should also have been discredited" (61).

[7]   Apparently this was not the case in English literature, as Gail Kern Paster emphasizes: "Childbirth is especially invisible in dramatic representation, where the act of giving birth has been an offstage event, as unstageable as the other forms of bodily evacuation it so embarrassingly resembles" (163).

[8]   In the "Aventura séptima" (Seventh Adventure) of Salas's masterpiece *Don Diego de noche*, we find the protagonist witnessing a woman giving birth in a cemetery while the

epistle dedicatory to his *Don Diego de noche* (Don Diego at Night): "los piden por impresos antes de estar perfeccionado el parto" (they ask to see them printed before one has finished giving birth to them); the image of *mantillas* (swaddling clothes) is one of those most widely used in the period when referring to the development of the theatre as inherited by Lope de Vega. However, this idea of *nacer al mundo*, being born into the world, is a dualistic image, imbued with the optimistic endeavor of personal creation as well as the pain of the process itself, of efforts that do not always come to fruition. Sometimes you sit with your elbow on the desk and your cheek in your hand, as Cervantes reminded us in the Prologue to his masterpiece, and on other occasions one wants to write "y el llanto no me deja" (but my tears won't let me), in the semi-burlesque confessional words of Lope de Vega disguised as Tomé de Burguillos. In some cases, childbirth leads to a fateful denouement, with tragic heroes such as Segismundo in *La vida es sueño* or Marcela in the *Quixote*, "diabolical" embodiments of the supreme sacrifice of a mother who died in the process.[9] In others, however, childbirth functions as a leitmotif of social satire, with the cuckolded husband attending to his wife only to see her lover's child being born; this is exactly what happens in Tranco II ("Stride II") of Luis Vélez de Guevara's masterly Menippean satire *El diablo cojuelo* (*The Limping Devil*): "Allí está pariendo doña Fáfula, y don Toribio, su indigno consorte, como si fuera suyo lo que paría, muy oficioso y lastimado; y está el dueño de la obra a pierna suelta en esotro barrio, roncando y descuidado del suceso" (There is Doña Fáfula giving birth, and Don Toribio, her unworthy consort, very solicitous and distressed, as if what she is giving birth to were his; and the author of the work is in another part of town, sleeping like a log, snoring and not giving a thought to the event) (22). We even find examples in Golden Age fiction of childbirth being used to express the idea of one author borrowing from another, as in *La torre de Babilonia* (*The Tower of Babel*) by Antonio Enríquez Gómez, when the Marqués de la Redoma (Marquis of the Flask), in Vulco (Section) XIII, begins his autobiographical narrative with this confession:

> Yo, señores míos, después que el milagroso ingenio de don Francisco de Quevedo me dejó en su redoma hecho gigote, salí della un martes veinte y uno de Julio, año de mil y seiscientos y cuarenta y siete. ¡Gracias a Dios que me libró de barriga de mujer! ¡Sea bendito el que me libró de zahorí de tripas y explorador de cuajares! Envidiarán muchos mi nacimiento, como si hubiera mucha diferencia de mujer a vidrio [...] Soy parto cristalino de una panza veneciana. (586)

> (Gentlemen, after the prodigious ingenuity of Francisco de Quevedo left me stewing in his flask, I emerged from the flask on Tuesday the twenty-first of July in the year sixteen hundred and forty-seven. Thank God for delivering me from

---

child's father desperately tries to find a midwife; Peyton comments on the effect of Baroque contrasts of light and shade and life and death (112).

[9] On *La vida es sueño* and the astrological prognostication that accompanied Segismundo's birth, see Lanuza's chapter in this volume.

a woman's belly! Blessings on him who delivered me from the gut-diviner and abomasum-explorer! Many will envy my birth, as if there were much difference between women and glass [...] I am the crystalline offspring of a Venetian belly.)

All of the variants of the childbirth motif exhibit a special syntax in which the subject or the object is emphasized rather than the verb itself; in other words, light is cast on the creator or the creation rather than the crucial event of the actual birth. And yet there are also many texts that establish—or occasionally *exalt*—the act of parturition as a quintessential element of a kind of fiction that very often penetrates the intricacies of allegory to explore the mysteries of human nature, and especially female nature.

The phenomenon of parturition has been approached in recent decades by feminist critics, as well as by those coming from psychoanalysis and queer studies. The last of these has been addressed in recent years by Hispanists like Sherry Velasco and Peter Thompson, who build on François Delpech's stimulating analysis of the seventeenth-century actor Juan Rana. Juan Rana was also the protagonist of a number of plays, including of one of the most controversial ones of the period: *El parto de Juan Rana* (*Juan Rana Gives Birth*).[10] But whether we speak of the representations of childbirth in *El parto de Juan Rana* or in the works of Vélez de Guevara and Enríquez Gómez, childbirth provides authors with an extremely delicate tool, as delicate as the lacerated body. Among the various reproductive tropes, a very common example is that of the serpent or snake, which, in Salas Barbadillo's beautiful lines, "muda con prudencia / la piel, entre las piedras resbalándose" (carefully sheds its skin, slithering among the stones) (802),[11] to be reborn from a solitary sacrifice. This is a birth in reverse, a fruitful variant of a trope often given to misogyny, used to represent the resurrection of the individual, whether beatific or diabolic.[12]

Gestation and delivery assume a body in limbo, transitory, under tension, which is only resolved on completion of a journey that is at once private and ceremonial, intimate and shared. However, the act of procreation, and particularly the climactic moment of birth, are also articulated in Golden Age fiction with an unmistakable air of mystery. Pregnant women gave rise to a whole series of concerns and mystifications, as Gail Kern Paster, Sharon Howard, Patricia Crawford, and

---

[10]   For a stimulating reading of this problem in colonial literature, see Kirk; for the European context, see Sanders's "Midwifery and the New Science."

[11]   In *Tratado poético de la esfera* (*Poetic Treatise of the Sphere*), included in Arnaud III: 798–804.

[12]   In his *Francisco Santos' Indebtedness to Gracián*, Hammond has written that "both Gracián and Santos, with very slight differences, make the same bitter comparisons between the birth of the man and that of the serpent. Because the female, on conceiving, bites off the head of the male, the young take vengeance at birth by tearing open the mother's body. Just so is the bad wife who causes her husband's death in order to enjoy his wealth, the son who worries his mother to death so that he may inherit quickly, and the younger son who kills his brother in order to become the sole heir" (57).

Linda A. Pollock have indicated with reference to England, Jacques Gélis for France, Cristina Mazzoni for Italy, Montserrat Cabré and Teresa Ortiz for Spain, Herman Roodenburg and Myriam Greilsammer for the Netherlands, and Ulinka Rublack and Jennifer S. Spinks for Germany. As the Baroque period advanced and the effects of social and economic decline were felt in Spain, the image of childbirth gradually took on what one might call more *sinister* overtones. By sinister I do not simply mean that authors showed particular relish for the realistic or natural aspects of birthing, I mean also that there was an aesthetic intensification that was identifiable in the taste for hyperbole, animalization, or grotesque carnivalization.[13] Francisco Santos's fiction bears witness to the moral exhaustion of the last third of the century and makes exceptionally frequent use of the image of parturition to narrate the miseries of Madrid.

Santos's Madrid is a swollen, moribund, contaminated social body. Óscar Barrero Pérez, for example, has written that "Santos lived through the last stage of the Baroque period, a time when the increasingly obvious decline of the country exacerbated the confusion between ideal and reality in the minds of Spanish artists; reality was no longer monolithic and unalterable, either in ideological or existential terms" (37), and he suggests that perhaps "to some extent these features of external reality govern the structural disintegration of seventeenth-century narrative art" (38). Santos, whose attitude is in some ways akin to that of the scientific *novatores* at the turn of the eighteenth century.[14] His fiction prompts readers to consider another kind of "gestation," one that gave birth to a new way of seeing literary expression as a network of multiple tensions, among which science was beginning to play an increasingly significant role.

Francisco Santos and the Novel at the Crossroads

Little is known of the life of Francisco Santos, apart from what the author himself tells us in his writings.[15] Born in 1623 near El Campillo de la Manuela, in the neighborhood of Lavapiés in Madrid, he lived in some of Spain's most important cities, such as Seville (1666) and Toledo. Not inconsequentially, he was a soldier;

---

[13]   There is an extensive bibliography on the phenomenon of the monster in Golden Age literature; see, for example, the recent studies by Del Río Parra 46, 59–62, 134.

[14]   Santos's interest in science has not gone unnoticed. Czyzewski 127–8 reminds us that his *El arca de Noé* (*Noah's Ark*), 166–72, displays a keen interest in medicine, astrology, alchemy, and magic, and that the author cites numerous cures, plants, and recipes. The same is true of *La Tarasca de parto* (*The Tarasque Giving Birth*), in the section devoted to St. John's Eve (Midsummer Night), since superstition and magic are two of the novel's major themes. In his novel *La verdad en el potro* (*Truth on the Rack*), Santos wrote that the best doctors are "médicos del alma" (doctors of the soul), following Gracián, who coined the expression "médicos del cielo" (doctors of heaven).

[15]   See especially Milagros Navarro Pérez's "Introducción," *Francisco Santos* ix–lxxiii; see also Winter; Arizpe.

this familiarized him with the criminal underworld, the sleazy circles, and the itinerant lives of active soldiers and retired ex-combatants, to whom he devotes many passages. As he himself mentions in the preliminaries to his pamphlet-novel *El no importa de España* (*The "Doesn't Matter" of Spain*), he was a "criado de su Majestad en la Real Guarda Vieja Española" (servant of His Majesty in the Spanish Royal Old Guard) (cited in Hammond, *Francisco Santos* 4). He lived in the Calle del Olivar (in the house of Juan Martínez), attended Madrid's theatres during the mid-seventeenth century, married María Muñoz in 1647, and had nine children, one of whom followed his father's vocation, though less successfully. We know that Santos witnessed the fire in the Panadería (Bakery) in the Plaza Mayor in 1672, about which he wrote the pseudo-journalistic *Madrid llorando* (*Madrid Weeping*). By his own account he was a family man, deeply attached to Madrid and to his neighbors. He suffered terribly from gout in the last years of his life and died in poverty in 1698.

Straddling the twilight years of Philip IV and the beginning of Charles II's reign, Santos's work continues to be relegated to a minor position compared with some of his contemporaries and immediate predecessors. The stature of more famous seventeenth-century figures has reduced Santos's oeuvre to little more than a curiosity, even for specialists in the fiction of the period. This is puzzling, given the enormous success Santos enjoyed in his own time and immediately afterwards; he was greatly esteemed by authors such as Diego de Torres Villarroel and the Mexican writer José Joaquín Fernández de Lizardi, who drew the inspiration for his masterpiece *El Periquillo Sarmiento* from Santos's *Periquillo el de las gallineras* (*Periquillo of the Henhouses*). Constant similarities between Santos's works and those of Juan Zabaleta, Francisco de Quevedo, and other, earlier prose writers, such as Vélez de Guevara, have called into question the originality of his works.[16] Perhaps for these rather misguided reasons, Santos's writings are largely unknown; as Phyllis Eloys Czyzewski explains in a recent doctoral thesis, only *Día y noche de Madrid* (*Day and Night in Madrid*) and *Periquillo* have received the attention they deserve. But this is only a small slice of his output. Between 1663 and 1697 Santos published 16 works. Their popularity may have peaked in the eighteenth century—the only collection of his complete works was published in 1723—and since that time, few editions have been published. Apart from some very specific contributions—a handful of critical editions and the odd general article—by Milagros Navarro Pérez, Julio Rodríguez Puértolas, and Víctor Arizpe, nothing of real depth has been produced in the last 30 years beyond half a dozen doctoral theses, all unpublished.

Santos's novels reveal his wide reading: in addition to echoes of the medieval poet Jorge Manrique in numerous invocations of a glorious past, one detects above all the influence of Francisco de Quevedo, Gonzalo Céspedes y Meneses, Antonio

---

[16]   See primarily the studies by Hammond on Santos's borrowings from his contemporaries, as well as from earlier figures such as Cervantes; for his borrowings from Saavedra Fajardo, not examined by Hammond, see Hafter.

Liñán y Verdugo, Cristóbal Suárez de Figueroa, Diego de Saavedra Fajardo, and especially Baltasar Gracián, from whom Santos borrows repeatedly. As a prose stylist, Santos's language recalls that of Alonso de Salas Barbadillo (at his most satirical) and Juan de Zabaleta (at his most sententious); his sentences are short, incisive, and full of highly Baroque liberties and registers. For this reason it has been said that his fiction stands at the intersection of the picaresque and *costumbrismo* (literary representations of daily life).[17] On the other hand, he has frequently been criticized for his excessive moralizing and the rigidity of his opinions, to the point that two of the leading specialists on his work have spoken of "una delirante concepción del presente" (an outlandish conception of the present) and of a "moralidad atosigante, obsesiva" (an importunate, obsessive moralism).[18] Alive to the decline and corruption that prevailed in Spain under Carlos II, Santos could not shy away from the political, social, cultural, and economic turmoil of the moment; his complaints—accompanied by occasional practical proposals and solutions—are almost more moralistic than didactic. And yet a reading of his depictions of urban subjects continually presents us with examples of well-chosen content, stylistic originality, attractive characters, and copious information on little-known festivities and backwaters of Madrid. More than one text, for example, complains of shopkeepers who raise the price of meat to take advantage of the heavy demand at the end of Lent. This gives the reader some idea of the social repercussions of the ecclesiastical calendar, to the point that "by an irony of fate," as Navarro Pérez has written, "Francisco Santos's righteous indignation and severe moralizing have given us the best documented account of Holy Week in Madrid" (*Francisco Santos* xli).[19]

No one appears in a more negative light in these merciless portraits than the ordinary citizens of Madrid. Inheriting the tastes of his predecessors, Santos subjects the body to the jurisdiction of the urban landscape, and flesh becomes a motif towards which much of his fiction gravitates: bodies that consume and are consumed by others, bodies that generate and degenerate. In many of Santos's novels, pregnancy is denaturalized and recast as a monstrous activity that turns the pregnant woman into an image that allows the author to reflect on the "bloated" nature of the city and the nation as a whole. Santos exploits this to complain about the grandiosity and pomposity that ultimately bear nothing but excess. Likewise, the lacerated body of parturition leads to bizarre scenes that recall the landscapes of Bosch (to whom Santos pays explicit tribute, as we shall see shortly) or the fantastic excesses of François Rabelais. The act of birthing is frequently linked to a very esteemed literary motif, that of the storm, and in this new blend the female

---

[17]   See, for example, Alfaro; Czyzewski; Melero Jiménez; Navarro Santos, "Bibliografía."

[18]   The first quotation comes from Rodríguez-Puértolas, "Introducción," III: 419–30 [419]; the second is from Navarro Pérez, *Francisco Santos* xxvi.

[19]   In this connection, see the interesting study by Simón Palmer, "La Cuaresma."

body evacuates quickly and violently. The perils of the flesh, in Santos, are both a social threat and an attractive fictional resource.

In the 18 "Discourses" of his first published work, which he significantly entitled *Día y Noche de Madrid. Discurso de lo más notable que en él pasa (Day and Night in Madrid: Discourse on the most notable things that happen there)* (1663), the perils and pleasures of the flesh are presented in an extraordinary catalogue of outlandish scenes and motifs running through the novel from beginning to end. Although its two *aprobaciones* (censors' approvals) describe it as "exemplary" and "useful," the fact is that the book's survey of urban life is peppered with scandalous anecdotes that frequently verge on the distasteful. *Día y Noche* deals candidly with all kinds of activities that the author censures as deviations from the norm or as proscribed practices. Prostitution, procuring, pedophilia, fraud, adultery, compulsive gambling, domestic violence, and veiled references to bestiality are defining features of many members of both the upper reaches and the lower depths of Madrid society.

In *Día y Noche* the body is subjected to a whole range of internal and external tensions. From the very beginning the protagonist, Juanillo, is introduced to us as the tragic result of a violent gestation, in which maternal parturition becomes the primal trauma, like being born to death. When speaking of his mother, for example, the young man provides a narrative that does not recall typical accounts of the effect of the maternal imagination on the infant's body, but something strikingly different:

> era el renombre que me daba de carísimo porque de mi parto pasó muchos dolores, y con gran pesadez me trajo en sus entrañas; parióme doblado y a mi entender fue dar fin a mis dobleces, que, aunque es fruta del tiempo, en mi vida la he usado ni tenido. Tuvo grande mal en los pechos, que la prolija enfermedad no la dejó hasta que la cortaron el uno, en cuya enfadosa cama vendió cuanto tenía. (18)

> (She called me her "dearest" boy because giving birth to me cost her great pain, and carrying me in her womb was a great ordeal for her; I was born doubled up, and I think that was the last of my duplicities, for although it is a seasonal fruit, I have never used it or had it in my life. She had a severe ailment in her breasts, and she was not rid of this protracted illness until one of them was cut off, and as she lay suffering in bed she sold everything she had.)

The passage has a scientific basis: as Elena del Río Parra reminds us (46), the idea that the mother's imagination is imprinted on the fetus is present in Avicenna, Hippocrates, and Galen, was transmitted by St. Augustine, and survived in authors like Paracelsus and Ficino. Juanillo is born crooked, both physically and morally, without the rectitude that would have preserved him from this picaresque life. The quotation also contains a highly original element of that Baroque medical culture which hardly ever reappears in the fiction of the period, namely cancer; the mother rapidly dies of breast cancer, which consumes and debilitates her, and through this motif Santos also invokes the idea of internal illness as a form of putrefaction, which rots the human body, the social order, and the apparatus of the State. Santos's intuition contains within it an important kernel of Freudian thought, in that the theme of suppression of the mother springs from the impulse for oral gratification, depriving the breast of its ability to produce milk as a mark of continuity.[20] Starting from this decisive break (decisive because it defines the young man's picaresque life), the phenomenon of birth as a rite of passage refers us, as Theresa M. Krier has written, to a nostalgia for origins which in this novel takes the form of an unceasing quest for a longed-for land, a non-existent Garden of Eden that is none other than this *Madrid perdido* (*Lost Madrid*).[21]

But separation does not mean loss, and the narrative itself (in terms of quest and circularity) operates as a pathway to finding oneself, culminating in an honorable ending for its protagonist. The novel is thus a long process of mourning in the form of a journey around the city, where love for one's mother, according to Juanillo, is a defining feature of decent men (those who are not "brutes" or "ingrates"), just as respect for the surroundings is a defining feature of an upright man. Readers are reminded that:

> sólo a la víbora se le concede esta crueldad, por ser venenoso aborto de la misma fiereza, pues en naciendo, acarrean la muerte a las entrañas que la avivaron [...] Sólo el mal hijo imita a la víbora o al rayo, que para nacer hace reventar a la nube que le congeló, sin corresponder con la mayor obligación. (171)

> (It is granted only to the viper to perpetrate such cruelty, being a venomous abortion of ferocity itself, for in being born they bring about the death of the womb that gave them life [...] Only a bad son imitates the viper or the bolt of lightning, whose birth sunders the cloud that froze it, ungratefully violating its greatest obligation.)

Rather than a possible idea of renewal, the quotation suggests, on the contrary, a feeling of vertigo at the obliteration of origin brought about by new urban realities. It is a desperate appeal to the order offered by certain fundamental structures, such as the family or the army, that come under threat in an environment moving unstoppably towards its own destruction.

The vertiginous images of Madrid consuming itself acquire a new dimension in the narrative trilogy on festivities. In *Las Tarascas de Madrid* (*The Tarasques of Madrid*) (1665) Santos moves from the picaresque to the allegorical.[22] He imagines a whole catalogue of fantastic creatures that allude disparagingly to the people of

---

[20]   The cultural value and literary function of breastfeeding as an intimate relationship between mother and child has been studied in sixteenth-century literature by Nadeau, "Blood Mother," among others.

[21]   See Krier, especially Chapter 1, "Cradle and All," 3–21.

[22]   A *tarasca* or *tarasque* was what we might call a parade float today, modeled in the shape of a monstrous serpent or dragon. *Tarascas* were a regular feature of Corpus Christi processions in many parts of Spain.

Madrid, who turn Holy Week into a stage for abuses and outrages: drunkenness, gluttony, debauchery, and prostitution (Bernáldez Montalvo). Focusing on the most familiar Baroque topoi of the human condition, Santos surveys the preparations and celebrations that give rise to social mechanisms of personal subversion and collective identification. In the second work of the trilogy, *Los Gigantones en Madrid por defuera y prodigioso entretenido* (*The Giants of Madrid from the Outside and Prodigious Entertainment*) (1666), Santos moves on from tarasques or dragons to *gigantones* (giants). *Gigantones* were monstrously costumed figures that, like *tarascas*, were featured in the festivity of Corpus Christi and its octave. In *Los Gigantones*, Santos denounces the evils and sins committed by the people of Madrid on these feast days, entering a fully allegorical world that blends the fantastic and the real. For example, he includes the tradition of traveling the four leagues from Madrid to the Franciscan monastery on foot; the use of wagons, horses, and donkeys hired from water carriers to carry provisions and utensils for a picnic in the oak groves on the palace grounds; and walking at nightfall to the Fuente de la Reina to continue the feasting, revelry, and amorous trysts.

Dragons and giants—the elaborate machinery and costumes of Corpus Christi processions—are ever-present elements in the popular imagination because they are associated with the feast day and they are representations of sin. *Las Tarascas* and *Los Gigantones* together function as a thematic gateway to the third novel in the trilogy, which, in my view, is the richest source of material on these obsessions: *La Tarasca de parto en el Mesón del Infierno* (*The Tarasque Giving Birth at the Inn of Hell*) (1672). In the dedicatory, Santos announces that he is going to write about "las noches de los festivos días de Madrid, que mejor fuera llamarle sueños del Bosco, que si él pintó espantosas sabandijas, más atroces los bosqueja la torpeza de mi pluma" (the nights of feast days in Madrid, which should rather be called dreams by Bosch, for while he painted horrible insects, my clumsy pen sketches even fouler creatures) (fol. 2v.). He narrates how a hurricane lashes and cracks the earth, giving way to a tarasque, beset by labor pains, which takes refuge in the Hell Inn, where it spawns "a los más viles pecados de la república, aquellos que se cometen con capa de entretenimiento" (the most depraved sins in the republic, those committed in the guise of entertainment) (fol. 2v.). The terrified author witnesses the multiple birth alongside Desengaño (Disillusionment), who acts as his counselor and guide on his long journey. I will concentrate only on the first Discourse of the novel, because although the opening storm is a motif it shares with many other works of the period (including some by Santos himself), it contains the most kaleidoscopic and nuanced vision of allegorical birth.

The start of the urban nightmare suffered by the narrator-protagonist reads as follows:

> Un espantoso huracán, brotando bramidos contra la tierra, con alientos de venganza de tan impía madre empezó a destrozar peñascos, formando en ellos espantosas bocas, solo a intento de manifestar sus duras entrañas echando esfuerzo en los más levantados y soberbios, porque se oponían a las estrellas,

sin mirar la humildad de sus fundamentos, cuyas seguridades eran fabricadas de sus mismas ruinas.

Uno, pues, bostezando alientos, rompiendo sus mitades con tan espantoso rumor, que sin duda el [*sic*] ausencia de sol solo fue por no ver tan horrible retrato del infierno, y quiso más su ocaso, y fin, que gozar de vista tan penosa.

Manifestó este Gigante de la tierra trancas sus concavidades, en cuyas sombrías partes se oyó un eco, que entre ansias y suspiros, con sílabas mal juntadas, repitió diversas veces: ¡Ay de mí, que me muero sin remedio! ¿Quién prestará alivio a quien jamás le dio? ¿Quién socorrerá a la misma ingratitud? ¿Quién amparará a la que así se desampara? ¿Quién asistirá a quien no es de provecho para sí propia? ¡Válgame mi soberbia, y válganme los hijos a que en ella he tenido, sin remedio estoy, pisando el umbral de la muerte! ¿Habrá quien llame [a]una comadre para que partee a una desdichada, cuyo triste vientre ocupan las más infernales sabandijas de la tierra? ¿Quién se moverá a socorrerme con algunas mantillas, en que recoger estos pedazos del infierno, pues mis entrañas lo son? (fols. 1r–1v.)

(A fearful hurricane, roaring at the earth, seeking vengeance on so heartless a mother, began to shatter crags, forming horrible mouths in them, bent only on revealing their hard innards, venting its fury on the loftiest and proudest of them for defying the stars with no thought for their lowly foundations, whose solidity was built from their own ruins.

Then one of them, with a yawning exhalation, broke in half with such a terrifying sound that no doubt the sun stayed away just to avoid seeing such a horrible picture of hell, and preferred its own setting and demise to the contemplation of so harrowing a sight.

This Giant of the earth laid bare its recesses, in whose somber depths an echo was heard, repeating again and again, with anxious sighs and faltering syllables: "Woe is me, for I am dying with no hope! Who will relieve one who has never given relief? Who will come to the aid of ingratitude itself? Who will protect one who leaves herself so unprotected? Who will help one who cannot help herself? May my pride, and the children I have borne in pride, preserve me; I am without hope, on the threshold of death! Is there anyone who will call for a midwife to assist the labor of a poor wretch whose miserable belly teems with the most infernal creatures on earth? Who will trouble to come to my aid with swaddling clothes in which to wrap these pieces of hell, for that is what I have inside me?")

The narrator-protagonist then describes the tarasque, "que parecía el retrato del Centauro, si el uno medio caballo y medio hombre, ésta medio demonio y medio mujer" (which was like the image of a Centaur; while this is half horse and half man, she was half devil and half woman). Santos goes on to immerse us in this infernal vision of Madrid, not very different from the famous madhouse used by other narrative writers of his century: "De este modo [la Tarasca] pasó al mesón, y fue recibida con una alegría bien extraña, pues era suspiros y lágrimas;

aposentáronla con fingido amor, cuando oí decir: Afuera, a un lado, que viene la comadre doña Fulana al mesón del infierno, a partear la Tarasca del mundo, preñada de los vicios, y en días de parir" (And so [the Tarasque] entered the inn, and was received with a very strange kind of joy, consisting of sighs and tears; they accommodated her with a feigned show of affection, and then I heard someone say: 'Get out, stand aside, for Mistress So-and-So the midwife is coming to the Hell Inn to deliver the children of the Tarasque of the world, who is pregnant with vices and in labor') (fol. 3r.). Santos concentrates on the midwife, the personification of envy, portraying her with bright, colorful clothes, though also as "una fiera mujer, muy vieja, y muy afeitada, el cabello hecho moño desproporcionado de alto, con sus guedejas que tapaban lo hundido de sus carrillos recostados encima de las encías, desiertas de todo hueso dental y molar [...]" (a fierce woman, very old and plastered with makeup, with her hair done up in a disproportionately high bun and locks covering her sunken cheeks, resting on her gums, which were devoid of teeth [...]") (fol. 3r.). The description recalls the association of the midwife with the witch (Gélis 107–11), since many of the women who practiced midwifery were also advanced in years. When she enters the inn,

apresuró el paso, aún ahí lastimoso, que arrojó la que paría, rematando con unas lastimosas palabras, que dijeron: ¡Ay de mí! Que he quebrado la fuente, afuera vivientes (dijo la pulida comadre) que se desembarcan en el puerto del mundo, de una vil tartana, los más viles pecados de la República, aquellos que le cometen con capa de entretenimiento, afuera vuelvo a decir, que vomita el infierno por el vientre del pecado, juguetes de la tierra, que de sus juntas hace el demonio lazos en el soto del mundo, que puestos en la boca de la víbora, cautiva las almas. (fol. 3r.)

(She quickened her pace, as the mother in labor continued to let out terrible cries, ending with these pitiful words: "Woe is me!" "I've broken water. Get out, all you living souls," said the refined midwife, "for the most depraved sins in the republic, those committed in the guise of entertainment, disembark in the port of the world from a contemptible little dinghy, get out, I say again, for hell spews forth playthings of the earth from the belly of sin, and from all of them combined the devil makes snares in the groves of the world, which he places in the mouth of the viper to capture souls.)

The Tarasque gives birth to seven Mayas (May queens), the seven deadly sins, discussed in detail just afterwards, which are none other than the seven festivities that brightened life in seventeenth-century Madrid: *Mayas* (*Maytime*), *Noche de San Juan* (*Midsummer Night*), *Noche del río* (*Night on the River*), *Noche de toros* (*Bullfighting Night*), *Nochebuena* (*Christmas Eve*), *Carnestolendas* (*Carnival*), and the *Fiesta del Prado* (*Prado Festival*).[23] Giving birth to a girl, in the folklore

---

[23]   The motif of the hurricane also appears, for example, in Juan Martínez de Cuéllar's little-known work *El desengaño del hombre* (*The Disillusionment of Man*) (1663), published by Luis Astrana Marín in *Los clásicos olvidados* (Vol. V, Madrid, 1928).

of Renaissance Europe and in this novel, is associated with the outcome of either a drunken carnal encounter (not infrequently, on a feast day) or from a certain imperfection in the sperm (Paster 172). Santos's novel also follows the tradition of representing parturition as evacuation; each birthed (or evacuated) creature is presented with great pomp and ceremony in what amounts to a foundational rewriting of the city-as-spectacle. An example of this is the Paseo del Prado: "Dejamos de atenderla, por [...] la ocasión de las fieras voces que despedía la horrenda boca del mesón, diciendo: bienvenido, el paseo del Prado, sea en buena hora su dichoso nacimiento, dichosa la madre que tal parió" (We stopped attending to her [...] because of the ferocious cries emanating from the hideous maw of the inn, saying: "welcome, Paseo del Prado, may this happy birth be propitious, blessed the mother who has borne such a child") (fol. 5r.).

On the orders of Disillusionment, the protagonist then visits each of these celebrations—Midsummer Night, Christmas Eve, Carnival, and so on—recounting the evils to which they give rise. The festivities are not a triumph of the sin as such, but an opportunity for that sin to be committed: pride, avarice, lust, envy, gluttony, wrath, and sloth are given their own allegorical expression in the last part of this first Discourse, together with a final gibe at the midwife from Disillusionment for "todo lo que ha cobrado" (all the money she has made) (fol. 8v.). The *Mayas* or May queens who open the second Discourse become an object of censure: girls dress up in their finery for the May festivity and entice wealthy gentlemen with the promise of sexual favors (a deplorable technique learned, Santos claims, from their own mothers). The festivity marks the passage from childhood to puberty in girls, and thus, as Laura Serrano reminds us (84–5), women indisputably play the leading role in a festivity that corrupts them, just as the body of the midwife was corrupt and hollow.

The conclusion of the multiple births gives way to a celebration depicting some of the customs of the court at the time, particularly among women:

> Prosiguió la bulla y la algazara, todo estruendo, y voces. Venga chocolate, decía, lo tomará la señora comadre antes que se vaya. No lo quiero, dijo con voz melosa, si es de lo que venden en estas tiendecillas, porque tiene cacao Guayaquín, y da hipocondría; Caracas, y S. Domingo es, replicaron, bien lo puede tomar, vaya esa jícara a la parida, que bien la merece. Con esta bulla, y brindis Indiano, se fue apaciguando aquel espantable estruendo, y salió fuera la comadre, mudado el traje, pues sacaba un vestido muy del uso, y muy viejo, con que conociera, pues le llevaba guarnecido de lenguas, y ojos, y la cara ambiciosa, macilenta, y amarilla. Pregunté al Desengaño, que pues la parida era el mismo pecado, y la partera la envidia, qué gente sería la que asistía dentro [...] (fols. 6v–7r.).

> (The raucous hubbub continued, with deafening cries on all sides. "Here's some chocolate," said one. "The midwife must have some before she leaves." "I don't want any," she said in a sickly-sweet voice, "if it's the kind they sell in those little shops, because it's made with Guayaquín cacao and gives you hypochondria." "It's Santo Domingo, from Caracas," they replied, "and you can drink it safely. Here's a cup to toast the new mother, who certainly deserves it."

After this riotous Indies-style toast, the appalling racket gradually died down and the midwife left, having changed her clothes, putting on a very ordinary, very old dress, which made her recognizable, for she wore it decorated with tongues and eyes, with a covetous, gaunt, sallow face. I asked Disillusionment what kind of people they were in there, since the mother who had just given birth was sin itself and the midwife was envy [...]).

This context of celebrations and fear gives way to a quickening pace in the material and symbolic interchanges of the urban world, and thus the savoring of the forbidden extends not only to all kinds of soups and viands, but also to other "less healthy" and more lustful foods. Tasting chocolate—and we have seen how the midwife distinguishes between different varieties—completes this first comprehensive portrait of urban vices. This depiction of celebrations with a "New World" flavor is complemented a little later by a description of a strange bloated figure with a wolf's mouth that represents "the dark night of Shrove Tuesday." On Shrove Tuesday, people ate and drank immoderately, playing *alfiler* (hunt the pin), which involved hiding a pin and looking for it among the clothes of those present, *palillo* (toothpick), passing a toothpick from mouth to mouth, and *caldero* (apple dunking), in which the victim had to pick up an apple out of a *caldero* or copper cauldron full of water; or else they played at make-believe scenes of childbirth or law courts, among other improvised entertainments which exhibited that change of roles so characteristic of Carnival.

The idea of giving birth to seven children is not without its significance, as Jacques Gélis (199–200) and Elena del Río Parra have reminded us. In Aristotle's view it was impossible to conceive more than five children at once, and Pliny regarded any more than three as a monstrous birth, although there are numerous accounts in pre-modern Europe of women bearing up to 20 children at a time. However, the number seven has esoteric resonances: it was believed that the womb had seven chambers and that the perfect parturition was that of a seven-month-old fetus, as had been postulated by scholars such as Pierre Boaistuau (Bovistuau), Claude Tesserant, and François de Belleforest in their *Histoires prodigieuses* (translated by the Seville printer Andrea Pescioni as *Historias prodigiosas y maravillosas* and published in Madrid at the presses of Luis Sánchez in 1603). In the case of *La Tarasca de parto en el Mesón del Infierno*, multiplicity is associated with the foundation of the festive city: the birth of the seven monstrous feast days marks seven moments in the calendar that determines the rhythm and structure of life in Madrid. But the Tarasque's parturition is also monstrous because it is incomplete, in the sense that there is no lactation immediately after the birth, but instead a rapid expulsion of these "playthings," these "pieces of hell," propelled by the colossal flood with which the narrative begins. The absence of this final element, lactation, not only sullies the dignity of the process but also eliminates the positive role assigned to the mother.[24] In this anti-parturition Santos therefore

---

24   Paster has also drawn attention to this issue in the English context: "misogyny is legible as discomfort with the fluids and processes of female physiology and, [...] with the

reverses a tradition that had remained unchanged for over a century, from Fray Luis, who argued that bearing children could not be uncoupled from raising them—"Es trabajo parir y criar; pero entiendan que es un trabajo hermanado, y que no tienen licencia para dividirlo" (165)—to Fray Antonio de Guevara, who claimed that a woman "becomes half a mother by giving birth and half a mother by raising her child": "la mujer es media madre por el parir y media madre por el criar" (511).[25] Gail Kern Paster's observation is apposite here: birth has more to do with the history of shame, for oneself and others, than with that of reproduction (163).

Birthing

Santos was writing at a crossroads for the social context of giving birth, witnessing the decline of the midwife in favor of other kinds of medical intervention. Santos comes from a tradition which equates femininity with maternity, and which sees the traumatic experience of giving birth in a positive light: the sacrifice of the mother who splits herself open and risks her life in a slow torture. Jonathan Sawday, for example, has spoken of

> a profound awareness of the conjunction between profane representation, empirical science, scripture, and ecclesiastical doctrine, circulating around the representation of the female body. This awareness, in turn, tended to stress the endless *divisibility* of the female body. The perfect body, of course, was male—entire, whole, complete—a harmonious union of form and matter. And the most perfect male body was that of Christ, who, despite (or rather because of) the mortification endured during the passion, and his depiction as the broken and passive object of contemplation in the numberless images of the *pietà*, nevertheless preserved his essential spiritual and aesthetic unity. (217)

But in Madrid—taken as the *mater* or *matrix* through a derivation as much spiritual as etymological—childbirth accrues a power which arouses all sorts of misgivings in men. Men cannot control the birthing process (or the *matrix*) and feel supplanted by the midwife, and this gives rise to what Sherry Velasco has called "paternity anxiety" (45).[26] Velasco emphasizes that in this period "the womb became a heavily contested battleground": "Women's bodies (and minds through

---

technical events of birth. In reproduction, the female body was not only different as usual from the male body but different from itself in a way that, at its most dangerous, threatened contamination of self and baby" (173; see also 181).

[25] This qualification is discussed in Nadeau, "Authorizing" 23–5, and in Bergmann 39–49.

[26] Sawday, for example, comments: "The observation and anatomical reduction of the female body explicitly confronted this masculine erotic desire while at the same time it claimed to master that desire within the fracturing impulses of science, or knowledge. [...] It was only through controlling this reproductive process that the male's name and property could be transferred from one generation to the next" (222–3).

the maternal imagination) were seen as potentially dangerous spaces that must be controlled by men to ensure the legitimacy of the offspring's identity" (xviii). And more than one manifestation of this paternity anxiety to which Velasco refers can be detected in Santos. In his novel *El Rey Gallo* (*The King Cockerel*), for example, the author defines men of his time as totally consumed by the pleasures of the city, effeminate in their tastes and indifferent to the common good; to convey this idea he uses the expression "diptongos de raras mezclas" (diphthongs of rare mixtures), coined by Gracián (*Criticón* I), which he expands into a very significant complaint in *Periquillo el de las gallineras*: "¡Oh, mujer muy del tiempo! [...] Pero creo que ya no eres mujer, sino hombre, pues ya son ellos los flacos afeminados y vosotras las fuertes. [...] Y ya es ella quien lo puede y lo manda; y el hombre, ni manda, ni puede. Ya se trocaron basquiñas por calzones, después de su mucha conversación [...]" (Oh woman, so typical of these times! [...] But I think you're no longer a woman, but a man, for they are now the effeminate, feeble ones and you are the strong ones. [...] And now she is the one that is capable and in command; and a man is neither in command nor capable. Skirts have now been exchanged for trousers, after so much intercourse [...]).

Continuing with this concern, the last part of Santos's novel *El escándalo del mundo y piedra de la justicia* (*The Scandal of the World and the Stone of Justice*) is devoted to women, and Santos here reflects upon the dangers of the women of his time, while also exalting a model of modesty that had virtually ceased to exist. While paternity prompts men to make sure that all their children really are theirs, that final process involves the intercession of an outside figure, who symbolically displaces the father to the periphery of events: the midwife. Indeed, Santos's period is one in which doctors, theologians, and lawyers had gradually gained ground at the expense of birth attendants and also mothers themselves, particularly as a result of the debates on the spontaneous abortions and miscarriages which sometimes caused the deaths of pregnant women as well. We are therefore dealing with a writer who stands between two centuries, living at a veritable crossroads.

For Santos, childbirth becomes an elastic, fertile motif, open to a whole range of interpretations: a multiple birth which lays bare those "lofty, proud" individuals who produce nothing; a multiple birth which expresses the vertiginous pace of change in the capital; a multiple birth which pollutes a landscape that was once venerated; a multiple birth that symbolizes a demographic explosion saturating the streets and squares with more and more unemployed people given over entirely to frivolity and feasting; a multiple birth that mocks the lack of heirs of a royal house in decline [...] And the midwife thus becomes the ideal, if never idealized, embodiment of a doubly abject lexis—the oral and the feminine—in a metaphor that bridges two spheres through her status as an intermediary. She is a translator who gives impetus to this "urban birthing," who ensures life, but a life which, in Santos, already carries within it the seed of its own destruction. And as an intermediary agent the midwife is ultimately a perverse translator, as untrustworthy as the Cervantine translator had been almost a century before Santos, in that sublime *offspring of the mind*.

Chapter 8
"Sallow-Faced Girl, Either It's Love or You've Been Eating Clay": The Representation of Illness in Golden Age Theater[1]

Maríaluz López-Terrada

Introduction: Illness on Stage

The seventeenth century was not a golden age for the writing of medical texts on the Iberian Peninsula, but it was the Golden Age for the representation of medicine in other textual and cultural genres. Perhaps this is one reason why the study of medical images and practices in Golden Age Spanish drama has a long tradition.[2] However, in many such studies the dramatic text is taken simply as a source from which to obtain data and information about the medicine of the period. The aim of this essay is not to treat early modern theatre as a source of information *per se*. Instead, my object will be to examine health practices (in a broad sense) alongside theatrical practices as cultural creations of society as a whole.

As Salomon pointed out, "the theatre has its own laws, but its sphere of reference is not unconnected with reality"; in other words, it offers historians a fascinating insight into the social image of medicine at a time when the theatre was more or less a national obsession (*La vida rural* 13). Moreover, the production and reception of a dramatic text is a cultural practice. Dramatists always write on the basis of their own concept of illness, and significantly what is represented on stage also appears in contemporary academic medical texts or is derived from a range of medical practices, some of them of an empirical nature. But, of course, a playwright's concept of a particular disease or therapy often includes an awareness

---

[1]   This work is an outcome of the research project HAR2009–11030-C02-02, which is funded by the Dirección General de Investigación of the Spanish Ministry of Education and Science.

[2]   For example, Picatoste y Rodríguez; and E. M. Wilson, "The Four Elements." From a different perspective, see David-Peyre; and Soufas. Moreover, there is a long tradition among Spanish historians of medicine of using literary texts from this period as sources of data and information on medicine in the period, concentrating almost exclusively on academic physicians and the Galenism they practiced; see Albarracín Teulón; Granjel, *La medicina*; Pérez Bautista; and Sancho de San Román.

of dramatic possibility; the course of a disease or therapy can become plot. In a sense, the dramatists and actors are intermediaries between medical texts or practices and the audience.

Reading plays from the seventeenth century, it quickly becomes apparent that playwrights and audiences must have shared basic concepts derived from Galenic humoral medicine. The audience and the dramatist also clearly shared a language drawn primarily from academic medicine, including terms derived from Galenism. The stage is the point of contact between the text and its public, because "it encodes the message [...] making it accessible to the audience" (Grubbs 2). So we find examples ranging from subtle intellectual Galenism in the dialogues of some texts and the allegorical titles of others, such as Calderón's *La cura y la enfermedad* (*Cure and Sickness*), to satire on healers and their modes of treatment or irony based on humoral theory in the *entremeses* (interludes), to total distortion of reality by putting a female doctor on stage at a time when women were strictly forbidden to practice.

As in many other areas, Lope included long lists of illnesses in his plays. As John Slater has observed in discussing plants, the fact that they were not only mentioned frequently "but were mentioned in abundance is a characteristic feature of Golden Age literature," and was the result of a rhetorical objective: copiousness becomes art (*Todos* 53; 55–7).[3] In a play like *Barlaán y Josafat* (*Barlaam and Josaphat*), whose plot does not initially lead one to suspect that it deals with matters related to medicine, a poor cripple appears in the first act and gives Prince Josaphat an account of the illnesses that exist in the world:

> ¿cojedades,
> anguinas, apoplexías,
> catocas, disenterías,
> grangenas, sarnalidades,
> podragas, fiebres y tisis,
> estrangurias, ramicosis,
> lepras, gotas, poliposis
> garrotillos, paralisis,
> estrumas y teriomas,
> flemas, hidrocephalias,
> licantropías y nauseas,
> tabardillos y escotromas,
> toses, y melancolías,
> reumas, y gotas corales,
> fimeras, y comiçiales,
> verminas, y hidropesias,

---

[3] Slater explains the presence of long lists of plants in Baroque literature (*Todos* 52–8). Montesinos, on the other hand, in his critical edition of *Barlaán y Josafat*, examines the presence of enumerations of this kind in many of Lope's works and their textual origin, basically the *Officina* of the French humanist Jean Tixier de Ravisi (c.1470–1524), known as Ravisius Textor (Vega, *Barlaán* 241–6).

hipocondríaca, alfón,
cánzer, tercianas, harpés,
sabañones, mal francés (Vega 32–3)

(lameness, / angina, apoplexy, / catocha [catalepsy], dysentery, / gangrene, scabies, / podagra, fever and phthisis [tuberculosis], / strangury, ramicosis [hernia], / leprosy, gout, polyposis, / croup [diphtheria], palsy, / struma [goitre] and therioma [ulcer] / phlegm, hydrocephalus, / lycanthropy and nausea, / typhus and scotoma, / cough, and melancholy, / rheumatism, and epilepsy, / one-day fever, and seizures, / vermina [stomach cramps], and dropsy, / hypochondriasis, alphos [psoriasis?], / cancer, tertian fever, herpes, / perniosis [chilblains], French pox)

What we find here, despite the comments of some critics, is a homogeneous list of entirely academic medical terms. The words that appear here are standard terms used by writers of medical works in Castilian to refer to illnesses, and they are not popular names, even though some of them (such as "fever," "nausea," or "cough") were part of everyday speech. Some of them would have been understandable or familiar to members of the audience; others would have been completely unknown to them. The dramatic effect of this list is produced in part by the fact that the meanings of each of these words are *not* explained. Two things need to be emphasized here. Firstly, all of these words refer to illnesses that are described with their signs, symptoms, prognosis, and treatment in texts on medical or surgical practice composed in Castilian in the late sixteenth century and the first decades of the seventeenth, the same period during which Lope wrote *Barlaán y Josafat* (1611). And secondly, this example of "Baroque abundance" serves to show that illness is abundantly represented in the Golden Age theatre as a means of producing rhetorical and dramatic effects.

The list of academic terms used by Lope in *Barlaán y Josafat* was only one tool that the playwright had at his disposal. We might name any number of ways of referring to disease: there were allusions to particular outbreaks of disease, such as the Lisbon plague, which is constantly present in the background in *El amor médico* (*Love the Doctor*);[4] lists like the one we find in *Barlaán y Josafat* and elsewhere;[5] and love, jealousy, and dishonor, which are frequently treated as incurable diseases. But there are two basic ways of representing illness, which largely depend on theatricalizing medicine according to the conventions of different

---

[4]   However, the plague as an illness is not represented on the Golden Age stage; it was usually just referred to, often together with *tabardillo* (typhus), and associated with death: "*Estefanía*: Causáralo, Señor, el tiempo que es malo, y engendra melancolía; dicen, que la peste asombra todo este reino" (The cause, my lord, must have been the weather, which is bad, and produces melancholy; they say that the plague is terrifying the whole kingdom) (Molina, *Obras Completas* 744).

[5]   For example, Pérez de Montalbán included lists of illnesses in three different plays: *A lo hecho no hay remedio, y príncipe de los montes* (*What's Done is Done, and the Prince of the Mountains*) (1635), *Don Florisel de Niquea* (1638), and *El valiente más dichoso, don Pedro Guiral* (*The Most Fortunate of the Brave, Don Pedro Guiral*) (1638).

dramatic subgenres, such as the three-act *comedia* and the brief interludes known as *entremeses*. On the one hand, the *comedia*, where illness and its treatment are represented, tends to dramatize textual transmission. The *comedia* is a dogmatic genre in the early modern sense, with rules, precepts, and conventions, the "laws of its own" to which Salomon refers. The great majority of the medical knowledge in the *comedia* comes directly from medical texts. The *entremés*, on the other hand, tends to dramatize reception. While the *comedia* is dogmatic, the *entremés* is empirical (also in the sense of the period); it is not concerned with rules, and what it represents on stage is not bookish medical knowledge but the various forms of reception and transmission of medical practice. Illness as such is not represented; either it is implied—by showing its treatment in plots concerning everyday affairs or the theme of "the world upside-down"—or concepts from the humoral theory of illness are used. Here we shall concentrate on how medical knowledge is experienced and transmitted rather than on its textual origin. Contrasting the *comedia* and the *entremés* permits us to speak of a visual taxonomy of the theatrical representation of illness in Golden Age drama.

The *Comedia*: Representation of Illness and Its Treatment

Illness is dramatized in *comedias* that feature a variety of themes, including "capa y espada" (cloak and sword) comedies, honor plays, and those with plots derived from history or legends. The point that unites them all is that the representation of illness—from its genesis to its definition and characteristics, its actual diagnosis or its treatment—is based on and strictly conforms to seventeenth-century academic medicine. Thus the subtle, intellectual, humoralist Galenism studied in universities and practiced by doctors, surgeons, and apothecaries is transferred to dialogues between actors on stage.

In *El amor médico*, a play about a woman who disguises herself as a university-trained physician, there is a good example of how Galenic doctrine and its terminology are presented on stage. Jerónima, the protagonist, answers a question from Gaspar, with whom she is in love, on whether health is opposed to beauty:

> de las cuatro calidades
> los cuatro humores dan forma
> a la belleza apacible,
> buen talle, y gentil persona.
> Esto es lo que llama, *ad pondus*
> nuestro Galeno, y del consta
> la igualdad y simetría
> saludable y deleitosa.
> De aquí nace la belleza (Molina, *Obras* 751)

> (With the four qualities / the four humours give form / to a gentle beauty, / a fine figure and a handsome presence. / This is what our Galen calls / *ad pondus*, and herein lies / healthy and delightful / equality and symmetry. / From this, beauty is derived.)

de modo, que cuanto mas
fuere elegante una cosa,
tanto más tendrá la sangre
delicada, y si se nota
por esta causa estará
mas expuesta y peligrosa
a cualquiera alteración
que la destemple y corrompa (Molina, *Obras* 752)

(so that the more / elegant a thing is, / the more delicate its blood / will be, and
if it is noted / for this reason it will be / more exposed and vulnerable / to any
alteration / that unbalances and corrupts it.)

Accordingly, since love is being treated as an illness, she explains how an
incorrect quality of the blood in women and children, according to ideas on the
different temperaments, gives rise to a greater propensity to suffer the effects of
fascination or the evil eye ("Por esto niños y damas tan fácilmente se aojan" (This
is why children and women are so easily put under the evil eye). She ends with
a definition of the Greek term *symptom* as being equivalent to *accident*, another
fundamental aspect of Galenic doctrine (it meant anything that arose during an
illness and could help the doctor to form an opinion of its nature and, on that basis,
provide a prognosis and treatment).

¿Ve, señor, vuesa merced,
cómo toda dama hermosa
está sujeta a accidentes,
que llama el Griego *simptomas*? (Molina, *Obras* 753)

(Do you see, sir, / how every beautiful woman / is prone to accidents / which the
Greek writer calls *symptoms*?)

To sum up, Jerónima's speech perfectly illustrates the dramatization of medical
knowledge and academic medical culture, putting on stage a female doctor
with extensive theoretical knowledge, but one who shares with the audience a
conventional and literary understanding of love as a kind of illness.

Diagnosis, taking the pulse, is also regularly represented. In *Don Gil de
las calzas verdes* (*Don Gil with the Green Breeches*), for example, the servant
Caramanchel says the following when describing the daily life of his former
master, a professional doctor:

considere el pío lector
si podría el mi doctor,
puesto que fuese de bronce,
harto de ver orinales,
y fistulas, revolver
Hipocrátes, y leer
las curas de tantos males. (Molina, *Don Gil* 107)

("let the pious reader consider / whether my doctor, / even if he was made of
bronze, / being tired of looking at chamber pots / and fistulas, used to pore over
/ Hippocrates, and read / the cures for so many illnesses.")

Although the servant Caramanchel portrays his former master in this fragment
according to the stereotype of doctors who prefer reading to looking after their
patients, in seven lines he conveys to the audience how doctors examined their
patients. The inclusion of Hippocrates among his reading signifies, among other
things, a textual resystematization of academic medical knowledge designed for
an extremely heterogeneous audience. Many authors have discussed the inclusive
nature of the theatre and the fact that every kind of audience had access to it.[6] For
example, Guillén de Castro's comment that "[…] las comedias, con razón […] son
admitidas y estimadas, y su fin es procurar que las oiga un pueblo entero" (plays
are rightly approved and valued, and their purpose is to get an entire populace to
see them) takes it for granted that the public understands the play, and the dramatist
writes within parameters that make his text comprehensible (*El curioso* II: 492).

Undoubtedly, therefore, humoralist Galenism must have been something with
which the public was familiar. For "an entire populace to see them," as Guillén
de Castro puts it, means that in some way or other the audience witnessing the
theatrical representation of an illness understood and knew what was being
dramatized. So there was a common language concerning the theory and practice
of medicine, largely based on Galenism. In other words, it is not just a matter
of popularizing certain kinds of knowledge, but of active appropriation of such
knowledge by dramatists and audiences.

As I have said, the ways in which illness is represented in the *comedia* are
many, almost as many as the illnesses represented. Indeed, there are plays in which
an illness and its treatment are not just an essential part of the plot but constitute
the actual plot itself. Obviously the number of Golden Age dramatic texts is so
vast, and we find illness appearing in them so frequently, that a detailed study is an
impossible task. However, there are certain examples that clearly show the ways
in which illness and its treatment were represented in the *comedia*.

Illness and the Course of Treatment as the Mainsprings of Plot

Lope de Vega's *comedia* entitled *El acero de Madrid* (*The Steel of Madrid*) is
a perfect example of a play in which an illness (oppilation) and its treatment
("steeled water": water in which red-hot iron has been doused) are one of the
mainsprings of the plot. It is a *comedia de capa y espada* (cloak and sword
comedy) set in the capital, and has features in common with other *comedias* by

---

6   A number of specialists have discussed the inclusive nature of the theatre, such as
Zamora Vicente in his introduction (36, n. 30) to Tirso de Molina's *Don Gil de las calzas
verdes*. From another point of view, for a good example of the extremely extensive reach of
theatrical performances in the rural world, see Davis and Varey.

Lope, such as the names of the protagonists. The play is well known and has been extensively studied by literary historians; even its medical aspects have been examined (Morley 166–9; Arata 30–35). Morley, for example, cited the medicinal use of steel for oppilations from Covarrubias and the *Diccionario de Autoridades*, as well as the text by Monardes to which I shall refer later, to try to explain why Lope gave the play this title (169). However, as far as I know, none of those who have approached this work by Lope from a medical point of view has analyzed it in any depth.[7] According to Arata, the phenomenon of taking steel gave rise to a short-lived but successful poetic theme, which we might call "false oppilation" (31). One of its earliest manifestations is the anonymous song "Niña del color quebrado" (Sallow-faced girl), published in 1598 in *Flor de varios romances nuevos y canciones*; the song's elements are precisely those that constitute the plot framework of *El acero de Madrid*. To quote Arata: "everything, from the girl with false oppilation to the doctor, from the season of love to the character of the aunt, is already present in this song, which is like a brief draft in verse of what was to be Lope's play" (32). Leaving aside the tradition and the extensive range of examples of this motif,[8] the crux of which is false illness and sexual transgression, what is of interest from our point of view is that a particular illness and its treatment become the title and the mainspring of the plot of a *comedia*. Even though the two key words *oppilation* and *steel* are constantly used with double meanings (literal and metaphorical), and the illness is feigned, the diagnosis and treatment of an oppilation in this play correspond exactly to what is prescribed in academic medical texts.

The term "oppilation" was used in medical texts to denote the obstruction or blockage of some organ. As for "steel," it is a multipurpose word which gives rise, from the work's very title, to a series of ambivalences between the meanings "a cure with steel-water," "intimacy with a lover," and "sword" (Arata 56). On the other hand, the use of steel was standard practice in Galenic therapeutics and had various applications, including as a deoppilative. At the end of his commentary on Dioscorides' text on iron flakes, Laguna says: "Drinking water or wine in which red-hot iron is doused constrains the bowels, consumes the spleen and dissolves every sort of oppilation" (Dioscorides, *Acerca* 529).

---

[7]   Albarracín Teulón (234–6) merely cites this play in passing when discussing oppilation.

[8]   There are many references in Golden Age literature to the oppilation caused by eating clay and its treatment with steel, for example in a *letrilla* by Luis de Góngora: "Que la del color quebrado / culpe al barro colorado, / bien puede ser; / mas que no entendamos todos / que aquestos barros son lodos, / no puede ser" (It is quite possible / that the sallow-faced girl / blames red clay; / but it is impossible / that we do not all understand / that these clays are really mud) (55). It also occurs in another Lope play, *Las bizarrías de Belisa* (*The Gallantries of Belisa*): "Mañanicas de mayo / salen las damas; / con achaque de acero / las vidas matan" (On lovely May mornings / the ladies come out, / and with an attack of steel-sickness / they take men's lives) (135).

The plot of *El acero de Madrid* is as follows: Lisardo is a young gentleman of limited means who spends his days in the company of his friend Riselo and his servant, Beltrán. Lisardo is attracted to a young woman from a wealthy noble family, Belisa, whom he sees every morning when she comes out of church. Lisardo, however, cannot approach Belisa because she is always accompanied by her aunt Teodora. Belisa suggests to Lisardo the following plan: she will pretend to be suffering from oppilation and an obliging doctor will prescribe that she take steel-water and go for long morning walks. The next day, the servant Beltrán passes himself off as a doctor, visits the young woman and, after examining her, prescribes two things to cure her oppilation: first, Belisa must take steel-water for four mornings, and second, upon drinking the steel-water, she must to go out and walk (literally "walk it") in a shady park lane:

> Y os salgáis a pasear,
> al Soto, Atocha, o al Prado,
> pero con mucho cuidado
> de que el sol no os ha de dar.
> Porque allá Galeno dice,
> que cuando acero *tometur*
> *sol in capite non detur*,
> que a la cura contradice. (Vega, *El acero* 115)[9]

(And you must go out and walk, / in the Soto, Atocha or the Prado, / but take great care / that you are not out in the sun, / because there Galen says / that when steel *tometur* / *sol in capite non detur*, / for that counteracts the cure.)

In Act II, Octavio, Belisa's cousin, arrives at her house and is attracted to her; he asks Belisa's father for her hand, and her father grants Octavio's request. Between Acts II and III several months pass. During this time Belisa's relationship with Lisardo continues in spite of the obstacles. The situation comes to a head on the day the papal dispensation arrives (a dispensation that would have allowed Belisa to marry her cousin). Belisa reveals she is pregnant, her father discovers everything and events reach their anticipated conclusion: Belisa marries Lisardo instead of her cousin.

In other words, the whole work dramatizes an illness—initially feigned by Belisa in order to be able to see her beloved Lisardo, and in the end not an illness but a pregnancy—and its treatment, which is the guiding thread of the plot and gives the play its title. Indeed, in medical texts of the time one of the most characteristic forms of female oppilation is the cessation of menstrual periods, not necessarily due to pregnancy. Moreover, one of the commonest remedies to cure it was to drink steel-water and "walk it." There are many examples of

---

[9]   According to a note to the text by Arata, this prescription, steel as a cure for oppilation, has a clearly sexual meaning in the context of ambiguous language typical of a love-doctor.

medical texts that prescribe this treatment. In 1574 no less a medical authority than Monardes wrote his *Diálogo del hierro y sus grandezas* (*Dialogue on Iron and Its Great Qualities*),[10] a monograph on the therapeutic use of that metal. Monardes's academic work, based on the strictest humoralist Galenism, contains the seeds of the plot I have just set out. The physician explains that "water or wine in which a piece of red-hot iron has been doused" is good for oppilations, among many other illnesses, and especially when he indicates the way in which this remedy is to be administered (*Diálogo* 141r–141v). First:

> Tomarán los polvos que más convinieren, de las tres cosas dichas del hierro, del azero, o de la escoria dellos, la cantidad que al médico pareciere, conforme a la edad, virtud, fuerças […] hanse de tomar por las mañana en ayunas.

> (They are to take the most appropriate powders of the three things mentioned, iron, steel or the slag of these two, in the quantity the doctor thinks fit, according to age, vigor and strength […] they must be taken in the morning on an empty stomach.)

And he continues:

> y luego en acabado de tomarlos, han de andar y hazer ejercicio dos horas, si uviere fuerças para ello, y sino bastara una, o el tiempo posible el andar sea de manera que no se canse mucho, y si lo fuere puedese se assentar a trechos, que como los que los toman [el hierro] están opilados de cualquier ejercicio por poco que sea se cansan luego, y todo trabajo es de los primeros dias, que después andaran muy bien, y no se cansaran tanto. Este ejercicio se haze mejor fuera de casa y por las calles, y por el campo, importa tanto el andar para que estos polvos se actuen y hagan provecho que si no se anda bien con ellos, no hazen el efecto que se desea." (145r–145v)

> (and then as soon as they have taken them, they are to walk and take exercise for two hours, if they have the strength to do so, and if not, one will be sufficient, or for as long as possible. The walking must be such as not to be too tiring, and if it is, they can sit from time to time, for since those who are taking them [iron remedies] are oppilated, any exercise, however light, will soon tire them, and all the hard part is in the first few days, for after that they will walk very well and not get so tired. This exercise is best taken out of doors, in the street and in the country. Walking is so important for these powders to work and yield benefits that if one does not walk properly while taking them they do not produce the desired effect.)

Similarly, the double meaning Lope gives to oppilation (illness/pregnancy), seen from Monardes's medical perspective, is as follows:

---

[10]   See Ralph Bauer's article in this collection.

> El uso del azero [...] principalmente aprovechan estos polvos a mugeres: porque por la mayor parte se opilan y padecen retención de menstruos, en lo qual cierto en ellos estos polvos hazen maravillosos efectos, sanandolas de las opilaciones, y haziendoles venir los meses. Danse assi mismo estos polvos so ay calenturas lentas, la mala color, de cualquier parte que provenga la quita. (*Diálogo* 146r–146v)

> (The use of steel [...]: these powders are mainly useful for women: because most of them become oppilated and suffer from retention of menstruation, for which these powders produce wonderful effects, curing them of oppilations and giving them regular periods. They are also given these powders when they have slow fevers, and they remove bad colour, wherever it comes from.)

Clearly, the same elements related to diagnosis, treatment, and precise therapeutic indications appear in Lope's *comedia* and Monardes's scientific text: the oppilation of an organ, a women's illness, is treated by taking steel-water in the morning, and after ingestion the patient needs to walk for it to take effect. In the same way, the term "oppilation" is used to refer to an absence of menstrual periods. We might say that Lope treats Monardes's *Diálogo del hierro* as if it were already a dramatic text, a primitive script to be adapted and embellished; at the very least, Lope finds dramatic possibility in Galenic cures.

It may also have been the conventional nature of the steel-water treatment that made it adaptable to the stage. A good indicator of how common the use of iron was in therapeutics is the polemic between Melchor de Villena (under the pseudonym Pedro Juan Jiménez) and Miquel Jeroni Romà, both professors of medicine at the *Studi General* in the city of Valencia at the beginning of the seventeenth century. This polemic centered on the use of iron filings and their therapeutic indications, including that of an oppilation such as amenorrhoea, and it gave rise to the publication of several short treatises in Latin.[11]

Dramatic Structure and the Course of Disease

In *El parecido* (*The Stranger*), by Agustín Moreto, feigning an illness is one of the basic elements of the plot, and the illness is dramatized in accordance with medical texts.[12] In this play the leading character, Don Fernando de Ribera, has

---

[11]   According to Chinchilla, the polemic between Villena and Romà was on precisely the same subject as the plot of *El acero de Madrid*. In commenting on two of Miquel Jeroni Romà's pamphlets, he says, "this little work (*Secundae satisfactoriae reclamationis castigatio*) recommends ('squame aeris' = iron filings) for curing amenorrhoea," and that the *Antipolegeticis* "seeks to prove that iron preparations were very suitable for curing serous cacochymy." He goes on to say that these ideas displeased Villena, who devoted several brief treatises to them (Chinchilla II: 323). According to Juan Bautista Peset, this polemic was started by Romà's work on "iron filings and their therapeutic indications" (198–9).

[12]   On Moreto's *El parecido*, see also Lanuza's chapter in this volume.

had to leave Seville after killing a man who was responsible for dishonoring his sister Juana. When he arrives in Madrid he is mistaken for a rich gentleman who was thought to have died in the Indies, Lope Luján, the brother of Inés, with whom Fernando has fallen in love. Though initially reluctant, he agrees to adopt this new identity when he realizes that Inés is betrothed. In order to carry out his deception, he pretends he has lost his memory through having suffered an attack of palsy, and is therefore unable even to recognize his own father. This leads to a series of complications and misunderstandings. As is common in this kind of play, the final scene takes place in an inn, where everything is cleared up, enabling the couples to marry.

The plot is not particularly original; indeed, it has been pointed out that it is a reworking of pre-existing dramatic material. The interesting point is that palsy, an illness that is not represented as often as oppilation, is used as a device to substantiate impersonation, a fairly common theme in Golden Age drama. Thus, in order to account for the fact that the protagonist does not recognize anyone, the *gracioso* (comic servant) Tacón describes the symptoms and effects of his master's illness on stage:

> Del mal más terrible.
> Oigan, que es raro el suceso.
> A él le dio una perlesía
> y della resultó luego
> un mal que manía se llama,
> de quien refiere Galeno
> que quita la voluntad,
> memoria y entendimiento.
> Él lo perdió todo junto,
> mas, como traía dinero,
> —que él ha estado en Filipinas,
> aunque no se acuerda dello
> y allá dicen que hizo cosas—
> pues no pasó caballero
> más bizarro a Nueva España
> desde que allá pasó el Credo
> se curó en fin, porque allí
> seis médicos le asistieron
> de cámara." (*El parecido*, no page no.)[13]

(Let me tell you of this most terrible malady, / for it is a strange affair. / He had an attack of palsy, / which then gave rise to / an illness called mania, / which,

---

[13]   This work was originally published in the *Segunda Parte de las comedias de Agustín Moreto*, Valencia, en la imprenta de Benito Macé, 1676, although it was composed in 1652, and there is a longer manuscript version known as *El parecido en la Corte* (*The Stranger at Court*). The differences between the two plays, which have the same plot, are immaterial to our object of study. The two are analyzed by Madroñal Durán ("Diferencias").

as Galen tells us, / takes away the will, / memory and understanding. / He lost them all at once, / but since he had money with him, / — for he has been in the Philippines, / although he doesn't remember it — / and they say he did things there, / for no more gallant gentleman / has ever been to New Spain / since the Credo arrived there, he was finally cured, / because six royal doctors / attended him there.)

As in the case of oppilation, the diagnosis and prognosis of the illness, put in the mouth of the comic servant of the play, coincide with what Dionisio Daza Chacón, one of the most distinguished doctors in the Hapsburg court, indicated in his treatise *Práctica y teórica de cirugía* (*Practice and Theory of Surgery*): "se llama en griego parálisis, y los latinos resolutio [...] y es quando se pierde el sentido, o el movimiento, no de todo el cuerpo, que entonces sería apolexia, sino del lado derecho, o izquierdo, o de algún miembro" (it is called *paralysis* in Greek, and *resolutio* in Latin [...] and it is when one loses sense, or movement, not in the whole body, which would be apoplexy, but in the right side or the left, or in one of the limbs) (68). Later on, when discussing the eight prognoses of this illness, he notes that the first is that although the illness is long-lasting, it is not acute and the patient nearly always recovers. The second of these prognoses describes precisely what supposedly happens to the protagonist of Moreto's *comedia*: loss of memory. Daza's indication is expressed as follows:

El segundo es [...] que es muy ordinario a los que le viene la perlesía universal morirse de presto, pero sino son arrebatados luego viven por más tiempo, pero muy pocas veces sanan, y el tiempo que viven, por la mayor parte, no solo toman el aliento con mucho trabajo, pero pierden la memoria. (70)

(The second is [...] that those who suffer a universal palsy very commonly die at once, but if they are not carried off, they then live longer, but they very rarely recover, and as long as they remain alive, for the most part, not only is their breathing very laboured, but they lose their memory.)

Memory loss turns out to be a central element of plot in *El parecido*. As in the case of Lope's *El acero de Madrid*, Moreto's play stages illness on the basis of the medical theory and terminology of the time. Moreto chooses an illness, palsy, which, according to medical treatises, causes loss of memory, in this case that of the protagonist, and this constitutes the basis of the whole intrigue of the play. Once again, medical knowledge is dramatized, and the dramatist is an intermediary between the academic medical text and the audience attending the performance. Whereas Lope's *El acero de Madrid* explores the dramatic possibilities of a particular therapy, in *El parecido* Moreto creates dramatic structure from the course of disease.

Illnesses Commonly Dramatized by Playwrights

The illnesses that most often appear in plays are not by any means those with the highest incidence at that time or those most commonly experienced by the populace (although we are dealing with a period for which no reliable figures are available). Illness in the theatre is, of course, a literary convention, and although it is not unconnected with reality, the two illnesses that constituted a veritable obsession in the *comedia*—melancholy, which is perhaps one of those most frequently represented, and dropsy—were not particularly common.

There are monographic studies on melancholy in Golden Age drama, and it has been studied both from the point of view of the history of medicine and in literary terms, though separately.[14] In *El bobo del colegio*, Lope describes melancholy—the malady—as very grave:

> la mayor enfermedad
> llaman melancolía,
> Porque no admite alegría
> y anda a buscar soledad (98)

> (they call melancholy / the most serious illness, / because it leaves no room for joy / and goes in search of solitude)

But melancholy was one of the four humors (an excess of which caused the disease). In *La prueba de los ingenios* (*The Test of Wits*), Lope, citing Galen himself, uses the same term in this other sense to refer to one of the four humors. The character Florela explains:

> sequedad, melancolía
> acompañan la grandeza
> del ingenio, aunque Galeno
> estas partes diferencia:
> melancolía con cólera
> y sangre pura gobiernan
> los ingenios altamente" (126)

> (dryness and melancholy / go together with greatness / of mind, although Galen / distinguishes these attributes: / melancholy with choler / and pure blood govern / the highest minds)

According to Galenism, as is well known, the balance and equilibrium of the four humors (blood, phlegm or pituita, yellow bile, and black bile or melancholy) determined one's state of health or illness. Thus a well-balanced, "natural" quantity of each of the four elements produced a state of good health. Illness was due to an abundance or imbalance of one of these humors in relation to the other

---

[14]   Notable among these studies are those of Bartra and Soufas. On melancholy and the saturnine temperament, see also Lanuza's chapter in this volume.

three, and curing it involved restoring the natural equilibrium through therapeutic treatment. The illness called melancholy was caused by an excess of that dry, cold humor. It is well established that Lope drew on a famous medical text—Huarte's *Examen de ingenios* (*Examination of Men's Wits*)—to write this play, albeit in opposition to that work (Heiple; Mochón Castro). However, in my view it is a magnificent explanation of the complex subject of the composition of the parts of the human body on the basis of humors, as well as their characteristics. Florela's explanation combines sophistication and naturalness. Although melancholy on stage is certainly a literary convention, its representation and transmission, and how the etiology of the illness is defined for the audience, also conform to the strictest humoralist-based Galenism. Even the similarity between the title of Lope's play (*La prueba de los ingenios*) and Huarte's book (*Examen de ingenios*) forces audiences to consider the medical text that functions as both antecedent and rival.

In addition to melancholy, dropsy appears on stage with great frequency. Dropsy was defined by Juan Fragoso as "an illness that never occurs without damage to the liver," and is characterized by swelling of the body (237). Although it is alluded to regularly, patients suffering from "textbook" dropsy are almost never represented; its effect on the liver is never mentioned, for example. Instead, mentions of dropsy are almost always a means to refer to one of its more well-known symptoms: a raging thirst. The term *hidrópico* (dropsical) is used in all sorts of contexts to denote an unbridled desire or a metaphorical thirst. Dropsy is a figure of desire, sexual desire, bloodlust, greed, and so on. Dropsy is also mentioned in the context of hatred and revenge, underlining their virulence.[15]

The French Disease or French Pox

Dramatization of the French pox (*morbus gallicus*) has features of its own, some exclusively literary, others shared with medicine. On the one hand, the French pox appears frequently and in much the same way as melancholy and dropsy; it is sometimes the case that dramatic representations of the pox have more to do with literary requirements than with medical orthodoxy. On the other hand, the French pox had a broad social significance that is not precisely comparable to dropsy, for example, making it difficult to compare it with other illnesses. The French pox is one of the few illnesses whose (comically spurious) etiology is dramatized; characters say it comes from catching cold, when everyone knows it is sexually transmitted. Similarly, it is one of the few diseases whose diagnosis, prognosis, and treatments are represented. While the etiology is almost always discreetly disguised with euphemism, treatments are represented in accordance with academic medical knowledge. The two most important treatments, for example, are mentioned: both with "wood" (guaiacum) and mercury compounds.

---

[15]   Albarracín Teulón examines the metaphorical use of the term *hidrópico* on the basis of twentieth-century medical concepts (204–5).

Lope even wrote a *comedia* whose title—*Juan de Dios y Antón Martín*—alludes to the name of a hospital in Madrid devoted to treating the French disease (the Hospital de Antón Martín).

Playwrights do not tend to draw on a single text for their dramatizations of the *morbus gallicus*. But the disease is often mentioned in the *comedia* and by a number of playwrights. Thus what we need to examine here is not only the representation and popularization of humoralist Galenism, but also an aspect of social reality directly connected with health and illness. Given the public health problem that the *morbus gallicus* represented in Spanish society in the sixteenth and seventeenth centuries, the extent to which dramatic representations coincide or diverge with the reality of the disease is "certainly instructive with regard to trends and tastes in the society for which dramatists invented their intrigues" (Salomon 13).

Juan Pérez de Montalbán's *Don Florisel de Niquea* provides a good example of the French pox on stage. In Act II, the footman Bretón, after listing a series of ways in which women cause men to suffer "como unos mismos cochinos" (like veritable pigs) and die, he explains what the world would be like if there were no more women:

> Porque a estar desmugerados,
> desnudos a puto el postre,
> nos anduviéramos todos
> como unos santos Onofres,
> y no hubiera finalmente,
> achaques, malos humores,
> bubas, gomas, resfriados,
> jarabes, emplastos, votes,
> zarzasparrillas, estufas,
> magistrales, y sudores,
> hasta las unciones perras
> del conficionado azogue,
> con que un hombre en sus salivas
> escupe sus tentaciones,
> porque todos estos males
> interiores, y exteriores
> nos vienen de andar con ellas,
> y somos tan moçarrones,
> que las compramos los axes,
> les feriamos los dolores,
> y nos vamos al infierno,
> pagando primero el porte. (298–9)[16]

---

[16]   I quote from Pérez de Montalbán's *Doze comedias* (1649?). The first edition of the play is Pérez de Montalbán's *Segundo tomo de las Comedias* (1638), in which the quotation appears on pages 49v–50r.

(Because if we were unwomaned, / we would all be / like so many Saint Onuphriuses, / naked, and the devil take the hindmost, / and finally there would be no more / ailments, bad humours, / bubos, resins, colds, / syrups, plasters, jars, / sarsaparillas, stoves, / potions and sweats, / right up to the abominable unctions / of the quicksilver compound, / which make a man spit out / his temptations in his saliva, / for all these internal / and external ills / come to us from being with them, / and we are such foolish lads / that we buy our cries of anguish from them, / we barter our pain with them, / and we go to hell, / having first paid our passage.)

This long speech from Bretón on women, beginning with the problems they cause for men of any social group that have relations with them, is really (in my view) an explanation of how men catch the French disease, what happens to them when they have caught it, and how it is treated. Let us take it in stages. He says that the source of the affliction lies in women; in other words, they infect men with the disease. Right from the earliest medical treatises on this illness, which appeared at the end of the fifteenth century, it was known to be sexually transmitted. Early in the passage, Bretón refers to the deplorable physical state of those suffering from the disease, through the image of Saint Onuphrius.[17] After describing the symptoms, Bretón goes on to enumerate the usual remedies for the *morbus gallicus*. His list is simply a summary of the customary treatment for this illness, consisting of either mercurial unctions or two medications of American origin, guaiacum and sarsaparilla. Both were basically applied topically with salves (the "abominable unctions of the quicksilver compound") or vapors (using fumigation stoves), in addition to the internal administration of compound medications in some cases (the syrups, resins, plasters, and potions listed here). Bretón even goes so far as to mention the salivation and sweating provoked by mercurial unctions ("which make a man spit out his temptations in his saliva"), ending with the internal and external symptoms of the disease and the pains suffered by those affected in the more advanced phases.

This same characterization of the French disease, that is to say, the infection and treatment, can be found in a completely different sort of text: a witness statement made before the Real Audiencia (Royal Court of Justice) in Valencia in 1590 by Pere Melchor Català (alias Renart), chief surgeon of the General Hospital in Valencia, explaining the transmission and treatment of the *mal de siment* (i.e. *morbus gallicus*) with the object of substantiating the need to enlarge the ward where patients suffering from the disease were treated:

Ya ha dicho y vuelve a decir, la gran estrechez del lugar y el gran número de pobres, y que en la época de las unciones, aparte de los que están en el Hospital, hay muchos enfermos que toman los jarabes que se les dan, y por no poder estar ni caber en el Hospital, se van por Valencia a dormir en hosterías y bodegones y otras partes, lo que redunda en notabilísimo daño para la república, por ser el

_____

[17]   A saint who is represented in iconography in a deplorable state of health and extremely thin.

dicho morbo gallico de los más contagiosos que hay entre otros males, porque se contagia al comer, beber, dormir, por la ropa, tocar, respirar y otras maneras. Y luego se sigue que los dichos pobres, habiendo tomado los jarabes, vuelven al Hospital a tomar la purga y las unciones, donde muchas veces no hay comodidad para acogerse, por lo que les han de dar la purga para que la tomen fuera.[18]

(He has already said and says again that space is very restricted and the poor are very numerous, and that when the unctions are administered, there are many patients, apart from those in the Hospital, who take the syrups they are given, and because there is no room for them in the Hospital they go off round Valencia sleeping in hostelries and inns and other places, which is extremely harmful to public welfare, since the said French disease is one of the most contagious of all illnesses, because it is spread when eating, drinking, sleeping, on clothing, by touch, by breath and in other ways. And so it follows that these poor people, having taken the syrups, return to the Hospital to take the purgative and the unctions, where there are very often no facilities for receiving them, with the result that they have to be given the purgative so that they can take it elsewhere.)

Comparing the two texts suggests that the way the illness is represented in the *comedia* is based not only on the theoretical Galenism of medical texts but also on dramatists' and audiences' experience of the disease. In both places, unctions, syrups, purgatives, and pain are mentioned, as well as ease of transmission and contagiousness. Bretón's understanding that a "fondness for women" leads in the end to "going to hell having first paid our passage" has the undeniable ring of personal experience. And, indeed, an awareness of the disease (a serious health problem in European cities at that time), the suffering it caused, and the measures taken to cure it were simply part of urban life during the seventeenth century.

The *Entremés*: The Reception of Illness

Unlike the *comedias* analyzed to this point, the brief dramatic interludes known as *entremeses* tend to dramatize reception rather than transmission. The focus in *entremeses* not on where the medical knowledge comes from, but rather on how people react to it. There are countless examples of how dramatists used terms designating illnesses to introduce comic elements into the humorous, satirical discourse characteristic of this genre.[19] Illness as such is not represented; the

---

18   Archivo del Reino de Valencia. *Papeles de Real Audiencia*. Apéndice no. 4155 (1590). This statement was made in a lawsuit between the General Hospital of Valencia and the Confraternity of Bethlehem of the same city over the land on which the "new *mal de siment* ward" was to be built, given the insufficiency of the existing wards to accommodate the patients admitted for this reason. See López-Terrada ("El tratamiento").

19   Eugenio Asensio says of Benavente: "Without any lapse in good taste, he managed to make courtiers and villagers laugh, satisfy both simple and refined viewers and bridge the gap between the actors and the audience" (124).

treatment of an illness may make its way into plots concerning everyday affairs or *entremeses* that employ the motif of the "world upside-down." Concepts from the humoral theory of illness sometimes appear, as well. But the brief allusions to cures or humors that one finds in the quick repartee of an *entremés* imply previous knowledge of the characteristics of the illnesses that were put on stage. Without previous knowledge, the jokes of a farcical or satirical *entremés* become meaningless. It makes sense, then, to focus on how medical knowledge is experienced and received, and not on its textual origin.

The Galenic Theory of Illness as Satire

The beginning of Quiñones de Benavente's *entremés* entitled *El murmurador* (*The Backbiter*) is a magnificent example of how the popular experience of Galenic theory of illness is dramatized to provoke laughter in an audience. As is well known, prognosis, when the doctor foretold the course of the illness after establishing the diagnosis, was one of the key elements of the doctor-patient relationship. It was normal practice in medical treatises, after describing the illness, to indicate the prognosis, which could be anything from an immediate cure to the death of the patient. *El murmurador* starts with a meeting between two friends, Quiteria and Estefanía, and the dialogue begins as follows:

> *Estefanía*: ¿De qué es tanta tristeza amiga mía? estás mala?
> *Quiteria*: Y muy mala Estefanía.
> *Estefanía*: ¿Duélete la cabeza?
> *Quiteria*: Peor amiga.
> *Estefanía*: ¿ante aojado?
> *Quiteria*: Peor.
> *Estefanía*: ¿Es calentura?
> *Quiteria*: Peor.
> *Estefanía*: Valgame Dios, ¿tienes modorra?
> *Quiteria*: Mucho peor.
> *Estefanía*: ¿Sin duda es tabardillo?
> *Quiteria*: Muchísimo peor.
> *Estefanía*: ¿Peor? ¿Es peste?
> *Quiteria*: Peor, y repeor.
> *Estefanía*: Ay tal desdicha.
> Dímelo tu, pues yo no acierto en nada,
> ¿qué tienes mi Quiteria?
> *Quiteria*: Soy casada. (2878)

(*Estefanía*: Why so sad, my friend? / Are you ill? *Quiteria*: Yes, very ill, Estefanía. / *Estefanía*: Have you got a headache? *Quiteria*: Worse than that, my friend. / *Estefanía*: Has someone given you the evil eye? *Quiteria*: Worse. *Estefanía*: Is it a fever? / *Quiteria*: Worse. *Estefanía*: Good heavens, have you got the staggers? / *Quiteria*: Much worse. *Estefanía*: It must be typhus? / *Quiteria*: Much, much worse. *Estefanía*: Worse? Is it the plague? / *Quiteria*: Worse, a thousand times worse. *Estefanía*: How terrible! / Tell me, for I can't guess / what is wrong with you, my Quiteria? / *Quiteria*: I'm married.)

This dialogue centers on a list of illnesses, all of which—as in the earlier example from Lope—are referred to by the Spanish names used in medical treatises of the period. The interest, however, lies in the fact that they are mentioned on stage in a very particular order. It is by no means just a set of ailments mentioned at random or reproducing a list from some humanistic *cento* or a book of commonplaces; on the contrary, they are arranged in ascending order of the seriousness of their prognoses according to humoral academic medicine, building up to *tabardillo* (typhus), an epidemic disease with very high mortality and incidence at the time when this *entremés* was written, and culminating in the worst of all, "plague," a term denoting an illness for which the only prognosis was the inevitable death of the patient. For Quiteria, worse than the plague—the most feared of all diseases with a fatal prognosis—was being married. In other words, we have here an example of the reception of academic medicine by the public, who knew its terminology (nowadays terms like *tabardillo* and *modorra* are not in common use), but also its content. This is one of the many ways in which Galenism was popularized on stage, because if one is not familiar with it the satire is obviously meaningless.

Wordplay and Satire

Most of the wordplay abundant in the *entremeses* has a clearly erotic content. Plays on words tend to be based, once again, on the humoral theory of the cause of illness: an imbalance of the humors, resulting in "cold" and "hot" illnesses. Allusions to sex as an illness, a topic that has been well studied by literary historians, are common in a genre like the *entremés*. As Huerta Calvo has pointed out, "metaphorically [sex] is registered as an illness to which someone—whether he is called a doctor or a barber—has to provide a remedy and give consolation: medicine for the wound, as a woman in an *entremés* literally says" ("Cómico" 18). In other cases, the terms designating illnesses are used with double meanings.

Indeed, some of Quiñones de Benavente's *entremeses*, such as *El doctor Juan Rana* or *El doctor*, are based on double meanings of both the illnesses and symptoms from which the patients say they are suffering and the remedies prescribed. In *El doctor Juan Rana*, the protagonist is a doctor who conforms to the stereotype of the literature of the period, that is, someone interested in money and with little real ability to cure people (Slater and López-Terrada; Bergman 138–42).

> *Juan Vivas*: De una ocupación de celos
> estoy, señor, reventando.
> *Juan*: Ese llaman *morbus tontus*.
> No piense, y quedará sano.
> *Juan Vivas*: Para ahíto de muchos celos,
> ¿qué remedio me da?

Juan: Volvellos.
Íñigo: Muy ahíto me siento de cierta hembra.
Juan: Échese dos ayudas de bolsa pliega.
Íñigo: Cada vez que compra, me sangra un criado.
Juan: Recupere la sangre de su salario.
Catalina Rosa: Un gatazo me enferma de carne y queso.
Juan: Tome nuez de ballesta, que es gran remedio. (Quiñones 415–16)

(*Juan Vivas*: I am so obsessed with jealousy / that I'm bursting, sir. / *Juan*: That's called *morbus stupidus*. / Don't think, and you'll get better. / *Juan Vivas*: What remedy can you give me / For sickness from jealousy? / *Juan*: Throw it up. / Íñigo: I feel sick because of a certain female. / *Juan*: Take two purgatives. / Íñigo: Every time one of my servants goes shopping, he bleeds me. / *Juan*: Dock the blood out of his wages. / *Catalina Rosa*: A thief is making me ill with meat and cheese. / *Juan*: Take some crossbow nut, for it's a great remedy.")

It is this doctor to whom the patients describe their ailments in Galenic terms, although they are really playing on the words' double meanings.

Among the diseases we commonly find in the *entremeses*, some were considered "new." Plague and typhus had been around for a long time. However, there are others, such as *garrotillo* (croup or diphtheria) and, again, the French disease, that were new.[20] *Entremeses* suggest that audiences were familiar with symptoms and transmission of a disease like *garrotillo*, which was not only new but also epidemic in the period. Quiñones's *El talego* (*The Money Bag*) is extremely interesting for its representation of a consultation of physicians; female doctors carry out the following diagnosis:

Frutos: ¡Ay, señoras, que es garrotillo!
Luisa Bordoy: Veamos la boca.
Luisa Cruz: A ver donde toca.
Josefa: Será garrotillo si siente embarazo.
Luisa Bordoy: *Gritillo.* ¡Ay, señoras, que es garrotazo!
Josefa: Garrotillo, y de madera, ¡guarda fuera!
Luisa Cruz: ¡guarda fuera!
Todas: ¡guarda fuera!
Josefa: Nadie se llegue, que es mal que se pega. (272)

(*Frutos*: Oh, ladies, it's *garrotillo*! / *Luisa Bordoy*: Let's look at his mouth. / *Luisa Cruz*: Let's see where the trouble is. / *Josefa*: It must be *garrotillo* if he feels stifled. / *Luisa Bordoy*: *(with a scream)* Oh, ladies, it's a bad case: a *garrotazo*! / *Josefa*: *Garrotillo*, and very severe; keep away! / *Luisa Cruz*: keep away! / *All*: keep away! *Josefa*: No one come close, for this disease is catching.)

In order to understand this dialogue the audience obviously had to know what *garrotillo* was, and they knew with good reason. Between 1583 and 1638 there

---

[20]   *Garrotillo*: a suffocating angina or squinancy of a diphtherial nature.

were six epidemics of *garrotillo* on the Iberian Peninsula; doctors such as Mercado had described the disease in 1574, and several monographic treatises had been published on it (López Piñero, *Ciencia y técnica* 354).

Conclusion

In the case of the *comedia* it is tempting to speak of three medical conventions. There is a theater of pathology, such as Moreto's *El parecido*, in which the course of the disease (palsy) provides dramatic structure. There might also be a theater of therapy, in which the course of treatment becomes the mainspring of the plot, as in Lope's *El acero de Madrid*. And we might identify an epidemiology of the stage, given the fact that the frequency of certain diseases represented in plays (and the rarity of others) is particular to theater. But there is a danger in applying systems of classification and categorization from medicine to theater too literally, even when playwrights borrow quite literally from medical texts. Our attempt has not been to explain early modern drama's debts to medicine or to "medicalize" the readings of plays by Lope, Moreto, Quiñones, and others. It is particularly clear in the *entremeses* and representations of melancholy or dropsy in *comedias* that doctors and dramatists play by different rules, even if they share an idiom.

Rather than consider debts, we have examined the ways in which the academic medicine, the medical knowledge represented in plays, and the experiences of audiences can be understood to overlap. As the production and reception of a theatrical text is a cultural practice, the various ways in which illnesses are named and represented in early modern drama correspond to those of Galenic medicine. Dramatists wrote on the basis of their own concept of illness and dramatized academic medicine, a point of contact with the public, since both sides shared concepts from the same Galenic humoral medicine. Without that point of contact, theatrical texts would not have been comprehensible to a heterogeneous audience.

Chapter 9
The Dramatic Culture of Astrological Medicine in Early Modern Spain

Tayra M. C. Lanuza-Navarro[1]

Introduction

The representation of astrological themes in early modern Spanish plays is varied and rich, and touches upon many aspects of the theory and practice of astrology. The most famous of these plays is *La vida es sueño* by Pedro Calderón de la Barca, in which the king, Basilio, makes decisions based on the natal chart or figure of his son and heir, Segismundo.[2] Other plays feature copious mentions of astrology—often predictions about the futures of other characters—and astrological imagery, as well as astrologers appearing as characters.[3] The presence of astrology in Golden Age plays has been the object of several studies, notably several by Frederick de Armas, which illuminate the role of astrology and classical myths on stage as well as in society.[4] The dramatic representation of astrological medicine, however, is an issue that has not received much attention from scholars.[5]

---

[1] Research for this chapter was funded by *La cultura médica ante su público: la representación de la medicina en el teatro del Siglo de Oro* [HAR2009-11030-C02-02], underwritten by the Spanish Ministry of Science and Innovation.

[2] There are a number of plays by different playwrights in which the plot hinges upon a king reading the stars or following the advice of astrologers. On the astrological plot of *La vida es sueño*, see Frederick de Armas, "Icons of Saturn," "El rey astrólogo," and "El Planeta más impío," and Nicolas M. Vivalda's "Basilio o el ocaso del monarca-astrólogo." On the use of horoscope motif as literary resources, see Christine M. E. Bridges, "El horóscopo y el vaticinio."

[3] On the representation of the Arab astrologer Albumasar in the several versions of the play *L'astrologo* by Giambattista della Porta (including Lope's), see De Armas's "Saturn in conjuction."

[4] See Frederick de Armas's *The Return of Astraea*, "El Sol sale a medianoche," *Heavenly Bodies, A Star-Crossed Golden Age*, and "The Saturn Factor." On astrology as an occult science in the plays, see Robert Lima, *Dark Prisms* and *Stages of Evil*; Pavia; and Friesen.

[5] There are references to medical astrology in Albarracín Teulón's *La medicina en el teatro de Lope de Vega* and in works about melancholy, such as in Teresa Scott Soufas's *Melancholy and the Secular Mind* or Berta Pallarés's "La melancolía como enfermedad" and "La melancolía en la comedia palatina."

During the early modern period, astrological theory and practice was closely related to medicine.[6] The medical function of astrology was to provide a tool for diagnosis and treatment, based on the astrological principle that certain positions of the stars and planets caused illnesses. Furthermore, certain planetary configurations were better or more auspicious than others for medical treatments, such as bleeding, purging, or taking prescribed medicines. The relationship between astrology and medicine was based on the Galenic idea of the human body and its health, ideas about sickness and the development of diseases, and the therapeutic measures to be taken by physicians. These were ideas shared by both astrology and medicine.

Astrological tools were appropriated by medicine without much controversy. There was, in general, little objection on the part of astrologers or physicians to the use of aspects of astrology that might indicate when to bleed patients, or how temperament might incline patients to particular diseases. There were always exceptions, but the general agreement between astrologers and medical practitioners meant that astrological medicine was to some extent isolated from other debates, frequently theological debates, about astrology. Physicians and theologians tended to react differently to the cultural status of astrology; consequently, theological and medical discourses about astrology diverged. One of the tendencies of dramatic representations of astrological medicine was to treat astrological medicine as if it were strictly a branch of astrology—with its own peculiar forms of etiology, diagnosis, therapy, and so on—not an unremarkable aspect of quotidian medical practice. There were two important consequences of treating astrological medicine as if it were a purely astrological and not also a routine part of medical practice. First, it made it seem as if astrological medicine was more controversial than it would have seemed to most medical practitioners and patients. Second, it made astrological medicine potentially available to theological polemics about astrology.

Although plays do sometimes distort aspects of astrological medicine, at other times, plays hew very close to its scholarly and non-scholarly traditions. Dramatists represent temperament, inclination, disease, and prognostication in ways that largely coincide with historical records concerning astrological medicine. The present chapter considers some of the ideas about astrological medicine and astrological themes that were represented in the plays of the period, and examines the way these ideas were characterized. Dramatic representation undoubtedly contributed to the circulation of some of the concepts of astrological medicine; the ways in which these concepts were staged—frequently with little explanation or context—suggest that the plays make reference to issues already familiar to

---

[6]   See, among many others, Anthony Grafton and Nancy Siraisi, "Between the Election and My Hopes"; Capp, *Astrology and the Popular Press* 180–221; Allan Chapman, "Astrological Medicine"; and Monica Azzolini ("Reading health" and *The Duke* 135–66). For the case of Spain, see Tayra M. C. Lanuza-Navarro's "Medical Astrology in Spain During the Seventeenth Century."

the public. Previous knowledge probably allowed the audience to understand, in addition to jokes, how the heavens might influence the physical and emotional traits of people; sicknesses and their development; and therapeutics. But plays can also distort aspects of astrological medicine or manufacture distinctions where there are none. Thus, what we find in the plays is not precisely a borrowing from or an attack upon or a misuse of astrological medicine. It is something unto itself: a dramatic culture of astrological medicine.

Physicians studied aspects of astrology as a regular part of their university training. Astrology, however, was not exclusively academic or scholarly: it had a broad impact, thanks to the astrological prognostications, lunar calendars, and similar pamphlets that were not written for scholars.[7] These widely disseminated texts may have been an important source of information regarding astrology for some audience members. Because the knowledge of lunar cycles was useful to farmers and shepherds—it might indicate when to plant, graft, reap, shear, and so on—astrology permeated the agricultural and pastoral life of much of early modern Spain. Thus basic astrological concepts of one sort or another could be found among illiterate laborers, the erudite, readers of cheap pamphlets, and so on. This makes it surprising that—although astrological themes appear regularly in early modern plays—astrology is not even more common on stage.

In this chapter, I am not primarily concerned with what playwrights might have known or believed.[8] Instead, this chapter considers the ways in which plays represent the medical utility of astrology in order to outline the dimensions of a dramatic culture of astrological medicine.

Representing Astrological Difference

The increasing interest of humanist physicians in the study of astronomy and astrology, the publication of a large number of textbooks explaining the principles of astrological medicine, and university curricula all demonstrate the importance of medical astrology during the Renaissance (Grafton and Siraisi 73).[9] The consequence of humanist interest in astronomy was an abundance of what we might call physician-astronomer-astrologers in Europe at the end of the sixteenth century; these practitioners used astrology in their interpretation of Hippocratic

---

[7]   The term used in Spanish works is *lunario*, meaning a general prognostication based on the lunar calendar, which as a genre of astrological texts can be read as an equivalent to the English almanac.

[8]   For studies on the attitude of several playwrights towards astrology, see Frank G. Halstead's "The Attitude of Lope de Vega toward Astrology and Astronomy" and "The Attitude of Tirso de Molina toward Astrology and Astronomy"; Augusta M. Espantoso-Foley's "The Problem of Astrology" and *Occult Arts and Doctrine in the Theater of Juan Ruiz de Alarcón*; and E. W. Hesse and A. Martinengo.

[9]   See also Siraisi, *Medieval and Early Renaissance Medicine*; and Lindemann, *Medicine and Society* 251–2.

texts (Navarro Brotóns, "La actividad"). It was widely known that astrological medicine was taught at the universities, but all sorts of medical practitioners used astrology in healing, too. This does not mean that a university-trained physician and a folk healer, for example, believed that they were both involved in a related enterprise simply because they both drew on astrology. In fact, plays help us trace the delineations among medical cultures, whether scholarly or non-scholarly.

Medical advice that draws on astrology, although not difficult to find, does appear less often than general astrological predictions in early modern plays. There is a straightforward representation of astrology as a therapeutic option in the discussion between the characters Casandra and Prince Alejandro of Alexandria in Lope de Vega's *Lo que ha de ser*. The plot of *Lo que ha de ser* is set in motion through an astrological horoscope (De Armas, "El rey astrólogo"). In one of the scenes of Act III, Alejandro declares his (love) sickness to Casandra, Princess of Athens, asking her to be his doctor. To avoid taking his pulse—and the physical contact that it would entail—Casandra tells Alejandro that she heals using astrology. In the scene Casandra is disguised as a farmer named Laura:

> *Alexander*: [...] give me your hand, Laura, for in the pulse and struggle of my love you will feel what an ardent fever has afflicted my will.
> *Casandra*: Do not order me to do so, for even if you persist, I heal using astrology [...]"[10]

In this case, Casandra suggests that "healing by means of astrology" would imply that the doctor would not use regular diagnostic methods, such as taking the pulse of patients. It is, of course, a pretext: Casandra/Laura is simply trying to avoid a potentially erotic situation. This does not mean that, as a rule, physicians who made use of astrology touched their patients less than physicians who did not use astrological knowledge. But even if audience members knew a physician-astrologer would likely have taken the patient's pulse, they would also have known that by making the patient's natal figure, or by making the figure of the skies in the moment when the patient fell ill, a physician-astrologer could learn about the sickness. And herein lays Casandra's stratagem: she hopes to avoid Alejandro's earthly seductions by claiming to look skyward.

But there is a second feature of Casandra's distinction between "normal" medicine and astrological medicine. To a certain extent, she uses medical astrology as a shorthand for practices that are out of the ordinary. This is because astrology in medicine had two faces. On the one hand, it was mainstream and unremarkable. For a scholar, such as Bartolomé del Valle, astrology was simply a tool that might be useful for academic medicine. Del Valle was a physician and a professor who taught at the University of Salamanca from 1612 to 1623. During this time, he wrote a prognostication on the comets of 1618 that included ideas

---

[10]   "*Alejandro*: [...] la mano Laura me dad, / que en el pulso del amor / conoceréis de qué ardor / enfermó la voluntad. / *Casandra*: No me mandéis que lo intente, / que en esta mala porfía / curo por astrología [...]" (Vega, *Lo que ha de ser* 396).

about astrological medicine (*Explicación*). And Del Valle's tenure at Salamanca was contemporary with *Lo que ha de ser*, which was written in 1624 (Bergman, "En torno" 365).

On the other hand, the medical astrology of non-scholar astrologers was often associated with magic or witchcraft. This non-scholarly tradition did not conform to Galenic and Hippocratic ideas but rather with practices of supernatural healing. There was not always a clear distinction between academic or scholarly medical astrology and its more popular, non-scholarly counterpart.

Evidence of the blurring between scholarly and non-scholarly astrological medical cultures can be found in the annual prognostications and *lunarios* or lunar calendars—containing general medical-astrological guidance—that could be found in all levels of society. As Mary Lindemann points out, the lines we draw today between "legitimate" and "alternative" medicine, or even superstition, were not as clear during the early modern period (Lindemann).[11] Differing approaches and beliefs might lead to conflict in some cases, but might not in others. As many contributions in this volume demonstrate, the coexistence of different forms of healing is a basic feature of the medical cultures of the early modern Spanish Empire; astrological medicine is no exception. And scholarly and non-scholarly astrological medicine had in common concepts concerning the human body and sickness.

Like *Lo que ha de ser*, Lope's *El bobo del colegio*, written between 1604 and 1610, plays with the idea that astrological medicine is something other than "normal" medicine.[12] In *El bobo del colegio*, the gentleman Garcerán is in love with a lady, Fulgencia. Garcerán's footman, Marín, in order to help his master, tries to convince Fulgencia's aunt Lisarda that, after trying everything Galen said (that is, after consulting several doctors), he turned to an astrologer. Marín explains that he did so because he was told that Garcerán's sickness was the result of a bewitchment. In this context, speaking in first person although referring to Garcerán, as he later explains, Marín says that an astrologer gave him an unusual cure: Garcerán had to be blessed for seven days by a pure lady.

> *Marín*: As I say, Lisarda, no remedy was found for my illness, although I tried everything Galen knew. A certain woman told me I was bewitched. [...] I grow thin and weak from amorous cares. An astrologer gave me a remarkable remedy [...][13]

Marín's account suggests that, in this case, the astrologer was not a regular physician who made use of astrology, but a practitioner outside of the Galenic

---

[11]   On medical pluralism in Spain, see López-Terrada's "Medical Pluralism."

[12]   On this play, see Kurtz.

[13]   "*Marín*: Como digo, no se halló, / Lisarda, a mi mal remedio, / aunque puse de por medio / cuanto Galeno alcanzó. / Díjome cierta mujer / que estaba hechizado, [...] Por amorosos cuidados / me enflaquezco, y debilito. / El remedio que me dio / un astrólogo es notable; / mas porque de veras hable / todo aquesto sucedió" (Vega, *El bobo* 33–4).

mainstream. The astrologer was to cure a supernatural malady, characterized as outside the purview of a physician. The use of supernatural remedies is presented here as coexistent with elite or academic medicine but, in Marín's account, distinct from it.

Although both *Lo que ha de ser* and *El bobo del colegio* exaggerate the differences between medicine and astrology, they are helpful because they represent, on the one hand, the notion that characters are able to choose from a wide range of treatment options for illness and discomfort, and, on the other, the process by which characters chose from among these options. That is, the plays represent the plurality of medical cultures of early modern society and show some of the faces of astrological medicine, with an insistence on its non-scholarly aspects.

Astrological Etiology: Sickness and the Stars

Seventeenth-century plays make use of the idea that astrological configurations could be the cause of sickness in several ways. There are some cases in which the representations are limited to a simple mention of the stars as the cause of or justification for a character's illness. In other cases, plays make reference to firmly established traditions that explained particular sicknesses or developments of the state of patients through the influence of concrete planets.

According to the principles of astrological medicine, sickness—in Galenic terms a result of *discrasia*, the loss of balance of the humors—could be caused by the influence of heavenly bodies.[14] This influence acted in several ways. The constellations and planets could affect the humors; the organs (parts of the body had heavenly associations—*melothesia*—from which the popular Zodiacal man derived); air, food, and drink (through the action of their occult qualities on some of the Galenic *sex res non naturales*); and the passions of the soul (i.e., spiritual and emotional conditions).[15] Most often the effect of the heavens on the health of a character is represented simply by attributing the onset of a sickness to "the stars." This is the case in Lope de Vega's *La dama boba*, composed in 1613.[16] The character Laurencio, who has decided to pursue the comically nitwitted Finea because of her dowry, tries to woo her by comparing her eyes to stars, telling her that he is affected by them. Finea, missing Laurencio's astrological/amorous conceit, understands only that he is sick. So she responds by telling him that his cold (*romadizo*) must be a result of "going with the stars" (i.e. traveling at night):

---

[14] See López-Terrada's chapter in this volume.

[15] On the *sex res non naturales*, see the chapter by Pardo-Tomás in this volume. Occult qualities are understood as they were in the early modern context, as qualities not perceptible by the senses; they were not supernatural or magical, but rather opposed to manifest qualities. On occult qualities, see Copenhaver; Henry; Hutchison; and Giralt.

[16] On this play, see Bruce Wardropper's "Lope's *La dama boba* 1–3; Holloway; Bergmann's "*La dama boba*" 409–14).

> *Laurencio*: Those famous stars, those night lights, have me out of my wits.
> *Finea*: If you go with stars, why are you surprised that you have a runny nose?[17]

In this instance, Finea exhibits a rudimentary, if excessively literal, understanding of the relationship between stars and disease. She completely misconstrues the compliment paid her, based on an analogy between, on the one hand, her eyes and the stars, and on the other, Laurencio's love and disease. But what she grasps, at least on a very literal level, is the relationship between stars and disease. Finea's answer, therefore, simultaneously demonstrates her ignorance and the notion that even the simplest person would know basic astrological concepts. Figures of speech are complicated; astrology is not.

Certainly, Finea does not demonstrate a sophisticated understanding of the relationship between the stars and the qualities of the humors or the parts of the body. As a general rule, certain planets were considered to have beneficent influences, and certain others, malefic ones. Planets were linked with humors and the properties (in a Galenic sense) of those humors; these properties might be active or passive, a concept common to medicine and astrology. Heat and moisture were beneficent because they were fertile and active, being forces of generation; dryness and cold were maleficent forces because they were destructive and passive. Hence Saturn, being the coldest planet, and Mars, the most dry, had malefic influences over human health (and in general, in human affairs of every kind); Jupiter and Venus, on the other hand, were beneficent because of their heat and moistness.

These relationships (e.g. Saturn/cold/maleficence) appear with some regularity in seventeenth-century plays, such as Lope's *La resistencia honrada y condesa Matilde*, written between 1596 and 1603 (Hochman 95). According to the character Tibalte, the king has a cold because he is subject to the influence of Mars:

> *Tibalte*: [...] he has not been well, he has a cold. He is very subject to the law of Mars [...][18]

Tibalte's comment draws on a number of associations with Mars. First, as a maleficent planet, Mars explains the king's illness. Second, Tibalte alludes to the notion that warriors are necessarily subject to Mars (because of the planet's bellicose associations in myth). But Tibalte's explanation does not go beyond this and the explanation of astrological medicine is not drawn out. Specifically, what he does not explain is how Mars had affected the king's yellow bile or his liver.

---

[17]   *Laurencio*: Esas estrellas famosas, / esos nocturnos luceros / me tienen fuera de mí. / *Finea*: Si vos andáis con estrellas, / ¿qué mucho que os traigan ellas / arromadizado ansí?" (Vega, *La dama boba* 1351).

[18]   "*Conde*: ¿Ha se levantado el Rey? / *Tibalte*: ¡Oh, señor Conde! No ha estado / bueno, que anda resfriado; / es muy sujeto a la ley / del fiero Marte [...]" (Vega, *La resistencia* 776).

In the system of Galenic astrological medicine, Saturn, for example, dominated the element earth; it was cold and dry, and thus it acted on black bile, which was also cold and dry (like earth). Jupiter acted on blood, because it was hot and moist (like air); Venus (and the Moon) acted on phlegm, being cold and moist (like water); and Mars, hot and dry (like fire), acted on choler or yellow bile.[19] Each humor was also associated with a major organ of the human body: blood was associated with the heart, phlegm with the brain, yellow bile with the liver, and black bile (often called "melancholy") with the spleen. The clearly articulated relationships among planets, humors, and organs meant that connections between human and heavenly bodies were explicit.

The person subject to Mars, as the king is said to be in *La resistencia honrada y condesa Matilde*, might suffer from a list of sicknesses associated with the planet. The physician Joan de Figueroa (c.1610–c.1670) explained, in his great work on astrology in medicine (1660), which illnesses Mars ruled. Figueroa was a councilor of Lima and a lay member (*familiar*) of the Inquisition; he explained that Mars had power over "acute and pestilent fevers, frenzy, *apostemas* which were unlikely to mutate into plague,[20] red jaundice, erysipelas,[21] carbuncles,[22] fistula, epilepsy, dysentery, tertian and quotidian fevers, empyemas,[23] *ignis sacro* or Saint Anthony's

---

[19] Popular works on astrology, as well as many academic texts, expressed the idea this way: planets did not share qualities with sublunar, corruptible matter, they only influenced it. Heavenly bodies were perfect, being made of the fifth element in the Aristotelian-Ptolemaic cosmology.

[20] *Apostema*, to where the term "abscess" was redirected, was defined in Blankaart's *Physical dictionary* of 1684 as "an exulceration left after a crisis" (26). In Andres de León's *Libro primero de annathomia* (1590), *apostema* is "a tumor against our nature where some matter is located" (Que apostema es tumor contra nuestra naturaleza donde está allegada alguna materia) (127r).

[21] Erysipela, in Blankaart, is defined as "wild-fire" and "a swelling in the skin or any other fleshie or membraneous part" (122). Andrés de León classifies them as a kind of *apostema*, namely, the one deriving from the humor choler: "Praeter naturam tumors are the four apostemas mentioned, corresponding to the four humours. [...] the second tumor is called erysipela, and comes from and is made of choler" (Los tumores praeter naturam son los quatro apostemas referidos, correspondientes a los quatro humores. [...] El segundo tumor se llama erisipila [sic], que se haze y compone de cholera) (88v).

[22] *Carbunculus*, says Blankaart, is the same as *anthrax* (48), defined as "a tumor that arises in several places, surrounded with hot fiery and most sharp pimples" (20). León says that "carbuncles are bad sanguine pustules" (carbunculos son unas pústulas malas sanguinas) (133r).

[23] An empyema is defined by Blankaart as a collection of purulent matter in the cavity of the thorax. It is defined by the physician Ramírez de Arellano in his *Cirugía* as "the collection of matter or blood *in cavitate toracis*" (empiema impropio es colección de la materia o de la sangre *in cavitate toracis*) (152).

fire,[24] causons,[25] sicknesses of the bile and all those coming from choler, excess of heat and dryness."[26] Notably, a cold does not appear on this list, which would seem to contradict Tibalte's diagnosis. Actually, the common cold was associated with illnesses related to the qualities of coldness and moistness, thus with phlegm and, consequently, with Venus or with the Moon. Figueroa stated that Venus ruled "on every frigid and humid intemperance, and in the sicknesses of this quality" and that the Moon ruled "phlegm," as well as "frigid and moist" complexions.[27] Like Finea, in Lope's *La dama boba*, Tibalte understands the basic relationship between stars or planets and disease. The finer points of this relationship (among them, for example, Mars, heat, yellow bile, liver, pestilent fever) are, unsurprisingly, beyond him. For Finea and Tibalte, astrological medicine is not a sophisticated web of resonances and linkages, but a rudimentary tool used to explain misfortune and, to a more limited extent, the place of human beings in the universe.

The Moon—a planet in the Aristotelic-Ptolemaic system—was of particular importance to playwrights and astrologers. From the standpoint of astrological medicine, the Moon had long been associated with health issues. The idea was based on the relationship established between the Moon and the tides, which supposed a corresponding relationship with fluids, including the four humors, particularly blood (Roos). According to this tradition, the Moon's waxing and waning regulated blood and humoral fluctuations, an idea developed in the Middle Ages that leaned on some assertions in the Hippocratic corpus (French, "Astrology in Medical Practice" 39). The Moon was cold and moist, and together with Venus it ruled phlegm, the fluid associated with the brain. One of the Moon's main effects was the moistening of bodies; moistening the brain could result in an excess of phlegm and thus lead to mental disorders. This was the medical-astrological basis for the popular idea that the Moon caused madness or lunacy.

The relationship between the Moon and mental illness is an idea that plays represent often. In Agustín Moreto's *El parecido*, written in 1652, Tacón, a servant, suggests that his master, Fernando, deceive Pedro, father of the lady he loves. The ruse is as follows: Pedro will be led to believe that Fernando is his son, Lope, who has just returned after a long stay in the colonies. This way Fernando will be able to be near his beloved. Because Fernando finds the lie distasteful, he occasionally denies being Pedro's son, Lope. Tacón, the *gracioso* in his role as a clown, tries to explain the contradictions about his master's identity by stating that Fernando

---

[24]   *Ignis sacer* is the same as erysipelas, says Blankaart (162).

[25]   Causons were ephemeral fevers. Blankaart calls them *causus* and refers to them as burning fevers with a greater heat than other continuous fevers (55).

[26]   "Marte […] de las enfermedades domina en las fiebres agudas y pestilentes, frenesí, apostemas, que no fácilmente mutarán en la peste, en la itiricia [sic] roja, erisipelas, carbuncos, fístulas, epilepsia, disentería, tercianas y cotidianas fiebres, empimas [sic], *ignis sacro* o fuego de San Antón, causones, enfermedades de la hiel, y todas las que proceden de cólera, exceso de calor y sequedad" (Figueroa 144).

[27]   "Venus domina […] de los humores en la flema natural […], y en todas las destemplanzas frígidas y húmedas, y en las enfermedades desta qualidad" (Figueroa 144).

suffered from palsy (*perlesía*), and therefore (as medical texts explain) his memory was affected.[28] The influence of the Moon is used to justify the periodic changes in Fernando's memory:

> *Tacón*: Ah! Now I remember. What phase is the moon in?
> *Pedro*: Today I think it is the new Moon.
> *Tacón*: Is it not the February new Moon?
> *Pedro*: Yes.
> *Tacón*: Well then, do not expect anything from Lope until it begins to wane.
> *Pedro*: Why?
> *Tacón*: Years ago he fell ill at this time, and this Moon affects him so violently that he behaves quite madly while it lasts.[29]

Tacón repeats this explanation, based on the influence of the Moon depending on its phase, on other occasions in the play:

> *Tacón*: You have really done it now, by God; are you going to give him that news knowing that it is a crescent moon? It will be all the harder to persuade him that you are his father. [...]

And later:

> *Tacón*: Jesus! Can you not see that it is because of the crescent moon?[30]

The ruse aside, from the point of view of astrological medicine, Tacón is not wrong to suggest that the phases of the Moon might play a role in Fernando's health. The astrologer Jerónimo Cortés—widely read among lay audiences—explains in his *Lunario* that "it must first be noted that the effects of the crescent Moon are very different from those of the waning Moon, and thus every prudent person takes into account particularly the waxing and waning [phases] of the Moon for many and varied issues related to agriculture and to corporal health."[31] According to

---

[28] For a full description of the argument of the play and the representation in it of medical knowledge related to palsy, see the chapter by Mariluz López-Terrada in this volume.

[29] "*Tacón*: ¡Ay, que ahora se me acuerda! / ¿En qué estado está la Luna? / *Pedro*: Hoy pienso que es Luna nueva. / *Tacón*: ¿No es la de Febrero? / *Pedro*: Sí. *Tacón*: Pues de Lope no hagáis cuenta / hasta que entre la menguante. / *Pedro*: ¿Por qué? / *Tacón*: Hace años en ella / que le dio el mal, y esta Luna / le entra con tanta violencia, / que hace en ella mil locuras" (Moreto, *El parecido* 46). The verses in the earlier version of the play *El parecido en la corte* are the same for this part (Moreto, *El parecido en la corte* 95–6).

[30] "*Tacón*: Por Dios que la has hecho buena; / ¿sabiendo que es la creciente / le vas a dar esa nueva? / Más habré de trabajar / en que por padre te crea. [...] / *Tacón*: ¡Jesús! ¿Pues no adviertes que eso / lo ocasiona la creciente?" (*El parecido* 49). The verses in the earlier version of the play *El parecido en la corte* are the same for these parts as well (100; 127).

[31] "Primeramente se ha de notar que los efectos de la Luna en creciente son muy diferentes que en menguante, y assí todas las personas de prudencia tienen cuenta particular

Figueroa, palsy fell under the Moon's dominion.[32] However, astrological rules were complex and the planets, in this case the Moon, were not the immediate causes of disease, but rather parts of an interactive system. This system included the planets, the Zodiacal signs, some of the fixed stars, and the astrological houses, among other factors. The phase of the Moon was a key element, and one with a popular tradition probably as long as the astrological ideas themselves. But the sign of the Zodiac where the Moon was placed, in relation to the illness, would have a major role. That is why Tacón's assertion that the patient's symptoms were particularly acute in February's new moon makes perfect astrological sense. The theory of astrological revolutions, that is, the annual return of the Sun to a given position, asserted that the astrological figure made for the anniversary of something (usually a birth) revealed the same content already present in the original figure, but with a focus on the year in question (Bouché-Leclercq 506–8).[33] The anniversary of the moment when Fernando fell ill with his palsy would be meaningful in this astrological context.

Part of the humor found in *El parecido* derives precisely from the sophistication of Tacón's astrological deception. Fernando's illness is feigned so as to correspond with official medical knowledge.[34] Tacón may use astrology as an explanation for symptoms that the audience knows to be false, but the astrology involved in the evolution of the sickness is drawn from scholarly sources. In this sense Moreto, the playwright, does not ridicule astrology, but hews very close to what might be found in academic works on general astrology and on the medical astrology of popular works such as Cortés's *Lunario*. The play simultaneously represents ideas shared by the public, such as the influence of the phases of the Moon on mental illnesses, and disseminates astrological knowledge.

Legitimating Astrological Medicine: Complexion, Inclination, and Free Will

The plays written, represented, and published during the last decades of the sixteenth century and over the course of the seventeenth century appeared at a time when the legitimacy of astrology was hotly debated. This debate took place mainly in the scholarly realm and involved university professors and theologians, censors and counselors of the Inquisition, and other intellectuals. One object of the debate

---

con los crecientes y menguantes de la Luna para muchas y diversas cosas tocantes a la agricultura y a la salud corporal" (Cortés, *El non plus ultra del lunario* 87–8).

[32] "La Luna domina [...] de las enfermedades, la epilepsia, passión de cólica, los menstruos, apostemas flemáticas, opilación de nervios, perlesía, hidropesía de viento, obstrucción de nervios, letargo, morbo caduco, temblores, distilaciones, conmoción de miembros, torturas y todas las que provienen de frialdad y humedad" (Figueroa 145).

[33] This theory of astrological revolutions was developed by Masshala and his disciples. Albumasar, also considered part of the Hermetic tradition, further explained how to make general predictions about the fate of the world.

[34] See Maríaluz López-Terrada's chapter in this volume.

was to establish which aspects of the discipline were acceptable in a Christian context and which were not. The discussion included religious arguments as well as arguments disputing the validity of astrology, either partially or entirely.[35] These arguments gained resonance among wider audiences through the lunaries and annual prognostications in which popular astrologers repeated simplified versions of scholarly defenses of their art. Plays were involved in this process because they represented some of the opinions expressed in the polemics. They dramatized the ideas that justified astrological medicine through the relationship established between Galenic complexions and temperaments and astrological inclination. Inclination included the tendency of a person to be, act, and feel a certain way, as well as a person's tendency to experience health or sickness as a result of the stars' influences.

Plays represented the two considerations that were the basis of beliefs about astrological inclination. The first of these was the idea of harmony between the microcosm of the human body and the macrocosm of the heavens, an idea that justified astrological medicine through the pre-Socratic tradition of mutually dependent parts of the cosmos. The second was drawn from Thomas Aquinas's teachings on the influence of the stars as inclinations that respected free will. This second idea—that the stars might incline us to certain behaviors or states without robbing us of free will—was one of the main arguments in the defense of astrology. Free will is a subject that appears frequently in early modern Spanish drama, and not exclusively in an astrological context.[36] At the beginning of the seventeenth century, Spain was in the midst of a dispute between Jesuits and Dominicans on the subject of human freedom and the power of Divine Grace— the *De auxiliis* controversy—and Lope de Vega and Calderón de la Barca studied in Jesuit institutions.[37]

The history of contentious debate about free will made astrological inclination a subject of particular interest to dramatists. Lope de Vega represents the harmony of heaven and earth as related to the balance or imbalance of the elements and humors (and thus, related to health). In perhaps his most famous play, *Fuenteovejuna*, two villagers, Barrildo and Mengo, refer to the need for "peace" among the elements as a requirement for health. This leads them to a discussion of the concord between the terrestrial and celestial spheres ("here and there"):

---

[35]   These debates dated to antiquity. See Thomas; Garin, *Astrology in the Renaissance*; Van Nouhuys, *The Age*; Vanden Broecke, *The Limits*; and Patrick Curry. For the case of Spain, see Pardo-Tomás, *Ciencia y censura*; and Lanuza-Navarro, *Astrología, ciencia y sociedad*.

[36]   There have been abundant studies on the dramatic representation of arguments concerning free will. See, among others, Sabik; Nadeau ("Star-Crossed Love"); Pan; DiPuccio; Soufas; Espantoso Foley (*Occult Arts*); E. H. Friedman; and Valbuena Briones 48–53.

[37]   On *De auxiliis* controversy in theater, see Antonini. On the controversy itself, see Egido López, et. al (196–204).

Mengo: [...] if the elements live in eternal discord, and from them our bodies receive nutrition, choler and melancholy, phlegm and blood, it is clear.
Barrildo: The world of here and there, Mengo, it is all harmony.[38]

This is actually a discussion about the nature of love. Mengo begins his reflections lamenting the "eternal discord" of nature (the elements and humors). Barrildo interrupts, stating that the terrestrial and celestial worlds are linked by cosmic harmony. This debate—whether the universe tends toward discord or concord—was ancient. But it was generally accepted that there was *some* relationship between heavenly and elementary bodies, whether the influences were due to occult qualities (only known via their effects) or to the shared primary qualities of stars and bodies. The debates on the legitimacy of astrology often made reference to Fathers of the Church. Defenders of astrology found their arguments in Thomas Aquinas's works, as in both the *Summa Theologica* and the *Summa contra gentiles* several passages posited the influence of the stars on bodies.[39] Whatever the cause of these influences, their existence could not, Aquinas asserted, be doubted.[40] This affirmation proved crucial for the defense of astrology.

Aquinas argued that the stars influenced the physiology of living things (Litt 240). This made his ideas particularly useful for the defense of astrological medicine. Influences on living bodies were explained through the astrological inclinations that were connected with the people's temperament (in Galenic terms). The humoral constitution of each person, generally referred to as complexion, determined temperament.[41] The temperament of a person should be understood in the sense of bodily dispositions, including proclivity towards certain illnesses, but also as tendencies (or inclinations) towards specific behaviors and emotional states. These aspects of Galenism were extremely close to the assumptions of natal astrology. According to the astrological doctrine of genethlialogy, the planets that had predominance in the natal chart of a person would have an influence on his temperament.

The temperament linked with Saturn is represented often in plays of the period. The popularity of the saturnine temperament stems from its relationship with the

---

[38]   *Mengo*: Yo no sé filosofar; / leer ¡ojalá supiera! / Pero si los elementos / en discordia eterna viven, / y de los mismos reciben / nuestros cuerpos alimentos, / cólera, y melancolía, / flema, y sangre, claro está. / *Barrildo*: El mundo de acá, y de allá, / Mengo, todo es armonía (Vega, *Fuenteovejuna* 62).

[39]   On Thomas Aquinas's position regarding astrology, see Thomas Litt's *Les corps celestes dans l'univers de Saint Thomas d'Aquin.*

[40]   Aquinas says that celestial influences act on men's bodies and not directly on their intellect and will, for instance in the *Summa contra gentiles,* III, Part II, Chapters 84–7, 149; and in the *Summa Theologica*, q. 115, a. 3–6.

[41]   Complexion, in Galenic terms, was the individual and natural combination of the four corporal humors and their qualities in specific proportions that resulted in the physical nature of the person. Complexion was a result of inherent innate qualities. See Groebner ("Complexio/complexion").

humor of black bile (that is, melancholy), which associated it with the sickness of melancholy. In other words, melancholy is a humor, also known as black bile. An excess of this humor causes a disease also called melancholy, and the tendency towards this disease is an effect of the saturnine temperament. Melancholy has been the object of numerous works, both from the point of view of the history of medicine and from that of the history of literature (Bartra; Flor, *Era melancólica*; Atienza). A comprehensive study of the complex manifestations of melancholy in early modern cultures is beyond the scope of this chapter.[42] However, I would like to make reference to the way the saturnine temperament appears on stage, if only to point out that it is usually accompanied by references to the sickness of melancholy. As I have mentioned, melancholy was caused by an excess of black bile, which was cold and dry (making the illness cold and dry in nature). From the astrological point of view, the saturnine person would be cold and dry, because of his temperament and the influence of Saturn at birth. All the elements—inclination, temperament, disease, and so on—were related and formed a system that made astrological medicine coherent with humoral Galenism.

These were such popular ideas that in a play like *De una causa dos efectos*, first published in 1682, Calderón only needs to stress several times that the character Carlos is of a cold and dry disposition, that he tends to sadness and his preference is to study rather than to be entertained by buffoons, to make the audience expect his description: he is a saturnine type.

> *Pernia*: One of them is a saturnine type, one of those that hardly make two statements you can understand, and those two after long meditation [...] he is a very truthful man, and is reputed in the world to be the cleverest man known in Italy today. The other is a fool [...][43]

Saturnines were, according to the popular *Lunario perpetuo* written by Jerónimo Cortés, "inclined to knowledge and studies, especially to philosophy, and things of understanding, because they are very studious and friends of knowing the secrets of nature and even mechanical and liberal arts."[44] Calderón's description of Carlos follows these ideas. The saturnine Carlos was intelligent and dedicated to study, as opposed to his brother Fadrique, "a fool." The predominance of one of the humors, in this case melancholy, was in this way represented along with its

---

[42]   Klibansky, Panofsky, and Saxl's famous *Saturn and Melancholy* inspired scholars to study the appearance in the plays of this particular temperament in its several natures (De Armas, "Black Sun" and "The Saturn Factor").

[43]   "El uno es un saturnino / de aquellos que apenas hablan / dos razones entendidas, / y essas dos muy ponderadas. / [...] es hombre todo de veras, / y tiene en el mundo fama / del hombre más entendido, / que hoy se conoce en Italia. / El otro es un majadero [...]" (Calderón, "De una causa" 219).

[44]   "Los saturninos son inclinados a letras y cosas de estudio, especialmente a la filosofía y cosas de entendimiento, porque son muy estudiativos y amigos de saber los secretos de naturaleza, y aún de las artes mecánicas y liberales" (Cortés, *El non plus ultra* 71).

astrological relative, the classification of characters according to the planet that ruled their births.

These ideas were not only present in popular contexts; on the contrary, they circulated among scholars, especially since the Neoplatonic revival. This revival was largely a consequence of Marsilio Ficino's translations of and commentaries on Plato, and Ficino is particularly relevant for astrological knowledge in the Renaissance. Ficino's *De vita*, widely disseminated in sixteenth-century Europe, explains at the outset that both Mercury and Saturn were of a cold and dry nature: "just like the melancholic nature, according to physicians. Mercury and Saturn impart this same nature to their followers, learned people, from birth and preserve and augment it day by day."[45] In Book III Ficino underscores the point made in Calderón's *De una causa dos efectos*: study and solitude were characteristic influences of Saturn (Peset Reig 85–9). Ficino explains, "By withdrawal from human affairs, by leisure, solitude, constancy, by theology, esoteric philosophy, superstition, magic, agriculture, and by sorrow, we come under the influence of Saturn" (*Three Books* 113, 253).

One of the ways of referring to the results of the predominance of one of the humors in a person's complexion was to speak about his "inclinations." In terms of humoral theory, inclination was the consequence of temperament. In terms of astrology, inclination was the consequence of the position of the stars at birth. That is why the term "inclination" (inclinación/inclinar) appears in the plays to refer in a general way to the influences of the stars, which "inclined" people to something.

From antiquity, "inclination" was a key term in the debates on the legitimacy of astrology. One of the main arguments in defense of astrology was based on the use of the term "incline," as it appeared in the aphorism attributed to Ptolemy, "astra inclinant, non necessitant" (the stars incline, they do not compel). The doctrine of inclination implied that humans retained the freedom to resist the influences of the stars; thus there was no determinism that would be objectionable to Roman Catholic theology.

Inclination is represented on stage mainly in plays that make reference to astrological predictions. Crisanto, the pagan character who becomes a Christian in Calderón's *Los dos amantes del cielo*, explains:

> Though the violence of a star has inclined me towards a deity, it has not forced me, for the stars do not force, but only incline. My will, soul and heart are free.[46]

---

[45]   See Tarabochia Canavero's "Il 'De Triplici Vita' di Marsilio Ficino," which traces editions and translations through 1650, as well as the introduction to her translation of Marsilio Ficino's *Sulla Vita* and Ficino, *Three Books of Life*, edited by C. Kaske and J. Clark. See also Zanier, *La medicina*; Garin, *Marsilio Ficino*; Cassirer; Allen, Rees, and Davies' *Marsilio Ficino*.

[46]   "Si de un astro la violencia / a una deidad me ha inclinado, / no me ha forzado, que no / fuerzan, sí inclinan los astros. / Libre tengo mi albedrío, / alma, y corazón" (Calderón, *Los dos amantes* 233).

Calderón's public was probably already familiar with the notion that "the stars incline, they do not compel." The phrase appears not only in plays, but also in almanacs and annual prognostications (the most popular astrological works). For instance, the popular astrologer Juan Casiano wrote that "in what concerns contingent futures, no celestial cause obliges, but merely inclines."[47] Writing for a more scholarly audience, albeit in the vernacular, the physician Joan de Figueroa concluded his treatise on the relationship of astrology and medicine by noting: "This is what can be deduced in a natural and discursive way from the inclination of the stars, and from so many universal causes as have come together in our era; I don't mean that all their effects must happen, nor that any of their influences make any imprint upon men's will, which is always free to choose at its discretion, because the stars incline, but they do not compel."[48] By using the same arguments and terms that were part of the controversies about astrology, plays form part of a much broader debate about the legitimacy of astrology.

Calderón's *Los dos amantes del cielo* hints at one further aspect of the debate concerning astrological influences. Crisanto says that his "soul," in addition to his "will," is free. Astrological medicine was careful to point out that any influence of the stars affects only the humors and not the soul. Aquinas established the principle that cases depending on human will, or in general the spiritual acts, could not be directly influenced by the heavens because they did not depend on the organs.[49]

Lope de Vega distinguished between the will and the body by using the metaphor of slavery. In *El hidalgo Abencerraje* the body is in bondage, but not the will:

> Consider, brave Cárdenas, that the body is merely a slave, and that is why the will is called free.[50]

This language of slavery and freedom corresponded to the terminology Aquinas used. The Galenic tradition that one of the non-natural things that affected health was the passions of the soul was linked in the Aristotelian-scholastic division of the faculties. The soul was intellective, not sensitive. This made the soul theoretically free from the influences of the stars, as Aquinas explained,

---

[47]   "Ninguna causa celeste en lo que toca a los futuros contingentes no obliga, sino sólo inclina" (Casiano 263).

[48]   "Esto es lo que de natural y discursivamente se puede colegir de la inclinación de los astros, y de tantas causas universales como han concurrido en estos nuestros tiempos, no que necessariamente ayan de suceder todos sus efectos, ni que alguno de sus influxos haga impresión en el albedrío del hombre, que siempre es libre para poder elegir a su voluntad, porque las estrellas inclinan mas no necessitan" (Figueroa 349v).

[49]   "Therefore, since it is clear that intellective understanding and willing are not acts of corporeal organs, it is impossible that the celestial bodies should be a cause of human acts" (*Summa Theologica*, q. 115, a. 4).

[50]   "Advierte Cárdenas bravo, / que el cuerpo solo es esclavo, / que por eso el albedrío, / se llama libre" (Vega, *El hidalgo Abencerraje* 207v).

because the stars affected only sensitive faculties (ruling inferior appetites and the knowledge derived from the senses). The expression that man is a "slave to his passions" was a way of referring to the vulnerabilities of sensitive faculties. Christian doctrine taught that bodily passions could be related to the stars (making astrological medicine theologically palatable), while the passions of the soul were not influenced by the stars. The will and intellect had to be free.

Astrologers had to make clear that the celestial influences acted only on the body. Tirso de Molina's *Amazonas en las Indias*—which dramatizes the Pizarro's conquest of Peru—explores the Thomistic tradition that the stars affected the bodily passions but not the soul. Menalipe, the queen of the Amazons, tells her sister, Martesia, that neither "plants and spells" nor the stars could affect the soul; because of this, Menalipe says, Pizarro could resist the stars' influence and turn Martesia's prediction into a lie:

> *Menalipe*: You are not wise in the cures you use, for the soul, which is pure spirit, is not subject to plants and spells as the body is; its substance is so perfect that wise men consider it to be free, confounding the force of your astrology, for omens and influences are indications, but are not decisive (si señalan, no ejecutan). Let the sovereign will of my valiant Spaniard not be swayed by them, and the stars shall have lied.[51]

In the notes to his critical edition of the play, Miguel Zugasti refers to the presentation of free will as a necessary element of Tirso's theology; the playwright juxtaposes the divine plan with ancient cosmological ideas. Zugasti explains that the expression *señalar y no ejecutar* is taken from the language of fencing (*Amazonas* 102). However, the words also carry astrological resonances, not unlike "inclinan y no fuerzan" (stars incline, but they do not compel). The Amazonian Menalipe uses an argument common in astrological works: that the stars were signs but not causes, that they incline and do not force.

Nevertheless, there was a second issue in Aquinas's doctrine on celestial bodies that allowed for limited influence on free will, an issue also often represented in plays. Aquinas explained that, even if their direct power was on physical matters, stars could indirectly influence the intellect: even if the will is not compelled to follow the inclinations of the body, men often surrender to them or decide (freely) to follow corporeal passions (*Summa Theologica*, q. 115, a. 4). Thus in the play Menalipe specifies that Pizarro's will is free, but there is a possibility that he might follow the inclinations of his body (his sensitive passions). If he is not swayed by the force of those inclinations, if he exerts his free will, the astrological indication would not be fulfilled and thus, "the stars shall have lied."

---

[51]   "No curas como discreta, / que el alma, espíritu puro, / ni a las yerbas, ni al conjuro / como el cuerpo se sujeta: / su sustancia es tan perfecta, / que por libre la reputan / los sabios, con que confutan / tus astrólogas violencias, / porque agüeros y influencias / si señalan, no ejecutan. / No se deje llevar de ellas el absoluto albedrío / del gallardo Español mío, / y mentirán las estrellas" (*Amazonas* 102).

The insistence on free will and the stars' effects on bodies is extremely relevant in the context in which the plays were written and represented. The Church, via Sixtus V's 1586 Bull, and the Spanish Inquisition, via the rules included in the Index of Forbidden Books of 1584, had sanctioned the use of astrology. They sanctioned not only natural astrology (that is, the aspects related to medicine, navigation, and meteorological-agricultural issues), but also some parts of judiciary astrology (related to the natural dispositions and inclinations of men).[52] Written in this context, plays reflect the idea that some aspects of astrology were allowed and other aspects forbidden. In Tirso's *El melancólico*, Rogerio is a wise man who knows all the sciences—among them, astrology—but his knowledge is limited to permissible subjects.[53] Pinardo tells Rogerio:

> You are subtle at dialectics, well versed in philosophy, you know about astrology, what is licit and no more [...][54]

Pinardo's claim—that Rogerio knows everything, and is proud of having the knowledge of all sciences—is repeated several times in the play. Rogerio is, of course, a melancholic, referred to as cold and dry (a saturnine temperament).

Almost everyone, even illiterate Spaniards, was familiar with the distinction Pinardo makes between licit and illicit forms of astrology. Although debates about astrology were carried out by intellectual elites—censors and expert advisers consulted by the Inquisition, many of them university scholars—a number of mechanisms made the distinction between licit and illicit forms of astrology widely known (Pardo-Tomás, *Ciencia*). The arguments appeared abridged in popular almanacs, lunar calendars, and annual prognostications that were widely distributed (Lanuza-Navarro, *Astrología*). Edicts published by the Church were read in every town and village in Spain. One such edict—forbidding, and at the same time explaining, judiciary astrology—specified that on the Saturday following its receipt, an announcement that the edict would be read had to be made. Villagers were obliged to attend church that Sunday to hear the reading; every

---

[52]   The prohibition reads: "Se prohiben [...] las partes de la judiciaria que llaman de nascimientos, interrogaciones y electiones. Y se manda y prohibe, que ninguna persona haga juyzio cerca de las cosas susodichas. Pero no por esto se prohiben las partes de la astrología que tocan a conocimientos de los tiempos y succesoss generales del mundo, ni las que enseñan por el nacimento de cada uno a conoscer sus inclinaciones, condiciones y qualidades corporales, ni lo que pertenece a la agricultura y navegación y medicina y las electiones que cerca de estas cosas naturales se hazen" (The parts of the judiciary called births, interrogations and elections are forbidden. And we order and forbid that no person does judgment about the said things. But for that we do not forbid the parts of astrology about knowledge of time and general events of the world, nor those that belong to agriculture and navigation and medicine and elections done about these natural things) (*Index et Catalogus* 3–4).

[53]   On the character of Rogerio, see Arellano, "El sabio."

[54]   "Sutil dialectico estás, / docto en la filosofía, / sabes de la astrología / lo que es lícito, y no mas [...]" (473).

citizen who was not present or did not denounce the activities mentioned would be excommunicated.[55] This made for a uniform message concerning the aspects of astrology that were deemed dangerous or unacceptable: popular astrological prognostications, lunaries, and almanacs, together with the edicts of the Inquisition and plays such as *El melancólico*, all communicated the same information. All of these media simultaneously denounced and popularized controversial aspects of astrology. It is important to point out, however, that while judiciary astrology was broadly condemned, medical astrology was not.[56]

Physiognomics: Representing a Knowledge Shared by Physicians and Astrologers

Natal figures or charts included among their astrological predictions a person's future characteristics; the position of the stars might indicate his or her intellective, emotional, or spiritual traits, such as intelligence, but also physical traits, such as the shape of one's face, stature, or the quality of one's hair. These assertions established a relationship between, on the one hand, the position of the planets and signs at the moment of birth, and on the other, physical appearance and character. In this way, astrology was connected to the knowledge traditionally known as physiognomy, or, in a more academic tradition, physiognomics or physiognomonics. In his Spanish dictionary of 1611 Sebastián Covarrubias defined physiognomy as the "art" with which one uses traits of the body and face to arrive at the knowledge of the nature of men, of their conditions and qualities (406v). An astrologer such as Jerónimo Cortés, interested in the topics where astrology and medicine met, defined physiognomy in terms of "complexion," the above-mentioned key term in Galenic medicine and in the astrological understanding of the human body, which defined the person's nature according to the combination of humors and their qualities.

When establishing that correlation between the art of physiognomy and astrology, in issues related to medical activity, astrologers were following a tradition derived from several works of the Hippocratic corpus, a spurious work of Aristotle's, and some works by Galen. This tradition was further developed in the medieval Arab and Christian worlds, and—as we can glean from the number of works dedicated to the subject—gained readerships across Europe (Caro Baroja 27–97). As one might expect, astrological physiognomy made its way into Spanish plays.

---

[55]   Letter that accompanied an Edict of Faith published in Cordoba during the seventeenth century, AHN. Secc. Inq. Libro 31. Fol. 238. On the edicts and instructions of the Inquisition, see Lea; and Pinto Crespo. For edicts related to astrology, see Lanuza-Navarro (*Astrología*).

[56]   An example is the *Index* of 1662, referring to a rule published in 1647, which was certainly in force earlier: "se notifique a los que escriven pronósticos lo hagan solo en quanto a la navegación, agricultura y medicina, que proviene necesariamente de causas naturales, como eclipses, lluvias, tiempos y pestes" (ÍNDICE.1662. MBN: fol. 202 and 63).

Physiognomy was of interest to physicians because the external signs of the body indicated the patient's complexion. Natal astrological figures were believed to provide information about innate qualities. The external aspect of a person was perceived as connected with the natural humoral constitution; therefore, by knowing physical characteristics, the doctor could determine the complexion of the person; the preponderant humor which defined his temperament; and the possible tendency to particular sicknesses that would be the consequence of complexion and temperament.

Astrology, medicine, and physiognomy come together in Guillén de Castro's *El conde Irlos*. In this play, Celinos addresses the magician Malgesi ironically, because Malgesi has just obtusely commented upon something that was plain to see: Celinos is in love. Celinos quips:

> *Celinos*: It must certainly have been an eminent doctor who identified the illness just from the expression of the face.[57]

Celinos shows some skepticism about physiognomy and its usefulness. As with astrology, attitudes towards physiognomy were diverse in early modern societies. Some doctors and scholars accepted physiognomy's usefulness, although others warned against placing too much faith in it (even if they accepted physiognomy's practical application in some cases). Covarrubias noted that "most times" physiognomy did not prove reliable (406v). But that left room for it to be at least occasionally useful.

One of the reasons physiognomy was rejected was its association with divinatory arts. Physiognomy was included in the list of superstitious divinatory disciplines that were condemned by the Church; a bull issued by Sixtus V included geomancy, hydromancy, aeromancy, pyromancy, onomancy, chiromancy, necromancy, and (as the Bull puts it) other sorceries and superstitions (*Coeli et Terrae*). These associations find an echo in Juan Ruiz de Alarcón's *La cueva de Salamanca*, concerning a legendary cave in which the devil himself gave lessons.[58] In the play, the Marquis of Villena makes a list of the arts he learned from Merlin, "the son of the devil." He begins with astrology, mentions chiromancy, and goes on with physiognomy:

> He taught me the effects and courses of the stars, as human understanding penetrates even the heavens. The chiromantic lines with which nature writes in the hand of everyone the events of his life. I knew the mute physiognomy, which speaks through signs, as through those of the face it tells the most secret inclination.[59]

---

[57]   "Sin duda será médico importante / el que la enfermedad ha conocido / en sólo los efectos del semblante" (Castro, *El conde de Irlos* 798).

[58]   On astrology in this play, see Espantoso Foley, *Occult arts*; on the Stoic elements and magical arts on this play see Whicker.

[59]   "Enseñóme los efectos, / y cursos de las estrellas; / que el entendimiento humano / hasta los cielos penetra. / Las quirománticas líneas / con que en la mano a cualquiera / de

Astrology, chiromancy, and physiognomy were the three most widely known divinatory arts. Physiognomy, the Marquis of Villena says, reveals the inclinations of people through the signs on their faces. Inclination, in this case, refers not only to individual preferences, but to the attitudes, behaviors, and diseases corresponding to humoral temperament. That temperament, revealed through the physical traits, was also related to astrology, as it was integrated in humoral Galenic theory.

Due to the association of physical traits with the astral influences at birth, knowledge of physiognomy was also expected of astrologers. The association of astrology and physiognomy can be seen in Lope de Vega's *El amigo por fuerza*, where the character Hortensio asserts that he only needs to look at his friend's face to know that he is in love.

> *Hortensio*: He is in love.
> *Lisaura*: Do you know with whom?
> *Hortensio*: I do indeed.
> *Lisaura*: Who is it?
> *Hortensio*: You, my lady.
> *Lisaura*: Are people speaking of it in the Palace?
> *Hortensio*: No, but I am an astrologer and understand physiognomy.[60]

The association of astrology and physiognomy could not be clearer; Hortensio is an astrologer, therefore he understands physiognomy.

An excellent example of the popularity of physiognomic ideas and their association with astrology and astrological works is found in Francisco Rojas Zorrilla's *Santa Isabel, Reina de Portugal*. In it, the character Tarabilla, who is making fun of astrology, makes a long speech that includes predictions for the year to come. After the predictions, and as if reading from a book, he lectures on physiognomy:

> *Rey*: And you say you are a great expert in this matter of astrology?
> *Tarabilla*: Very much so, and to show you, here are some prognostications. [...]
> The third chapter is on physiognomy.[61]

As in Lope's *El amigo por fuerza*, physiognomy is treated as nearly a sub-discipline of astrology. Tarabilla not only pokes fun at astrological-physiognomic assertions, but also parodies the style of astrologers' annual prognostications. The object of this parody can be found in works such as Jerónimo Cortés's popular

---

su vida los sucesos / escribe naturaleza. / Supe la fisonomía, / muda que habla por señas, / pues por las del rostro dice / la inclinación mas secreta" (Ruiz de Alarcón, *La cueva* 88).

[60] "*Hortensio*: Amores tiene. / *Lisaura*: ¿Sabéis vos dónde? / *Hortensio*: Sí, a fe. / *Lisaura*: ¿Quién es? / *Hortensio*: Vuesa Señoría. / *Lisaura*: ¿Dícese en palacio? / *Hortensio*: No, que soy astrólogo yo, / y entiendo fisonomía" (Vega, *El amigo por fuerza* 967).

[61] "*Rey*: ¿En esto de astrología / diz que sois grande sujeto? / *Tarabilla*: Notable; y porque lo veáis, / pronósticos son aquestos. / [...] Va el capítulo tercero / de fisonomía" (Rojas Zorrilla, *Santa Isabel* 40, 42).

work on physiognomy, *Fisionomía y varios secretos de la naturaleza.* The book, first published in 1595, went through at least 15 editions during the sixteenth and seventeenth centuries. The first chapter of the work explains: "Those who have a very high forehead are liberal with their friends and connections; they are usually kind, happy, virtuous, and of good intelligence." Those with a low forehead, Cortés explains are, "naturally simple," "covetous," and "cruel." A wrinkled forehead indicates shamelessness and irritability.[62] Comparing Cortés's earnest *Fisionomía* with Tarabilla's verses, the parody becomes patent:

> *Tarabilla*: Marcelio says that those who have a small, wrinkled forehead will have a monkey's face, if they have small features. Those who have a syrupy mouth (I mean wet, like a pool), who sends pellets here and there, raining arguments and spitting concepts [...] if he was speaking about irrigated lands, he will end up in dry land. Item, those who are cross-eyed are worth two one-eyed persons, because you don't know which of the eyes is the blind one.[63]

The reference to "Marcelio" is a corruption of the name of Marsilio Ficino, whose *De vita* was also popular as a reference for physiognomic knowledge. References to Ficino in Lope de Vega's work, particularly in his novel *La Dorotea,* have been pointed out by Edwin S. Morby and others (Vega, *La Dorotea* 267–70, 327–8, 404, 406–8, 410).

The dramatic representation of questions related to astrological medicine and physiognomy contributed, undoubtedly, to the diffusion of concepts; even passages such as Tarabilla's parody reinforced the authority of texts on physiognomy by authors such as Marsilio Ficino and Giambattista della Porta. But the way the ideas appear on stage—without an extensive explanatory apparatus—suggests that the plays make reference to themes already known by the public. Whether or not the public was familiar with the particularities of a text by Ficino or Cortés, they probably knew a parody when they heard one.

---

[62] "De la frente. Los que tienen la frente muy levantada son liberales para con sus amigos, y conocidos, suelen ser tratables, alegres, virtuosos y de buen entendimiento. Los que tienen los extremos de la frente pequeños, naturalmente son simples, codiciosos y cortesanos, aunque de poco se ensañan presto, y son fáciles en el creer. Los que tienen la frente arrugada y entrada en medio son desvergonzados, enojadizos y de grande corazón, aunque simples y de varia fortuna" (Cortés, *Fisonomía* 5v).

[63] "El que tuviere el aspecto / con frente chica, y arrugas / en ella, dice Marcelio, / que tendrá cara de mico, / si tiene pequeño el gesto, / el que tuviere la boca / en almíbar (decir quiero / en humedad, como balsa) / con perdigones a trechos, / que va lloviendo razones, / y ya escupiendo conceptos, [...] si hablaba de regadío, / hablará en secano luego. / Ítem, el que fuere bizco / viene a valer por dos tuertos, / pues no se sabe de qué ojo / de los dos viene a ser ciego" (Rojas Zorrilla 42, 43).

Conclusion

As we have seen, astrological medicine was sometimes represented as an alternative to "normal" medicine, and sometimes treated as unremarkable. It could be satirized and parodied or considered seriously. But what references to medical astrology in early modern plays most clearly show is that there was a dramatic culture of astrological medicine. In some ways, this dramatic culture diverged from what we recognize as routine medical or astrological practice. At times, dramatists borrowed heavily from scholarly and non-scholarly astrological traditions. But consistently, the dramatic culture of astrological medicine is recognizable as such: part textual allusion, part reference to daily practices, and always part invention. It contains enough of what audiences might be expected to know about medical astrology to confirm their expectations; it diverges sufficiently from the quotidian realities of medical practice to avoid being tiresome.

By exploring the points of convergence and divergence between astrological medical practice and the dramatic culture of astrological medicine, I have tried to give a sense of the issues that appear with the greatest saliency in early modern plays: the question of free will, the influence of the stars on temperament, the origin of disease, the cultural status of specific astrological practices, and so on. Like the edicts concerning astrological prohibitions that were to be read before popular audiences, dramatic works reached a very wide audience: they were represented in streets, squares, theaters, and at court (Davis and Varey; Salomon). Understanding the ways in which astrological medicine was represented provides us with one more tool to gauge the diffusion of astrological concepts.

But the significance of the dramatic culture of astrological medicine does not lie in the degree to which it adheres to astrological or medical orthodoxy. It would be pointless to fashion an index of astrological literacy for playwrights based on their plays or criticize them for a lack of realism. The stage does not owe loyalty to the astrolabe. This is not to say that the dramatic culture of astrological medicine did not contribute to ongoing debates about astrology. By representing astrology as potentially distinct from medicine, plays such as *Lo que ha de ser* may have focused attention on the astrological practices of physicians in unwelcome ways. In other words, the dramatic culture of astrological medicine may have been antagonistic to the daily practice of astrological medicine, at least in some instances. Creating a distinction on stage could lead the audience to differentiate the practices. Plays such as *El bobo del colegio* emphasize the supernatural aspects of astrology, placing it in the traditions of popular medical culture but out of the realm of "official" medicine. A number of plays raise the possibility that there could be medicine without astrology. In other instances plays reinforced the claims of astrologers and physicians. By assuming that there were parts of astrology that were *natural* and that stars influenced the complexion of the bodies, as in *De una causa dos efectos*, plays reinforced the basic idea that there was a relationship between astrological influences and medical knowledge. What playwrights such as Lope de Vega, Pedro Calderón de la Barca, and others do consistently, however, is disseminate the terms of the debate about astrology that was taking place among cultural elites. This continues to be the function of these dramatic works today: living in the twenty-first century, we are probably more likely to learn that the "stars incline, they do not compel" from Calderón than from Ptolemy.

The second thing that we find consistently represented in plays is the cultural ambiguity of astrology. Astrological medicine was a medical culture with many literary faces, just as it had many faces across social and scientific contexts. Early modern astrology walked a fine line between acceptance and rejection, between legitimate science and esoteric superstition. It is significant that what we see in the plays is a similarly ambiguous cultural status. Astrology, placed in between the realms of academic knowledge and popular culture, can be represented emphasizing one or the other aspect.

Of course, plays are not under any obligation to rescue astrological knowledge or portray scientific reality for us. The dramatic needs of the plays—and not scholarly agendas—determine the particular ways in which astrological medicine is represented. But simply because drama trumps science does not mean that the way science is represented is *necessarily* inaccurate. In a limbo between academic knowledge and popular culture, astrology could be represented in many ways. Sometimes the ideas of astrological medicine are related to divinatory arts and popular practitioners, to magic and the supernatural. Sometimes the astrological information is treated as trustworthy and authoritative, making reference to scholarly works. Depending, of course, on the temperament of the playwright.

Chapter 10

The Theological Drama of Chymical Medicine in Early Modern Spain

John Slater

Introduction

In November of 1681 a touring actor named Damián Polop arrived in Zaragoza with a painful ulceration in his side that was inflamed by the journey. He made his way to the hospital of Nuestra Señora de la Gracia, where surgeons told him that the cure—to be achieved by repeated bleedings—would take two and a half months. Polop must have panicked at the thought of weeks of lost wages. He was already a relatively important actor; earlier in 1681 he spent July 6–17 at court staging three plays for the king and queen (Shergold and Varey 145). Polop communicated his plight to Jaime Fernández de Híjar, Viceroy of Aragon. Híjar took an interest in the case, but did not send a renowned surgeon. Instead, he sent Juan de Vidós y Miró, a parish priest and, many would say, an ignorant empiric who proclaimed loudly that he was a follower of Oswald Croll (Crollius) and other early modern proponents of chymical or alchemical medicine. Vidós cured the actor in only five days; three days after that—on November 26, 1681—Polop was back on stage. Polop went on to enjoy a brilliant career, staging plays at court by Calderón and Francisco Bances Candamo (well known for his "chymical" plays, such as *El gran chymico del mundo* and *La piedra filosofal*).[1] For his part, Vidós continued practicing medicine—although he had no formal training—and published an account of Polop's cure in a book that vigorously attacked the methods of academic physicians and proposed new "chymical" remedies, entitled *Medicina y cirugía racional y espagírica* (1691).[2]

---

[1] By November 1681, Polop had already appeared in Pedro Calderón de la Barca's *Los alimentos del hombre*, and either *El tesoro escondido* or *El segundo blasón del Austria* (Arellano and Pinillos 12). By June 26, 1690, Polop was staging Calderón's lavish spectacle *Fieras afemina amor* for King Charles II and his new wife, Mariana von Neuburg. Polop must have become a favorite with the queen, because he staged *La púrpura de la rosa* for her birthday on October 28, 1694 (Wilson 19).

[2] There are two sources for this account. One is a brief pamphlet entitled *Súplica de Juan de Vidós al Justicia de Aragón* (no page no.), written sometime after 1681; and second, a markedly less detailed but more widely disseminated version in Vidós y Miró's *Primera parte de Medicina y Cirugia racional y espagirica* [...] (225–6).

The story of Polop's cure and Vidós's role in it was familiar enough in Spanish presses at the time: self-proclaimed paladin of chymical medicine triumphs over credulous exponents of an obsolete, rational-dogmatic Galenism. The antagonism between proponents of chymical medicine and Galenists, such as Vidós's great rival Nicolás Moneva, was the great medical drama of the 1670s and 1680s. It was a clash of medical cultures. But the fact that Vidós publicized his cure of an actor is not inconsequential: the language of the Paracelsians that Vidós favored could be overtly theatrical, if often in a conventional way. Croll, for example, called the "universal spirit" the "The Theater of the secrets of all Natur's Light" (*Philosophy Reformed* 203).[3] Vidos was more interested in the way that Croll articulated the centrality of chymistry to medicine than the dramatic possibilities of Croll's sometimes overheated rhetoric. Among Vidós's supporters in Zaragoza, however, the idea that in this theater of the world the "spiritual nature" of substances—what Juan Bautista Juanini, echoing Croll, called "the soul of the World," or the "universal spirit"—was theatrically disguised, even costumed in vestments, had the value of a chymical and *theological* truth (Juanini 129).

The three parties involved in Polop's cure—the viceroy, the priest, and the actor—represent the three fields—political power, religion, and drama—that come into uneasy contact in the controversies surrounding chymical medicine.[4] The practice of chymical medicine touched upon the privileges of civic and ecclesiastical powers in ways that are more or less clear; kings and municipal officials alike concerned themselves with the regulation of all sorts of medical practice—academic and extra-academic—and a confessor's concern with the spiritual health of his charge naturally led to at least some interest in the means by which physical health might be preserved. The role of drama in all of this, however, is somewhat more complicated.

As Félix de Lucio Espinosa y Malo pointed out, stagecraft was a perfection of natural philosophy; it was natural magic (241). But apart from the science of dramatic illusions, the stage provided a metaphysical model that could be used to explain the nature of matter and Eucharistic theology just as easily as it did the vicissitudes of life. As Fernando R. de la Flor suggests, interest in the Stoic notion of the "world as stage," placed in the service of an attempt to elucidate

---

3   "Theatrum secretorum Luminis Naturae totius" (Croll, *Basilica chymica* 195).

4   The intersections of power and alchemy and the dramatic implications of alchemical imagery are well understood, thanks to Mar Rey Bueno and Frederick de Armas, among many others. Less understood is the crucial role that priests and friars played in enabling the practice and, in some instances, the development of chymical medicine in early modern Spain. Mar Rey Bueno's scholarship on alchemy at the court of the Hapsburg kings is a tremendous influence on my work; see, for example, *Los señores del fuego*; to name but two of Frederick de Armas's extraordinary studies of alchemical imagery in seventeenth-century Spanish drama, see "El sol sale a medianoche" and "The King's Son and the Golden Dew."

the operations of nature, was one of the defining features of seventeenth-century Spanish theology and philosophy (146–7). Ecclesiastics in Spain and chymists across Europe drew on a lexicon of costuming, representing, and dramatic revelation to explain the material world; theology and chymical medicine found common ground in the language of theater. So, preachers were drawn to chymical medicine because it offered a symbolic and metaphysical lexicon that they found useful.[5] Their interest, however, went beyond the rhetorical. Working largely behind the scenes, preachers such as Luis Pueyo y Abadía played an important role in legitimating the claims of serious physicians who advocated chymical medicine, as well as the work of flamboyant empirics that appropriated some of chymistry's more esoteric claims.

The texts of empirics and serious physicians alike give us evidence that priests and friars, in their capacity as confessors and convent officials, were able to promote chymical remedies, give practitioners of chymical medicine access to patients, and facilitate the publication of works on chymical medicine. In this chapter, I argue that they did so largely because the language of chymistry had a theatrical dimension that resonated with contemporaneous theology. We know that during the late seventeenth century, preachers and friars were fascinated by the language and imagery of alchemy and hermeticism. Juan de Mora nearly makes Hermes the patron of preachers, explaining that the etymology of "Hermes" was "sermón" (195), and Raymundo Asensio, a friar of the Order of Our Lady of Mercy, claimed that the etymology of "mercy" was Mercury (6).[6] What has not been explored is how the theological or rhetorical inclinations of preachers related to the practice of chymical medicine.

There is still a tendency to understand the Spanish Baroque as obsessed with "desengaño" or disillusionment, and for this reason opposed to scientific modernity, quantification, and so on. Representative of this line of reasoning is Sigmund Méndez's contention that the characteristics of the Spanish Baroque, and particularly the allegorizing bent in Spanish philosophy and theology, condemned Spain to "live apart from scientific and industrial modernity, in a paralyzing limbo distant from the terrestrial paradise of progress" (159).[7] Where strains of scientific modernity did make inroads into Spain, however, they were abetted by the very tendencies of the Spanish Baroque that have too often been labeled anti-scientific.

---

[5]   Ralph Bauer's chapter in this volume explores sixteenth-century uses of alchemical language, specifically in the context of American natural history.

[6]   Asensio's work is of interest not only because he places Mercedarians under a Hermetic sign, but also because the *aprobación* is written by Jerónimo Monterde, whose exercises in gematria were exceptionally well developed.

[7]   "vivir fuera de la modernidad científica e industrial, en un limbo inmovilizador fuera del paraíso terrenal del progreso."

Setting the Stage: Sermons and Science

During the first half of the seventeenth century, Spanish authors of devotional and theological texts sometimes responded to scientific and medical controversies with little more than a shrug. Hortensio Félix Paravicino dispassionately preached on the corruptibility of the heavens, citing the supernova in Cassiopeia famously observed by Tycho Brahe in 1572; the preacher said that the Church, like the heavens, once seemed inalterable and now, in the wake of Luther, was known to be altogether mutable (16v). Paravicino found it sad, but incontestable. Considering the differences between Aristotelian and alchemical physics, Juan Eusebio Nieremberg phlegmatically declared that the varying models could be easily reconciled; if the Aristotelians claimed there were four elements (earth, air, water, and fire) and the alchemists claimed three (salt, mercury, and sulfur), then it was simply best to add them up and say that there were seven (318).[8] Nieremberg's argument was actually fairly subtle—the elements of the philosophers were modes of the alchemists' *tria prima*—and his ideas were perhaps not so far from those of "heretics" such as Croll, but Nieremberg saw no need to gin up debate by naming controversial figures.[9] On the whole, and with notable exceptions, the texts motivated by religious devotion published during the first half of the seventeenth century treated developments in science and medicine as adiaphora, neither heretical nor orthodox. As Víctor Navarro Brotóns showed in the case of the Spanish reception of Copernicus, readers by and large took what they found useful and "passed over" the "controversial aspects" (53).

The last decades of the seventeenth century would find an important change in the works of Spanish preachers and theologians. Rather than coolly considering scientific ideas, many authors of religious texts, particularly preachers, enthusiastically explored the more arcane areas of scientific, mathematical, and medical inquiry. In an earlier study, I demonstrated the rhetorical similarities between the sermons of Manuel de Guerra y Ribera and Juan de Cabriada's chymico-medical polemic ("Rereading"). Far from being limited to a narrow conception of alchemy and chymical medicine, however, early modern Spanish sermons explore nearly every manifestation of what Michael T. Walton has called "chemical philosophy": "the conjunction of alchemical, Neoplatonic/ Neo-Pythagorean, Kabbalistic ideas developed by Paracelsus and like-minded

---

[8]   Ralph Bauer's chapter in this book examines the relationship of Aristotelian and alchemical natural philosophy in greater detail.

[9]   As I explain below, Croll would become a highly controversial figure in the last decades of the seventeenth century. Nieremberg's argument also recalls the work of Quercetanus (Joseph Duchesne), who may have endorsed ideas that were officially considered heterodox in Spain, but who never incited much actual controversy. In the *Plaza universal de todas las ciencias y artes* (1615), for example, Cristóbal Suárez de Figueroa lists Quercetanus as one of the reliable authorities that apothecaries should consult, alongside Galen, Pliny, Nicolás Monardes, and Pietro Andrea Mattioli (304).

natural philosophers" (xii).[10] Félix de Aguirre preached on mathematical conceits deeply influenced by Christian Cabbala in his *Enigmas Sacros Panegiricos* (1689) and structured another sermon—*Mesa soberana del sol y de las aves* (1690)— around alchemy and geometry.[11] Manuel Sánchez del Castellar y Arbustante, for his part, specialized in sermons built around concepts taken from mathematics and gematria; gematria and Christian Cabbala feature prominently in his *Gramática consagrada* (1676) and *Triángulo de Perfecciones* (1691), while his *Sacro enigma* (1679) contains a detailed explanation of perfect numbers. Perfect numbers, Arbustante explains, are integers equal to the sum of their factors or divisors; 6 is a perfect number because the sum of its factors (1, 2, and 3) is 6.[12] Arbustante correctly cites 6, 28, 496, and 8,128 as perfect numbers. Given the complexity and abstruseness of these sermons, one might reasonably think that their recondite mentions of science and medicine impinged very little on the world of scientific and medical practice.

But the activities of priests, friars, and other church officials have long been central to the way that we understand the medical and scientific developments of the final decades of the seventeenth century (Rey Bueno, "El debate").[13] Throughout the seventeenth century, friars contributed serious works to the body of alchemical and medical literature, such as Esteban Núñez's *Miropolio general y racional de botica*, made available in a marvelous edition by Miguel López Pérez and Mar Rey Bueno. The work of ecclesiastics is easy to caricature, however, and the reasons for this are not difficult to understand. During the 1680s and 1690s, many earnest physicians—most famously Juan Bautista Juanini and Juan de Cabriada—struggled to introduce recent developments in chymical medicine to Spain. These modernizing physicians came to be known as *novatores*. The repercussions of their efforts extended far beyond medicine because new chymical understandings of the human body and its functions implied changes to classical models of nature and its operations. At the fringes of the efforts of the *novatores*, a number of empirics, many of whom were priests or friars, seized upon the growing

---

[10]   Walton's "chymical philosophy" is more akin to Hugh Trevor-Roper's notion of Paracelsanism as a "total philosophy" (195) than Allen Debus's more focused (i.e. more specifically "chymical") notion of "chymical philosophy" (*The Chemical Philosophy*).

[11]   To mention one instance of Aguirre's alchemical enthusiasms in the *Mesa soberana*, he explains Christ's statement in Matthew 5.13 that "you are the salt of the earth" in alchemical terms: "according to the alchemists (Quimicos) salt is the origin of all minerals [...]" (13). The influence of the Hermetic Corpus on this sermon is pronounced.

[12]   The anonymous *Aplausos al día seis de Noviembre, natal de Carlos II* [...] (c.1673) makes the explanation of perfect numbers sound positively mystical: "Goza el Número seis, por la igualdad que en el se considera, o dividido en dos medias partes, o en ternos, de la calidad de perfecto integralmente. Por lo qual lo señalado con él, se juzga siempre y se experimenta feliz" (no page number).

[13]   Rey Bueno makes the important point that Alderete's detractors, such as Juan Guerrero and Andrés Gámez, knew a great deal more about Hermetic philosophy than Alderete himself ("El debate," 351–2).

popularity of chymical language and used it to promote "universal remedies" and nearly miraculous cures.

Figures such as Buenaventura Angeleres, a Franciscan, and Luis Alderete y Soto, a lay official of the Inquisition, combined the esoteric language of traditional alchemy and the fervent anti-classical critique of the *novatores* to create a discourse of popular, pseudo-chymical mysticism. Neither Angeleres, nor Vidós, nor Alderete were trained physicians, and their medical claims ranged from the relatively modest (in the case of Vidós) to the decidedly extravagant (in the case of Alderete). Frequently, their motivations were ostensibly to aid the poor by offering home remedies that could be made cheaply and used for a variety of purposes.[14] But these wholesome impulses were almost always leavened with a strong dose of self-promotion (Rey Bueno, *Los señores* 15).

Vidós is often seen as simply a *pseudoquimico* and an "ignorante curandero," lumped together with some of the more flamboyant mountebanks of his day (Hernández Morejón, VI: 86). In reality Vidós was an extra-academic medical practitioner who published a collection of medical recipes—some chymical, some not—and anecdotes that we would today recognize as a book of secrets (Leong and Rankin). Some of his recipes, such as Queen of Hungary's Water, are classics of the genre (Vidós, *Primera parte* 428–32). At the same time, Vidós made it very clear that he was the intellectual heir to the French Paracelsians, Johannes Hartmann, and especially Oswald Croll.[15]

Vidós calls Croll "mi maestro," but the content of the citations amounts to little more than unremarkable defenses of chymical medicine, taken from Croll's *Basilica chymica* (Vidós, *Primera parte* 201). Some of the citations of Croll are accurate enough to make one believe that Vidós actually consulted the *Basilica chymica* with some care. Other citations are impossible to locate verbatim. The same passage—beginning "*Medicina & Chimica no possunt separari* […]"— appears three times (12, 244, 393). In the end, there is no reason to doubt Vidós's assertion that he consults Croll in manuscript—"mi maestro dice muchas veces en sus manuscriptos […]"—but the decision to do so in such a public way is telling (244). Attacks on Alderete's "agua de la vida" had already singled out mentions of the "heretic" Croll for special censure, so Vidós could be sure that even his perfunctory citations would engender hostility (Delgado de la Vera 28).

---

[14]　　Enrique Perdiguero explains that works such as Vidós's *Medicina y Cirugía Racional y Espagírica* responded to "charitable motives" because they provided "easy and inexpensive methods for self-treatment of illness" (170).

[15]　　The passage that Vidós cites most often is considerably altered from Croll's original. Vidós, in a number of instances, attributes the following to Croll: *Medicina & Chimica no possunt separari, hoc opus, hic labor, quia absque Chimica cognitione, nec Theorica, neque Practica medicina esse potest.* Croll's original is: "Absque Alchymiae cognitione neque Theorica neque Practica Medicina esse potest" (*Basilica Chymica* 84). The "hoc opus, hic labor" passage—which Croll took from Virgil—appears earlier on the same page; it may be that Vidós liked the allusion enough to summarize Croll freely.

What is most surprising about Vidós's interest in Croll is what Vidós does not cite. As a rule, Vidós is not interested in mystical speculation, the promise of universal remedies or panaceas, divination, or prognostication, and demonstrates few of the rhetorical excesses of some of his contemporaries (most obviously Alderete). In fact, Vidós disputes the assertion—made by Croll and Alderete—that there might exist a universal remedy or miraculous panacea; Vidós declares flatly that "it is impossible to cure all disease with a single remedy": "con un remedio [...] es imposible curar todas las enfermedades" (*Manifiesto* no page no.). Vidós does, however, invoke a more esoteric tone when he speaks of the sources of his knowledge. In addition to the mysteriously mentioned manuscripts, Vidós claims to have spent from May 27 to June 11, 1671, with an unnamed French chymist, who taught him many of the remedies listed in the *Medicina y Cirugia racional* and many others that remain secret: "otros muchos que no ha manifestado" (*Manifiesto* no page no.). It is at least possible that Vidós did in fact meet someone of the generation of Moyse Charas (1619–1698) or Sébastien Matte La Faveur (1626–1714). What is easier to confirm is that Vidós began practicing medicine shortly thereafter (by 1672) and was awarded a papal dispensation to continue practicing without a medical license as an act of charity on February 4, 1673.

There is very little evidence that Vidós sought money, but he did seek fame; in this sense he can be compared to another author of books of secrets: Leonardo Fioravanti. Of course, Vidós was neither as successful as Fioravanti nor as talented, but what William Eamon says of Fioravanti is true of Vidós as well: "there is reason to believe that Fioravanti's main aim was not to garner patronage, but to craft a public image" ("How to Read" 31). Eamon goes on to explain that Fioravanti was "a genius at it." It would be a mistake to think of Vidós as a genius. But like Fioravanti, Vidós published recipes that demanded "equipment that only a specialist, such as a pharmacist or an alchemical adept, would have access to" ("How to Read" 32). Vidós takes some pride in making secrets public; his cure for gangrene had been held as a "grande secreto." But the word "secret" itself is used sparingly, as are terms such as "miraculous" or "nearly miraculous" (*Primera parte* 419).

Theology and Theater in a Chymical World

By 1679 at the very latest, one could buy chymical remedies at established prices in Zaragoza. The *Tarifa y arancel de medicinas* published prices for chymical medicines and products ranging from "Olaei tartari" to "spiritus vitrioli," "spiritus salis nitri," "salis tartari," and even potable gold: "Auri potabl[is]" (no page no.). Despite the existence of an established, regulated market for chymical remedies, the intransigent Galenists of Zaragoza, particularly Nicolás Moneva, continued to protest in print and in the courts.[16] Rey Bueno and López Pérez show that the debates over alchemical and chymical medicine in Madrid and Seville were frequently unrelated to medical practice; chymical remedies had been used throughout Spain without controversy for decades (López Pérez and Rey Bueno, 282). The spirited pamphlets published in the course of medical debates—many of which are held at the Biblioteca Histórico-Médica in Valencia—make it easy to forget that Juan de Vidós was advocating the use of chymical remedies that, far from being strange or exotic, were already familiar goods for sale.[17] At the same time, the fervent, even reactionary Moneva—who at least for a time served in the capacity of substitute first physician (*protomédico*) of the kingdom of Aragon—maintained a sustained attack on Vidós, in part because of the chymical nature of the therapies Vidós advocated. It was across this uneven topography of acceptance and resistance that Vidós made his way.

One of Vidós's most direct confrontations with Moneva occurred in 1682. In late July of that year, Michaela Verges, a Carmelite nun living in the Convent of the Incarnation of Zaragoza, fell gravely ill (Vidós, *Memorial* 5–7). For over a week she suffered from terrible abdominal pain, diarrhea, and nausea. She was unable to sleep. Verges was attended by two physicians, one of whom was Moneva. But neither physician was able to do anything to ease Michaela's discomfort. Finally, on the morning of July 29, Moneva spoke privately with a representative of the Carmelite Order and advised that sister Michaela's confessor be called. The physicians spoke frankly with the confessor, who was Luis Pueyo y Abadía, telling him that sister Michaela was suffering from incurable, internal inflammation. But Pueyo did not do what we would expect and certainly did not do what Michaela's physicians expected. Namely, he did not prepare his charge for extreme unction. In fact, at this point in the story there is a very curious lapse, but it appears that Pueyo himself asked for the assistance of Vidós. This must have infuriated Moneva.

Thanks to Pueyo, Michaela was provided with an oil or balsam of Vidós's making, which was to be rubbed on her stomach. Later that same day, Vidós himself visited sister Michaela for the first time and declared that she was not suffering from internal inflammation, as Moneva claimed, but from *external* inflammation. Pueyo's role in the drama would subsequently become even more complicated. The two physicians returned, but declined to see their patient while Vidós was present. So Pueyo tactfully called Vidós away, stating that there were other nuns he wanted Vidós to visit. This began a back and forth between Michaela's physicians and

---

[16]   To be sure, Moneva's dispute withVidós had at least as much to do with the fact that Vidós practiced medicine without formal education—in violation of physicians' guild protections—as it had to do with *res chymicae*.

[17]   The marvelous volume bound as "Coleccion de Documentos Relativos a los Medicos, Cirujanos y Boticarios de Aragon" (call number C-31) at the Biblioteca Histórico-Medica contains many of the printed documents that are relevant to this study. As always, I am indebted to the generosity of the staff at the Instituto de Historia de la Medicina y de la Ciencia López Piñero who facilitated my access to the documents.

Vidós, each visiting the patient and prescribing contrary medicines, each warning that the treatments of his adversary would lead to death. The written account of this medical duel ends shortly thereafter and, oddly enough, without resolution. We are told simply that because the convent was so large, the events were well known and do not need to be recounted. The case history of Michaela Verges served Vidós as yet another example of the contest between old and new, between his own modernizing, humane medicine and the recalcitrance of Moneva and the Galenists bent on bleeding patients at every opportunity. But while the account ends here, the larger story continues in illustrative ways.

These events became the basis for a case history in a book written by Vidós himself, the *Memorial y manifiesto*, published in 1683. The publisher of the book was Gaspar Martínez, a former patient of Vidos's who went on to become the "Impressor en el Hospital Real y General de N. Señora de Gracia," or the official printer of the very hospital where Polop had been treated.[18] Pueyo himself wrote the *aprobación*. This means that not only was Pueyo a major character in sister Michaela's particular case history, but he also represented, at least in part, the legal authority by which the book was then published. Pueyo makes it possible for Vidós to treat the patient in the first place and then to publish the account.

Pueyo was a significant figure in the intellectual life of Zaragoza during the late seventeenth century (De la Flor, "La máquina"). In 1687, Pueyo signed an *aprobación* for the physician Francisco de Elcarte (who was a student of the renowned physician José Lucas Casalete). In other words, during the 1680s Pueyo had a history of helping Vidós and those we have become accustomed to calling "pseudo-quimicos," as well as Elcarte, Casalete, and the *verdaderos yatroquimicos* or true students of chymical medicine. Pueyo probably knew beforehand that he was running a risk in helping Vidós. In the medical debates of the period, every aspect of a published work was examined and subject to attack. Josef Martínez de las Casas had been vehemently criticized by Justo Delgado de la Vera simply for having signed an *aprobación* to a work that defended Alderete.[19]

---

[18]   Vidos reveals that Martínez was his patient, as well has his publisher in the *Súplica*. Although the *Súplica* does not contain explicit publication information, Vidós explains that Martínez walked without a limp after having his toes crushed, thanks to Vidós (4). It does not seem that Gaspar Martínez becomes the official printer of the hospital until the eighteenth century, when he publishes Martín de Ezpeleta's *Libro de cuentas extraordinarias* in 1704. Manuel Jiménez Catalán explains that being the hospital's printer could be very lucrative (34).

[19]   The work defending Alderete was Luis Amigo y Bertrán's *Apologia en defensa de la medicina substancial y universal del Agua de la Vida* (1682). Delgado de la Vera does not name Josef Martínez de las Casas, but he gives us enough information about Martínez to place him, noting that he is "Examinador Sinodal" (a position Martínez held) but faulting him for failing to "examinar algunas proposiciones fundadas en autoridades de la Sagrada Escritura" (28). Delgado de la Vera's critique is meticulous and withering; he begins by examining the first of Martínez's citations (Sixtus of Siena) and analyzing the aptness of the quotation.

So what inducements could there have been for a theologian and preacher like Pueyo to get caught up in the medical debates of his time?

Pueyo is very clear that part of his distaste for Galenism—and his corresponding interest in chemical medicine—has to do with language. Pueyo points out that the new way of curing was also a new way of talking; gone was the violent language of "cutting," "pulling out," "cutting open," "sawing," "lancing," and so on, to be replaced with the sweet, peaceful language of chymistry: "moistening," "washing," "refreshing," and "calming."[20] In this sense, Pueyo's medical and linguistic sensibilities were very like those of Joan Baptista van Helmont, one of the most influential chymists of the seventeenth century. Van Helmont, explains Allen Debus, rejected the Galenic model based on the "warfare" of "opposites to produce a mean." "Rather," thought Van Helmont, "we should seek health in harmony [...]" (Debus, *The French Paracelsians* 114). So chymical medicine represented a lexical shift that might be attractive to chymists and theologians for the same reasons: it permitted a language of gentleness rather than brutality.

Other, even more suggestive reasons for Pueyo's support surface in the published attacks on Vidós. Hippocrates had denounced bad physicians and those who would pose as doctors by saying that they were "like tragic actors." Hippocrates explained, "Many are physicians by reputation and in name, but few are physicians in reality."[21] One anonymous attack on Vidós extended this commonplace in the language of the contemporaneous stage:

> An actor takes the stage dressed as the emperor and for the time that he walks the boards in this guise we take him for Cesar. He exits. The same actor enters again and plays the role of lawyer, physician, or notary. He exits and enters, playing different roles all the while and the actor is neither emperor, physician, lawyer, nor notary; such are these doctors of whom Hippocrates complains, who see themselves as now a surgeon, now an apothecary, and now a physician [...].[22]

---

[20]   "Ya en adelante no será horroroso el vocabulario de la Cirugía; pues por aquellas vozes de cortar [sic], arranca, abre, sierra, pica, punza, abrasa, se oirán otras halagüeñas de moja, lava, limpia, refresca, enjuga, templa. En el vocabulario antiguo, solía ser más terrible la Cura que el tumor [...]" (Vidós, *Primera parte* "Aprobación"). This passage is actually a paraphrase of one of the more famous commonplaces of Spanish medical satire. The original is by Francisco de Quevedo: "corta, arranca, abre, asierra, despedaza, pica, punza, ajigota, rebana, descarna y abrasa" (*Sueños* 321). This passage would not only be repeated nearly verbatim by Francisco Santos—studied by Enrique García Santo-Tomás in this volume—but also would be cited in the entry for "rebanar" in the *Diccionario de autoridades* (Santos, *El rey gallo* 126). In essence, Pueyo harnesses the language of medical satire in order to authorize new practices.

[21]   "Simillimi enim huiuismodi Medici sunt personis, quae tragoediis introducuntur [...] Sic et medici fama quidem, et nomine multi, re autem, et opere valde pauci" (Fonseca 71).

[22]   "Un comediante ya sale vestido de Emperador y el rato que pisa las tablas con esta representación le tenemos por la Magestad Cesárea. Vase. Sale el mismo y haze papel de Abogado, Médico o Escribano. Enojase y sale otra y otras vezes con diferentes papeles y ni el representante es Emperador, Médico, Abogado ni Escribano, pues así son estos Médicos

In this comparison, theater is a place in which seeming is opposed to being and Vidós is nothing more than an actor. But Pueyo believed that theater reflected a metaphysical reality and that *no one* is anything but an actor. "What do you think the world is?" asks Pueyo, as if in response to the attacks on Vidós. "It is a great theater. And men, what do you think they are? Different roles played on this great stage of the world."[23] Pueyo even goes on to mention Calderón, the playwright behind so many of Polop's successes (*Proporciones predicables* 131). Pueyo developed his ideas extensively, explaining that Mary might be the mother of Christ and a queen in heaven and at the same time the handmaiden of God: "What do actors do in the theater? They are private citizens and they play the role of king. They are free and represent slaves. This is what Mary does in the mystery of the Incarnation: she was queen and mother [...] and played the role of handmaiden."[24]

Pueyo and Vidós's anonymous detractor are quite obviously talking about different things when they speak of the stage. But whether theater was likened to falsehood or a transcendental reality, acting and representing became central to the way that debates about chymical medicine unfolded. This went deeper than a consideration of the spectacular aspects of medical practice. For many ecclesiastics who supported the new medicine—whether it was peddled by mountebanks or authorized by physicians—chymistry offered an appealing stock of images that emphasized the unreliability of sensory perception and a reality beyond our direct knowing.

In the medical works of Joan Baptista van Helmont and others, chymistry revealed efficient principles by stripping away "vestments" and "masks." For example, Walter Pagel summarizes Van Helmont's thinking in strikingly dramatic terms: "Gas becomes manifest when a solid body is made to relinquish its 'vestments,' the husk or shell that conceals its essential (spiritual) nature. This is accomplished by burning the vestments away, *per ignem,* an 'undressing' performed by the chemist or by nature [...]" (62). This language was not very different from Pueyo's characterization of Mary as handmaiden. For many seventeenth-century theologians, theatricality could be imagined to pervade matter itself. When Croll explains that the universal spirit is "The *Theater* of the secrets of all Natur's Light," he deploys a dramatic idiom that to Spanish theologians would be one of chymical medicine's most intriguing features (*Philosophy Reformed* 203; emphasis mine). Pueyo tacitly acknowledges his own chymico-dramatic fascinations while praising Vidós's "discovery" of chymical medicine; calling Vidós the Columbus

---

quien se queja Hipócrates, que ya les verán Cirujanos, ya boticarios, ya Médicos [...]" (*Respuesta a las razones* no page no.).

[23] "¿Qué pensáis, que es la tierra? Un teatro grande de Comedia. ¿Qué pensáis, que son los hombres? Diferentes papeles de este Comedión grande de el Mundo" (Pueyo, *Proporciones predicables* 119).

[24] "¿Qué hazen los Representantes en el teatro? Son personas particulares, y representan la persona del Rey. Son libres, y representan la persona de un Esclavo: pues assí obra MARIA en el Misterio de la Encarnación: era Reyna, y Madre [...] y MARÍA representa el papel de Esclava" (*Proporciones predicables* 119).

and Vasco de Gama of his time, Pueyo conspicuously cites a verse from Francisco Bances Candamo's play entitled *Sangre, valor y fortuna*.[25] This is at roughly the same time (c.1690) that Bances Candamo is composing *La piedra filosofal* (*The Philosopher's Stone*).

Central to discussions about the theatricality of matter was the Eucharist. The consecrated Host, when taken not as exceptional but as a concrete object that was illustrative of humankind's perceptual limitations, was a source of frequent preoccupation for philosophers and theologians alike. Considering the Eucharist led Descartes to consider the "surface" (superficie) of objects a substantial mode; the surface of an object might be only the sensible boundary of the object, but the surface or attribute, according to Descartes, has the properties of substance, such as extension and duration (Bourg). Leibniz's explanation of transubstantiation—and the *vinculum substantiale* superadded to monads in order to constitute compound bodies—is another attempt to explain the how the material properties of bread might substantially obscure the body of Christ (Look).

Religious leaders had always found it hard to explain the nature of the Eucharist to believers. It was the material locus of mystery and faith, particularly after Trent. Pedagogical texts and devotional enchiridions such as Francisco Bermúdez de Pedraza's *Historia eucharistica* (1643) usually stressed two related problems. First, the real presence of Christ's body was hidden. (There was, however, continued reluctance on the part of philosophers and theologians alike to accept that there was nothing substantial or material in the means by which Christ's presence was hidden.) The second problem was related to believers' knowledge of the real presence; it was always taught that Christ's transubstantiated body could not under any temporal circumstances be made available to rational apprehension. Aquinas even argued that the living Christ himself could not see his own presence in the Eucharist (FitzPatrick 167–8). Bermúdez addressed these two problems—how Christ's presence was hidden and how we could know—in representative ways. To explain how we might understand transubstantiation, Bermúdez, like Aquinas, distinguished between reason and intellect; we could not arrive at knowledge about the consecrated Host through reason or the senses ("no es misterio que alcanza la razón"), but the Host could be the object of intellection (Bermúdez de Pedraza 7v). His answer as to *how* presence was hidden indicates a developing trend during the seventeenth century. He says, with a curiously material image, that Christ was hidden "beneath a white veil of bread" (7v).

---

25   Pueyo's citation of Bances is the italicized octosyllabic line in the following: "ya hoy ha descubierto *El Cabo de esta Esperança* tantos siglos oculto este nuevo vasso [sic] de Gama de la Cirugia [...]." Other than the title of the book, mentioned at the beginning of the *aprobación*, and one citation in Latin, these are the only italicized words. My citation of *Sangre, valor y fortuna* is from Ignacio Arellano's "El entremés de *Las visiones* de Bances Candamo" (31). This passage does not appear in García Castañón's edition of *Sangre, valor y fortuna*.

This "bread as veil" was represented by Calderón a number of times; for example, Cupid veiled before Psyche became an allegory of the Eucharist.[26] While it might simply seem as if the material prop (the veil) allegorized an accident (the species of bread) that was without substance, the language of seventeenth-century theology and religious instruction muddies the water. In fact, Calderón was only representing a theatrical trope that was already widely used in devotional texts. As the Eucharist increasingly served as an example of all substance, the matter that illuminated all matter, the metaphors that theologians chose to explain the species of bread and wine became accordingly material (as they did for Descartes and Leibniz).

The idea that Christ was "disguised" (*disfrazado*) as bread in the Eucharist was already present in Teresa of Ávila's *Camino de perfección* (1585), and the terminology of disguise, especially the use of the word "disfrazado," had grown in popularity by the time Cristóbal Moreno published his *Jornadas para el Cielo* some 10 years later (265). By the 1630s, the remarkable editorial success of Diego Niseno's *Asuntos predicables*—José Simón Díaz counts 18 editions and reissues between 1627 and 1634 alone (64–6)—marked a turning point in the popularity of the language of disguise. For Niseno, the Eucharist was not only "*disfrazado*," under veils (*velos*) and covers (*reboços*), but also had taken on more explicitly theatrical language: Christ awaited the faithful behind a curtain (*cortina*) of bread (Niseno 40). The theatricalization of Eucharistic language was fully realized by 1695, when Pedro Ortiz de Moncada could say that human spirit, itself a kind of non-rational apprehension, was capable of stripping itself of the effects of materiality in order to draw back the curtain of bread and reveal the divine "leading man" (*galán*), who was no longer disguised by the accident or species of bread.[27] What Calderón brought to the stage was the literal representation of explanations of Eucharistic theology such as this; the idea that Christ played the part of bread was as much a theological as a dramatic convention.

Pueyo dedicated two sermons to the theatricality of human existence and the idea that identity was illusory in a *theatrum mundi*. Both appeared in his *Proporciones predicables en fiestas de María Santíssima, y del Patriarca San Joseph* (1694). The arguments he presented for the importance of theater ranged from the pedestrian— that actors venerated Mary—to the ambitiously philosophical. He was particularly interested in the entrapments of fame and position, which he said were nothing more than shadows or costumes:

---

[26]   The image of the veil as allegory for the accident of bread in Calderón's plays has been studied by Vincent Martin (82–3; 109–14) and by Arellano (*Estructuras dramáticas* 217–18).

[27]   "lo que los sentidos no pueden por sí, como tan materiales, y groseros, el espíritu [...] se desnuda de toda la materialidad, corre la cortina, y le quita el emboço a este divino galán, disfraçado con los accidentes del pan [...]" (Ortiz de Moncada 147–8).

Christian Philosophy will not permit you to say that Charles V is king, because the royal person is only a visual and earthly representation that lasts no longer than it takes to represent a play, the play in which we are all present in the world, each of us playing the roles that divine providence has given us. Being a man is one thing, and being a duke is another. To be a man is to be ashes. To be a duke is only a bright and resplendent appearance.[28]

For Pueyo, as for Van Helmont, vestments that nature will one day strip away only temporarily hide a spiritual nature.

Even those who had little affection for theatergoing as a social phenomenon found utility in the language of the stage to describe the Eucharist. Juan Cortés Ossorio—who was an outspoken critic of theatrical spectacles—explained the Eucharist much as others did:

The wise philosopher cannot doubt that in the same way that vestments are distinct from bodies that clothe them, accidents are distinct from substances that adorn them; and if an earthly king might disguise himself by putting on the clothing that a field worker took off, why couldn't the king of heaven, if He liked, remove the accidents of bread from its substance, and dressing Himself in the accidents, represent the appearance of bread? Just look at how often those who represent something in the Theater of the World change their clothes [...][29]

The idea that substances disguise themselves in vestments, dressing and undressing according to the demands of the *theatrum mundi*, leaves us with the sense that the world and everything in it masquerades before our eyes.

The changing of accidents or appearances almost at whim is far from Van Helmont's chymical undressing of bodies through fire (*per ignem*), and no one would suggest that the husk of bread might be stripped away in the laboratory in order to yield the body of Christ. At the same time, however, it is not difficult to understand why Cortés Ossorio might be fascinated by the notion that Christ put on the accidents of bread as he might a suit, on the one hand, and the idea that the

---

[28]   "Pero nunca la Filosofía Christiana permitirá, que digas el hombre de Carlos es Rey, porque el ser de Persona Real es solo una vistosa representación temporal, que dura no mas, que lo que se extiende el tiempo de representar la Comedia, que estamos presentando en el Mundo con la diferencia de papeles, que repartió la Providencia Divina entre nosotros. Es ser hombre es una cosa, y el ser Duque es otra. El ser hombre es ser ceniza [...] El ser Duque es tener solo una lucida y resplandeciente apariencia" (Pueyo, *Proporciones predicables* 125).

[29]   "No puede dudar el Philosopho Sabio, que como los vestidos se distinguen de los cuerpos, que abrigan, assi los accidentes se distinguen de las substancias, que adornan; y como un Rey terreno se disfraza tal vez, vistiendose del trage, que desnudó un labrador; porque el Rey del Cielo no podrá, si gusta, despojar a la substancia del Pan de sus propios accidentes, y vistiendose con ellos, representar la apariencia del mismo Pan? Mira las vezes que mudan de trage todos los que representan algo en el Theatro del Mundo [...]" (Cortés Ossorio 366).

world was a place of transformation and change brought about "through chymistry (la Chymica)," on the other.[30]

Once we have in mind the notion that Spanish theologians and medical practitioners might use related language (the removal of vestments) to describe limitations of sensory perception, two more similarities come into focus. First, Spanish theologians and chymists understood transmutation in similar terms. One of the representative explanations of transmutation is found in *Sueños mysteriosos de la escritura* (1687) by Pedro Rodríguez y Monforte, who, as royal chaplain and officer of the secret *juntas* of the Inquisition, was the embodiment of orthodox authority. Monforte says that there are four kinds of transformation: false (i.e. that only appears to happen); natural (such as the birth of satyrs studied by M. A. Katritzky in this book); supernatural (as when men appear to be changed into beasts); and true mutation of the substance and essence of things wrought by divinity. There is a useful, if slippery, set of synonyms at work in Monforte's explanation; he says that "mutación," "transformación," "transfiguración," "metamorphosis," and "transubstanciación" are all related processes of change. This means that he can understand the Eucharist as the prototype for all changes of appearance (even changes that are false), changes of state, and substantial change (Rodríguez de Monforte 351–2).

In this model the Eucharist is, again, the model of what for Van Helmont would be the "chemical undressing" of substances. As Pagel explains, Van Helmont believed there to be a "eucharistic parallel with transmutation" and that this parallel was a "heavenly prologue to a natural process" (117–18). For Monforte and for Van Helmont, the Eucharist was a special sort of object that permitted—if not experimentation—then a particular kind of speculation about how transmutation and even less dramatic changes might happen.

At this point, we have Van Helmont contemplating the chemical undressing and Spanish theologians contemplating the vestments of bread in the Eucharist as parallel intellectual projects. I do not mean to say they are the same, but rather that both camps acknowledge similarities with the other and both draw on the same corpus of metaphors and terms to make comprehensible the perceptual limitations they face. It is in how they attempt to overcome perceptual limitations that someone like Monforte or Pueyo shares the most with Van Helmont or Croll. For centuries, the way that theologians had tried to solve the problem of knowing about the Eucharist was to differentiate between reason and intellect (as Bermúdez does above). Reason was a faculty dependent on the senses; intellect was not. Intellect could "reach out" beyond the limits of the senses. In the seventeenth century, dreaming increasingly came to be understood as an act of intellection. As Monforte says, in dreams "the intellect operates" but "without the rules that constrain reason"; this is

---

[30]   "Este globo de tierra que pisamos, como los demas elementos de que vivimos, se transmutan y se transforman unos en otros, como si todo este universo se conservase con la Chymica."

achieved through an "embargo of the exterior senses."[31] As Newman and Principe explain, Van Helmont shared this "oneiric epistemology," which they describe as "the intuitive revelation of knowledge" through dreams (57–8).

For intellectuals of Pueyo's stripe, chymistry and theology were related in three ways: they framed perceptual limitations similarly and used the Eucharist as a kind of epistemological touchstone; they shared a dramatic idiom to talk about these limitations and describe how they might be overcome; and they had models of transmutation and change that ran parallel to one another. Specifically in Pueyo's case, we have seen that the gentle language of chymical medicine was more appealing than the violent language of Galenism and that an allusion to Bances Candamo's play was playfully inserted into an encomiastic passage on Vidos's pioneering medicine.

Conclusion

For Pueyo and many of his contemporaries, theater served as a place of shared terrain between theology and the discursive possibilities of chymical developments in seventeenth-century medicine. Although theologians, as a rule, did not share Van Helmont's enthusiasm for experimentation, they had in common a fascination with a chymical world theatrically disguised by vestments and masks, a belief in the revelatory power of dreams, and what we might call a shared aesthetic. We have also seen that for Pueyo, these interests were translated into action through direct assistance to and collaboration with Vidós.

The advent of chymical medicine in Spain may have been socially disruptive and an open challenge to established ways of understanding sickness and health, but from a strictly theological point of view, chymical medicine *sounded* conservative. De la Flor contends that Pueyo was particularly interested in a "superficial appropriation of the language of the hard sciences" (158). I cannot disagree. Ecclesiastics' primary interest was not the advancement of science and medicine, even if they were frequently recruited to assist in the efforts of *novatores*. Instead, preachers and other religious authors were concerned with promulgating a theologically coherent, broadly synthesized understanding of a divinely created universe. For this reason, it was not particularly important whether Vidós was considered dangerous by physicians. For Pueyo, the language and the practice of chymical medicine served a particular theological end.

Pueyo's enthusiasm for the stage was not simply metaphysical, however. He also defended the propriety of the stage, urging students to attend: "to come to the university is good, and going to plays is not necessarily bad, but together university

---

31   "[…] pues aunque tal vez en Sueños parece que actua el entendimiento, es sin aquellas reglas que dispone la razón, guiada de la advertencia y executadas despues por un libre consentimiento. El extasis es un embargo de los sentidos exteriores dejando las potencias de la porcion superior del Alma […]" (Rodríguez de Monforte 5).

and theater, study and plays, make of a student a rational entity."[32] In this sense, Pueyo's thinking about theater, his work supporting chymical medicine, and his belief that the world was a place of illusion and deception mirror the writings of a contemporary, Manuel de Guerra y Ribera. Guerra preached on alchemical subjects, including those as dear to Van Helmont as a universal menstrum or solvent (Slater, "Rereading" 75). He also defended Calderón's theater, publishing a controversial *aprobación* to the *Verdadera quinta parte*, a volume of the playwright's *comedias*.[33] Furthermore, Guerra was a member of the circle of Juan José de Austria, the viceroy of Aragon, which included the "novator" Juanini. And Guerra had his own "oneiric epistemology," speaking of dreams as "a retreat from the false images of the world to the interior preserve of the intellect where understanding lies."[34] The interest in alchemy or chymical medicine, in theater, and in dreaming as a form of supra-rational apprehension constitutes a triad that was reproduced numerous times in Spain during the last decades of the seventeenth century.

There is very little evidence that Croll or Van Helmont might have been thinking of the stage, per se; but the chymical means of expression, this theatrical aesthetic, was also an important vehicle of chymical content. In other words, what was partly responsible for the successes of chymistry and the support for someone like Vidós was precisely the identification of chymical medicine as theatrical (even if only in a metaphorical sense). Vidós's rather humble rendering of chymistry made medical modernity accessible to a broad network of supporters, allowing him to recruit the viceroy (Jaime Fernández), the publisher of his book (Gaspar Martínez), an important preacher and theologian such as Pueyo, and so on. The *Medicina y Cirugia racional y espagirica* delivered some modern ideas, at times deformed, in a package that appealed to the Baroque theological sensibility.

As we have seen, linguistic borrowings, shared fascinations, and appropriation of medical ideas, as well as rivalry and animosity among varying medical factions, typified the medical cultures of early modern Zaragoza. Pueyo's case was very similar to many of the studies in this volume; he seized upon a particular set of medical ideas for reasons that were not entirely medical, even if his actions had important implications for the history of medicine in Spain. Neither Pueyo's efforts to support the work of Vidós nor Guerra's writings about alchemy, dreaming, and the stage were practically related to Van Helmont's chymical medicine. Neither is it the case that Vidós's book of secrets can be confused with the work of serious chymists. What is true, however, is that there was enough

---

[32]   "[…] venir a la universidad es bueno, ir a la comedia no lo tengo por malo, pero la junta de Universidad y Teatro, de lición y Comedia, haze un estudiante Ente de razón" (*Dialéctica económica, política, moral* 14).

[33]   On Guerra's defense of Calderón's theater, see the various studies by Herzig and that of García Lorenzo.

[34]   "[…] un receso destas imágenes del Mundo; al interior retrete de la inteligencia, entendimiento. Un abstraerse destos aparentes objetos, para contemplar con mas quietud las verdades" (Rodríguez de Monforte, "Aprobación").

similitude in the contemporaneous discourses of theology and chymical medicine, in the language itself, to inspire ecclesiastics across Spain to involve themselves in the debates about chymical medicine. For Cortés Ossorio, Pueyo, Guerra, Monforte, and many others, the principle attractions of chymical medicine lay in the evocative, dramatic qualities of its language. This led many ecclesiastics to act, too: to preach, to declare publicly their support in *aprobaciones*, to work behind the scenes to help Spain's chymical drama unfold.

Epilogue
The Difference That Made Spain, the Difference That Spain Made

William Eamon

Eighteenth-century Enlightenment critics of Spain almost always made pointed reference to Iberia's "difference," its "otherness" with respect to the rest of Europe,[1] beginning with the French *philosophe* Montesquieu, who asserted in 1741 that the grip of the Inquisition rendered Spain "incapable of any degree of light or instruction" (II: 56). Montesquieu's statement would prove to be only a contemptuous prelude to the question the famous French polymath Nicolas Masson de Morvillers polemically asked in 1792: "What do we owe Spain?" European intellectuals rebuked Spain as a backward nation and its people as ignorant, superstitious, and alien to all that modernity stood for. Particularly with regard to science, Masson asserted, Spain had become "the most ignorant nation in Europe." After all, he asked dismissively: "What can we expect of a country that needs to ask priests for permission to read and think?" In the eyes of many educated Europeans, Spain was different.

The image of Spain as barbaric and despotic took hold throughout Europe in the eighteenth century from Italy to England. Few authors did more to fashion the stereotype than Montesquieu (Iglesias). His *Esprit des lois* helped to set the fashion of depicting Spain as the land of fanaticism and ignorance. Like many others, Montesquieu attributed Spain's stagnation to the exaggerated Spanish tradition of honor that valued idleness over labor. Thus in the eighteenth century, the perception of the Spanish state gradually shifted from that of a benevolent Christian monarchy to that of an oriental despotism (Padgen, *Spanish Imperialism*; *Lords of All the World*).

In fact, all sorts of things—including Catholicism—were blamed for Spain's supposed degradation: sloth, climate, bad government, the stars (MacKay 108). According to the construction of Spain that emerged in the eighteenth century, the Spanish people were governed by barbaric institutions, engaged in pagan religious practices, and subjected to bloody tyrants. The contrast with other European nations seemed stark and absolute. Northern European travelers to Spain, such as John Armstrong, an English engineer who was stationed in the island of Minorca in the 1730s and '40s, reinforced these negative images of Iberia. "There is no

---

[1] I treat this theme in greater detail in my essay "Nuestros males," where a more complete bibliography may be found.

degree of superstition into which these people have not been led," Armstrong reported (Hontanilla 9).

Spanish observers—some indignantly coming to their country's defense and others joining in the chorus of criticism of Spain's supposed "backwardness"— also insisted that Spain was different from the rest of Europe. The satirist Juan Pablo Forner took Masson's article as representative of French libertinism and used his reply to Masson (*Oración apologética por la España y su mérito literario*, 1786) as a pretext for attacking the *philosophes* in general (Gies; Herr 123–4). Denouncing the article as typically Anglo-French, Forner pronounced: "We have not had famous dreamers like Descartes and Newton, but we have had the most just legislators and excellent practical philosophers" (qtd. in Herr 224).

Yet the idea that Spain was, by nature and misfortune, exceptional predates the eighteenth-century controversies about the state of Spanish science that came to be known as the "polémica de la ciencia espanola."[2] Already in the seventeenth century, and particularly during the reign of Philip III, a group of writers called the *arbitristas* put a name to Spain's predicament, as they saw it: *declinación*, or decline. Their reform proposals, covering all manner of problems from taxation to morality, called for a *restauración*, or restoration, of a bygone kingdom and, for that matter, bygone days of glory (Elliott, "Self Perception and Decline"). Some argued that the root causes of Spain's backwardness were sexual depravity and religious hypocrisy; others blamed luxuriant living, overindulgence in food and drink, and the effeminate fashion among men of wearing their hair long. (The cure, of course, was moral reform.) Others sought more "scientific" explanations. Was Spain's decline an irreversible part of some cosmic, cyclical process, they wondered? Or, applying the model of astrological determinism, was it somehow the result of the movement of the planets? Medical metaphors were abundant: Spain was just sick. Diseases, of course, can be diagnosed, but the cures proposed by the *arbitristas* were, frankly, not very helpful.

The Difference That Made Spain

Spain's critics, both from within and outside of Spain, as well as her defenders, were, however, right about one thing: Spain was different—though not for the reasons advanced by those on either side of the polemic. The difference that was Spain had nothing to do, of course, with the character of its people or its supposedly degenerative environment, but instead had everything to do with the most obvious fact about its early modern situation: it possessed the largest empire the western world had ever known, an empire that under Hapsburg rule reached from Madrid to Potosí and from Naples to Antwerp, not to mention the distant Philippines—the first empire in world history over which the sun never set. The Spanish Empire even included in its orbit Rome, where tens of thousands of Spaniards settled,

---

[2]   See López Piñero's *Ciencia y técnica* 15–27 and Nieto-Galán's "Images of Science."

colonizers for a kind of "informal" Spanish imperialism that until recently has received little attention (Dandelet).

During the heyday of the Spanish Empire, the sixteenth century, the Iberians confidently saw themselves as the first "moderns," surpassing the ancients. Yet it was not just Spaniards who saw themselves this way. The English, always creative borrowers, were among the first to recognize Spain's superiority and to imitate the scientific institutions created by the Iberians (Cañizares-Esguerra, "Iberian Science" 86). The Italian philosopher Tommaso Campanella thought that Spain was destined to rule the world before the final days: "The monarchy of Spain," he wrote, "which embraces all nations and encircles the world is that of the Messiah, and thus shows itself to be the heir of the universe" (qtd. in Pagden, *Spanish Imperialism* 50). Spain was a rising giant that would become the world's first modern global empire and would produce the first worldwide scientific network (Barrera-Osorio, *Experiencing Nature*).

Spain's possession of a vast global empire set it apart from the rest of Europe in a number of important ways, many of which are highlighted in the essays in this volume. Above all, the Spanish were the first Europeans to grapple with what was, from their perspective, the strangeness and novelty of America, its environment, its exotic flora and fauna, and the diversity of its peoples and cultures (Elliott, "Same World, Different Worlds" 195–7). For starters, the Spanish were the first Europeans who had to contend with the question of the humanity of aboriginal cultures (Pagden, *The Fall of Natural Man*). As José Pardo-Tomás's careful analysis of the medical content of the *Relaciones Geográficas de Indias* demonstrates in Chapter 2 of this volume, Spaniards wrestled with the most basic aspects of the character of indigenous peoples (including whether or not the Indians were rational humans or irrational animals).

The Spanish experience in America was entirely unlike that of the English in this regard. Although there were some points of similarity in the ways in which the Spaniards and the English responded to the challenges that confronted them in the New World, with respect to the treatment of the indigenous population, the differences offer a stark contrast (Elliott, "Britain and Spain in America"). "It is a melancholy reflection," wrote Henry Knox, the American Secretary of War to President Washington, in 1794, "that our modes of population have been more destructive to the Indian natives than the conduct of the conquerors of Mexico and Peru. The evidence is the utter extirpation of nearly all the Indians in most populous parts of the Union. A future historian may mark the causes of this destruction of the human race in sable colors" (qtd. in Elliott, "Britain and Spain in America" 150). To be sure, there was plenty of cruelty on both sides, but simply by demographic measures, a far greater percentage of Indians survived the conquest in the Spanish territories than in the English colonies.[3] The reason was

---

[3]   Elliott estimates that while 56 percent of the original Indian population in Hispanic America survived into the eighteenth century, only 6 percent of Indians in North America survived ("Britain and Spain in America" 150).

that the British lacked the driving impetus to convert the indigenous population that motivated so much of the Spanish enterprise in America. That powerful motivation, evident from the very first generation of friars in the Indies, inspired a remarkable and unprecedented attempt to understand the character and customs of the indigenous peoples of the New World. Millions of non-Europeans, whose very existence was completely unknown only a generation earlier, were suddenly thrust into the European consciousness. In short, as Anthony Pagden has shown, the Spanish experience in America created a new kind of opportunity for systematic ethnographic study and gave rise to the science of comparative ethnology (*The Fall of Natural Man*).

The questions the Spaniards asked during this process were so fundamental as to challenge existing assumptions about the nature of humanity. By studying strange men in alien environments, the Spanish asked questions that were at the same time creative and disturbing: What were the essential characteristics of humanity? What constituted a civilized man, as distinct from a barbarian or an animal? Were the natives, indeed, human or animal? Even if the answers were sometimes inadequate and ill-informed, merely asking them served, in the words of John Elliott, to "widen the boundaries of perception" ("Discovery of America" 43). It was, above all, José de Acosta's remarkable *Historia natural y moral de las Indias* that brought the nature of the aboriginal cultures of America to the attention of Europeans. Acosta's work, which was translated into several different languages, served as a major conduit of information about the Incas and Aztecs in the early modern period. In one sense, Acosta contributed to a process already well underway. Works such as Fernández de Oviedo's *Historia general y natural de las Indias* and, above all, Bartolomé de las Casas's *Brevísima relación de la destrucción de las Indias* touched off a Europe-wide dispute over the nature of aboriginal cultures. Spanish efforts to come to grips with the humanity of American natives were sometimes problematic, but they nevertheless opened up entire new ways of seeing humanity.

Related to this, the Spaniards were the first to grapple with the demographic catastrophe that afflicted the Americas during the colonial period. As Pardo-Tomás shows in his essay in this volume, Spanish officials made concerted efforts to understand the nature of the epidemics that swept through New Spain. Even more enlightening, however, are the native voices that echo throughout the *Relaciones Geográficas de Indias*, revealing a population whose health and numbers had declined steeply, whose indigenous healers had been killed off by diseases of unknown origin, a people desperate to understand why, in the words of one: "In the past they lived very healthy and died old, [...] and now they are few." The discourse between natives and oppressors took place in a context that was completely, or almost so, independent of metropolitan debates. The *Relaciones* reveal a hybrid medical culture unlike anything known in Europe, a culture, as Pardo-Tomás puts it, comprising "the diversified world of lay folk who were the authors and creators of their own medical culture, cultures that only entered the discourse of the experts in an impoverished and schematic form."

Then there was the matter of seeing America for the first time: its environment, its exotic flora and fauna, its peculiar environment, climate, and terrain, all so unlike anything that Spaniards had ever experienced. In the immediate wake of the first encounter with America, Europeans too often saw what they wanted or expected to see. It was all too easy to merely assimilate the strangeness of the New World into the familiar (Pagden, *European Encounters with the New World* 17–50).[4] Yet it was not long before the Spaniards realized that inherited preconceptions were inadequate to describe the New World, and that there was a wide divergence between image and reality (Elliott, *The Old World and the New* 21). Sometimes the problem of description reduced voyagers to despair. There was too much diversity, too much to describe. Gonzalo Fernández de Oviedo, who spent a total of 43 years in the Antilles and Central America—and who with some justification imagined himself as the "American Pliny"—was one of the first chroniclers to try. As Oviedo wrote to his patron, Charles V: "there are such great kingdoms and provinces, and such very strange people, of different customs, rites and idolatries, far removed from anything which has been recorded, *ab initio* up to our own time, that the span of a man's life is hardly sufficient [either] to see it, to begin to comprehend or [even] to conjecture upon it" (qtd. in Myers 146).

The more we learn about the Spanish experience in the New World the more we come to understand the significance of seeing American nature for the first time. A number of scholars, in particular Antonio Barrera-Osorio, have recently argued that the knowledge-generating practices of Iberian institutions, such as the Spanish Casa de Contratación, created a model that was emulated elsewhere in Europe, ultimately transforming natural philosophy from a discipline based upon deductive argument into one that increasingly emphasized the *experience* of concrete events. The power of this model is exemplified most famously by the research reports by the Fellows of the Royal Society of London, found in countless contributions to the *Philosophical Transactions*. Natural philosophers increasingly used reports of singular events anchored in a specific time and place (including "experiments" modeled on recipes found in books of secrets) as a way of constructing experiential statements.[5] Barrera has convincingly argued in works such as "Empiricism in the Spanish Atlantic World" and *Experiencing Nature* that fact-gathering became an essential component of Spanish imperial practices. The Spanish monarchs knew that to rule Spain's vast empire, they needed to know what that empire contained and where its sources of wealth came from. That meant taking inventory, which Philip II and his successors did time and again by sending agents such as Francisco Hernández to the New World to collect and codify the things of the Indies.

This kind of empirical information gathering, codification, and utilitarianism was pivotal in the development of European science, because, as Harold Cook

---

[4]   Pagden labels this strategy "the principle of attachment." See also Ryan, "Assimilating New Worlds."

[5]   See, for example, Peter Dear's *Discipline and Experience* 25.

pointed out, natural history was *the* empirical science of the early modern period (*Matters of Exchange* 411). Natural history, and particularly botany because of its practical use for *materia medica*, became pivotal sciences in Spain's pursuit of colonial wealth (De Vos, "An Herbal El Dorado").[6] It also provided a model for imperial information-gathering that was based on a close relationship between state support, scientific knowledge and practice, and commercial aims. Moreover, there is considerable evidence that many of the practices instituted by the Spanish generated keen interest among other Europeans, particularly the English. Further research is needed to trace the routes of communication between Spain and northern Europe, but one thing is clear: it is hardly an accident that "the so-called Scientific Revolution occurred at the same time as the development of the first global economy" (Cook, *Matters of Exchange* 411).

The Spanish naturalists were made constantly aware of the newness of the New World. At the outset of his *Historia general*, Oviedo lamented: "I am at the very end of my life, and yet I perceive that I am only just at the beginning [of my understanding of] the marrow of these great and innumerable secrets, which remain to be discovered in this second hemisphere and in these parts which were unknown to the ancients" (qtd. in Pagden, *European Encounters* 58). Oviedo's resigned lament raises the question: who makes the best witness? Who was best qualified to report on the novelties of the New World? Was it the philosopher who comes to nature with preconceived notions? Or was it someone like the "simple, crude fellow" who told Montaigne of the strange customs of the New World Indians? Montaigne seemed to believe the latter. His informant had lived for some time in Brazil, and it was a combination of experience and simplicity that, for Montaigne, made him fit to bear true witness. In order to get reliable reports about things we have not seen for ourselves, wrote Montaigne, "we need a man either very honest, or so simple that he has not the stuff to build up false inventions and give them plausibility" (152).

Spanish chroniclers may not have been as innocent of preconceived notions as the "simple, crude fellow" of Montaigne's essay. Yet, as Ralph Bauer argues in his essay in this volume, exotic American flora entered the early modern literature of natural history not only decontextualized from their meanings in Native American cultures, but also stripped of the layers of analogies and signatures that had encrusted them for centuries. The European encounter with the New World struck an irreparable blow to the doctrine of signatures. The plants and animals of the New World were entirely new. They had no known similitudes. Anteaters and sloths, tobacco and chocolate, are all missing from the writings of antiquity. As William Ashworth writes: "They come to the Old World naked, without emblematic significance (318). Hence naturalists could not approach the new flora and fauna in the manner of earlier humanists. Instead, they were forced to limit their descriptions to discussions of appearance, habitat, food, and reports gathered from native people.

---

6   See also De Vos's "The Science of Spices."

In shaking off the "crust of analogies" that had accreted in natural history over centuries, thereby making objects "naked," the sixteenth-century literature of the discovery and conquest of the New World represents an important step towards a natural history in which nature's specimens instead become objects of inquiry instead of vehicles of religious and philological meaning. Moreover, there can be little doubt that the experience of New World natural history stimulated the collecting impulse that was so characteristic of Renaissance natural history (Ogilvie 269).[7] Of course, the "curiosities of art and nature" that made up the princely *Wunderkammern* were not collected for strictly scientific purposes, but instead served as a testament to one's power, status, and authority. Nevertheless, they were ultimately deployed in the construction of the modern scientific "object" during the Scientific Revolution. Although the origins of objectivity are still not fully understood, it seems clear that seeing the New World for the first time will have a place in that history.

Finally, there was the matter of what may be called the "everyday Atlantic" (Elliott, "Illusion and Disillusionment" 133). In other words, if you were a Spaniard living in the sixteenth century, it would have been impossible to ignore the presence of the empire, in one guise or another, in almost every aspect of everyday culture. It is likely that you would have known someone who had gone to the Indies, or had returned from there. By the end of the sixteenth century, travel to New Spain was relatively common and affordable, even for average Spaniards. In growing numbers, Spaniards had the option of emigration. More than 2,500 Castilians took passage for the Indies each year in the sixteenth century, and at least 4,000 per year in the first half of the seventeenth century. The Jesuit chronicler José de Acosta reported that exit was as easy "as for a laborer to travel from his village to the town" (qtd. in Elliott, *Spain, Europe, and the Wider World* 133). One could buy passage to the Indies for a mere 20 ducats, about a month's pay for a skilled worker in Madrid. The passage was neither easy nor undertaken without trepidation, as the letters analyzed by Mauricio Sánchez-Menchero in this volume suggest. Yet, as Hernán Sanchez assured his brother Diego Ramos in 1569: "[I]t has been many days since one of the fleets has suffered an accident; because the route has been heavily traveled, and there are many skilled pilots" (qtd. in Elliott, *Spain, Europe, and the Wider World* 133).

Moreover, New World products, from tobacco and chocolate to maize, cochineal, and sassafras, were everywhere in sight. Visitors to the ports of Lisbon or Seville would have been made immediately aware—by sight, sound, and smell—of a strange new world of goods arriving from distant parts of the world. The first European dyers to work with cochineal, the exotic red dyestuff from Mexico, were almost certainly Spanish, although soon Spain's monopoly on the dye was broken by the Italians (Greenfield 72–3). Pharmacies, too, which stocked everything from guaiac wood to bezoars, put exotic plants and animals on display for the public, like natural history museums.

---

[7]   In addition, see De Vos's "The Rare, the Singular, and the Extraordinary."

The everyday Atlantic was also evident in popular literature and culture. The empire and the New World turn up frequently, almost as characters, in the popular literature of the period. In Francisco Santos's novel, *Las Tarascas de Madrid*, tasting chocolate is represented as one of the urban lusts to which women, in particular, were supposedly most susceptible.[8] Even on the theatrical stage, arguably the most popular literary form of Golden Age Spain, the empire asserted its presence—for instance, in the dramatization of syphilis or the French Pox, which was widely regarded as being a gift of the New World to the Old.[9]

Imperial priorities were also behind the search for local medicines in New Spain. Keeping planters alive in the colonies was an urgent concern for the Spanish Monarchy. In a recent study, José Pardo-Tomás has examined in detail the creole physician Juan de Cárdenas's appropriation of the books of secrets, a largely European genre, for the purposes of promoting local medicines and native medical knowledge in Mexico. Cárdenas not only presented his creole readers with a rational scientific knowledge (in contrast to the purely empirical knowledge traditions of native practitioners), but also vigorously defended local medicines and native practices. Similarly, the Spanish *encomendero* Antonio de Villasante learned about the virtues of native plants in Hispaniola from his Christianized Taino wife, Catalina de Ayahibex (a *cacica*). One of Villasantes's discoveries was a native balsam, for which he received a monopoly from the Crown (Barrera-Osorio, "Local Herbs, Global Medicines"). Of course, Europeans tended to think of the New World medicinal plants predominantly within a Galenic explanatory model of disease and therapy—perhaps confirming the notion that, in Guenter Risse's words, "travelers never leave home, but merely extend the limits of their world by taking their concerns and apparatus for interpreting the world along with them" (32). Nevertheless, a new creole scientific culture was being constructed within the Spanish Empire from materials on both sides of the Atlantic. Moreover, as Antonio Barrera-Osorio has argued, the empirical practices first put into play in the Spanish empire eventually became institutionalized both in the Spanish context and in the wider European scene (*Experiencing Nature*).

The principal problem with our current historiography of the Scientific Revolution, insofar as it regards the Spanish experience at all, is that it has been framed largely within the domain of intellectual history, thus keeping it safely within the comfort zone of the Anglo-French axis. A case in point is the most recent attempt at a broad synthesis or master narrative of the Scientific Revolution, Stephen Gaukroger's erudite work *The Emergence of a Scientific Culture: Science and the Shaping of Modernity, 1210–1685* (2006). In a book ostensibly about "the shaping of modernity," Gaukroger, surprisingly, does not include so much as a mention of some of the most obvious aspects of modernity, such as globalization, colonialism, and the expansion of the European system to

---

[8]   See Enrique García Santo-Tomás's article in this volume.
[9]   See, in particular, Slater's *Todos son hojas*.

distant parts of the world. Neither the words "exploration" nor "discovery" merit inclusion in the book's index, where alchemy gets fewer pages of notice than the Italian philosopher Francesco Patrizi. Medicine gets short shrift, despite the volumes of work coming out in recent years by scholars such as Harold Cook, who has sharply challenged existing interpretations of the Scientific Revolution and argued forcefully for the need to include medicine in our interpretation of it—or, alternatively, to dispense with the concept entirely. To be fair, Gaukroger devotes a sentence to José de Acosta's "pioneering work of New World natural history," but the opportunity to engage seriously with the far-reaching consequences of that work, or the work of Francisco Hernández, Nicolás Monardes (neither of whom are mentioned in Gaukroger's 500-page monograph), and countless others, is completely lost. Gaukroger does engage with natural history, but in an oddly detached and cerebral way, and only insofar as it leads to Baconian inductivism (359–67).

It is clear where Gaukroger's priorities lie when it comes to understanding the Scientific Revolution, and they do not include understanding science and medicine as having global significance, but only as local developments within the sphere of European philosophy. To Gaukroger, the problem of "science and the shaping of modernity" is, essentially, a problem simply of intellectual history. No wonder that Spain gets short shrift in this kind of historiography. Fundamentally, insofar as it includes Spain, the current historiography of science and medicine is Eurocentric in the most obvious and puerile sense, which is that, in general, it neglects the broader context of the Spanish experience. As the essays in this volume suggest time and again, to interpret early modern Spain without including its vast colonial empire seems, at best, strangely surreal, or, at worst, doggedly perverse.

Fortunately, this situation is changing, and changing rapidly. As a result of recent studies such as those in this volume, we are a long way from a situation in which, in 1961, a historian as distinguished as John H. Elliott could ask: "Why was it that science and technology failed to take root in Spain, at a time when they were beginning to arouse considerable interest elsewhere in Europe?" (*Spain and Its World* 234). Such a comment is all the more surprising coming from a historian who has, perhaps, contributed more to interpreting imperial Spain than anyone else. That Elliott should have gotten things so wrong with regard to science only underscores the underlying, fundamental problem with the current historiography of early modern Spanish science and medicine. It is not that "science and technology failed to take root in Spain"; it is rather that science, technology, and medicine were deployed for very different purposes in Spain than they were in the rest of Europe. Those purposes had everything to do with the relations between colony and metropolis.

The Difference That Spain Made

Scholarship on early modern Spanish science and medicine has a long history.[10] However, it has been only within the last decade or so that historians of science and medicine outside of Spain have begun to take Spain and its empire seriously and to include them in the larger picture of the Scientific Revolution.[11] What, then, was the difference that Spain made? Or, to rephrase the question in Masson's derogatory words: "What do we owe Spain?"

One could plausibly argue that we owe the modern idea of scientific discovery to the early modern Iberian experience. Prior to the Renaissance, discovery—in the sense of the discovery of new phenomena—was not a priority in natural philosophy. Instead, natural philosophy was conducted as a sort of hermeneutics—"natural philosophy without nature," as John Murdoch aptly characterized it (Murdoch 171). However, it was not very long before a new generation of intellectuals began thinking of science as a search for new and unknown facts, or of causes concealed beneath nature's outer appearances.[12] This conception of science rested, in turn, upon a redefinition of what constitutes scientific knowledge. In medieval natural philosophy, factual knowledge (or knowledge of individual, isolated events) did not qualify as science unless it could be demonstrated that such facts occurred by logical necessity. Medieval natural philosophers "had not dwelt upon phenomena and objects that did not fit within existing theories" (Daston 465). Facts were tucked snugly, and invisibly, under the blanket of *scientia*.

In the Renaissance, scientific inquiry was increasingly conceived as the discovery of *new* things rather than as attempts to demonstrate the known, as had been characteristic of Scholastic natural philosophy (Eamon, *Science as a Hunt*). Indeed, the themes of newness and novelty appear repeatedly in the scientific literature of the early modern period. During this period, the *Ne plus ultra* ("Do not go beyond") inscribed on the ancient Pillars of Hercules became a favorite device to illustrate the tyranny of ancient philosophy over creative thought. The growing awareness that reverence for antiquity hampered progress aroused a sense of the importance of new discoveries and of the value of novelty for its own sake. Oviedo articulated the idea explicitly and repeatedly. The very newness of the New World meant that no ancient models, not even Pliny, could serve as a guide. Comparing his eyewitness reports to Pliny's bookish accounts, Oviedo wrote: "I have not culled them from two hundred thousand volumes I might have read, as Pliny wrote [...]. I, however, compiled what I here write from two hundred

---

[10] Some of the most important works have been produced by José María López Piñero and his students, including Victor Navarro Brotòns, José Pardo-Tomás, Marialuz López Terrada, and many others.

[11] One of the earliest studies of early modern Spanish science from a non-Spanish historian was David Goodman's pioneering *Power and Penury*, although in that work Goodman focused mainly on Spain under Philip II and not on Spain and the Scientific Revolution.

[12] See also Rossi, "The Aristotelians and the 'Moderns.'"

thousand hardships, privations and dangers in the more than twenty-two years that I have personally witnessed and experienced these things" (qtd. in Myers 150).

Certainly the most important event contributing to Europe's heightened consciousness of novelty was the discovery of the New World. News of the discovery, which revealed regions completely unknown to the ancients, raised Europe's awareness of the sheer immenseness of the world. The explorers brought back specimens of exotic plants and animals, hair-raising tales of adventure, and accounts of completely new peoples and cultures. Above all, the new geographical discoveries demonstrated that ancient philosophy and science were not eternal verities. The relations of the voyagers to America seemed to confirm, in the words of the Spanish historian Francisco López de Gómara, that "experience is contrary to philosophy."

The New World itself became a metaphor for the ignorance of the ancients. As Thomas Browne put it, ancient philosophy was so fraught with error that the "untraveled parts of Truth," what Browne called "the America" of truth, still awaited discovery (5). In the mid-seventeenth century, the English virtuoso Joseph Glanvill still envisioned the opening up of an "America of secrets and an unknown Peru of nature" (178). Like the New World, nature stood before investigators as uncharted territory.[13]

These considerations lend new perspectives on our thinking about the origins of the Scientific Revolution and, in particular, the role of medicine within it. Where and when did the Scientific Revolution begin? Jorge Cañizares-Esguerra and Antonio Barrera-Osorio have both argued persuasively that the roots of the Scientific Revolution are, in fact, Iberian (Cañizares-Esguerra, "Colonial Iberian Roots"; Barrera-Osorio, *Experiencing Nature*). Harold Cook and others have convincingly argued that during the first period of globalization, "a worldwide natural science rooted in descriptive natural history developed for the first time" ("Global Economies and Local Knowledge" 101). Historians who have looked closely at the patterns of knowledge acquisition germane to the early modern global economy—including several of the contributors to this volume—have noted that the most important means for acquiring new information involved contact with other people on the global stage. As the essays in this volume demonstrate, that is precisely the pattern we see with regard to the medical cultures of the early modern Spanish Empire.

The personal interactions that are documented in many of the essays in this volume are examples—which could be multiplied many times over—of the exchanges that took place within the "trading zones" that brought together "experts" (Spanish physicians and local healers, naturalists, and native informants, etc.) from different disciplines or fields of activity.[14] Pamela O. Long defines

---

[13]   On these themes, see my essay "Science as a Hunt."

[14]   The term (and its usage here) is from Pamela O. Long (borrowing from Peter Galison) in *Artisan/Practitioners* 94–126. Long does not, however, consider the concept of trading zones in relation to colonial interchanges such as those examined in the essays in this volume.

such trading zones as "arenas in which the learned taught the skilled, and the skilled taught the learned, and in which the knowledge involved in each arena was valued by both kinds of 'traders'" (*Artisan/Practitioners* 95). Long gives examples of several kinds of trading zones, such as arsenals, princely courts, and print shops. Yet arenas of knowledge exchange among the learned and skilled were also located in the distant reaches of the Spanish empire, where metropolitan and colonial expertise intermingled, and in the institutions created by the Spanish monarchy that were designed to process empirical information, such as the Casa de Contratación.[15]

In a series of classic articles published in the 1940s, Edgar Zilsel argued that the empirical and experimental values that emerged in the early modern period were born from the union of academic learning and the practical activities of artisans. Zilsel linked the convergence of these previously alienated traditions to the collapse of the social barriers that had kept craftsmen and intellectuals apart. The breakdown of the barriers between artisans and men of learning, he argued, was a consequence of the rise of capitalism and the decline of craft guilds. The expansion of industry and commerce during the Renaissance opened up new opportunities for "superior craftsmen" to ascend from the ranks of guildsmen into the emergent middle class, and thereby to rub elbows with humanists. Such individuals, Zilsel claimed, "were the real pioneers of empirical observation, experimentation, and causal research" (551).

Zilsel focused on the interaction of artisans and humanists as the crucial interchanges that gave rise to the emerging empirical values of the early modern period. Building on Zilsel's insights, other historians have suggested that just as critical were the interchanges that occurred within medicine and natural history. In an article published in 1993, Harold J. Cook made reference to the seventeenth-century Dutch naturalist Jan Swammerdam as an example illustrating the point.[16] Swammerdam was the son of an apothecary whose shop bordered the Amsterdam dockyards, where ships from around the world unloaded their wares. Thus from an early age Swammerdam became interested in "things," collecting them in a natural history cabinet that grew to an impressive size, including more than 1,200 dried and mounted insects. Such curiosity about nature was not uncommon, especially among physicians, who, for reasons pertaining to both the art and science of medicine, took a keen interest in natural history. For their art—the cure of disease—they needed to know about the medicinal uses of plants, animals, and minerals that they used in their practice; for their science—the knowledge of health and disease—physicians shifted their focus from philosophical debate to investigations of nature (H. Cook, "Physicians and Natural History" 91). Physicians, leaders among those

---

[15]   See, for example, the chapters by Angélica Morales Sarabia, José Pardo-Tomás, Ralph Bauer, and Mauricio Sánchez-Menchero in Part I of this volume; as well as Pardo-Tomás's "Natural Knowledge and Medical Remedies."

[16]   Cook was one of the first historians to make this argument in a convincing way ("The Cutting Edge of a Revolution?")

who pursued knowledge of natural things, took an active role in the promotion of natural history and were critical participants in the development of the new philosophy of the early modern period. In the long run, to borrow a term from Gaukroger, natural history facilitated a kind of "focusing" on the particular rather than upon the underlying physical structure of things, thus facilitating a new kind of natural-philosophical approach that increasingly emphasized experimentation (356). The methodology advanced by Francis Bacon, who himself was an avid reader of Spanish colonial literature, exemplifies the new approach.[17]

Virtually all of the interchanges and new interests that historians have regarded as critical to the development of early modern natural philosophy were visible in the Spanish Atlantic empire: the coming together of scholars and craftsmen, the renewed interest in natural history, the emphasis on collecting, and the development of institutions to organize empirical knowledge. Added to these was something perhaps uniquely Spanish or, at any rate, uniquely Iberian. As is evident from even the most cursory reading of a work like José de Acosta's *Historia natural y moral de las Indias*, Spaniards were obliged by imperial mandate to convert the natives to Christianity, to document and understand native practices and beliefs, to account for the origins of the inhabitants of the New World, and to explain how they got there. Thus Acosta's work was a "natural and *moral* history" because it took into account the local and cultural. Medical practice, too, had to be *moral* because, as the essays in this volume illustrate, medicine in the Spanish empire was always the result of negotiations at the local level. Local practices and beliefs about the body and about sickness and health intersected and interacted with ideas and practices on the global stage.

Early modern Spaniards—both those who made the crossing and those who remained at home—were the first Europeans to construct, in their own imperfect and uncertain way, hybrid medical cultures that were cut loose from the strictures of academic medicine. They did so because they had to: there was no other choice.

---

[17] Spanish works on natural history and New World medicine circulated widely, both on the European continent and in England. For a variety of reasons, however, they had particular appeal in England. As early as 1577, the English merchant John Frampton translated Monardes's work on natural history and published it under the title *Joyfull Newes out of the New Founde Worlde* (London, 1577). Acosta's natural history appeared in an English translation by Edward Grimstone in 1604.

Bibliography

Abraham, Lyndy. *A Dictionary of Alchemical Imagery*. Cambridge, UK: Cambridge University Press, 1998.

Abulafia, David. *The Discovery of Mankind: Atlantic Encounters in the Age of Columbus*. New Haven, CT: Yale University Press, 2008.

Acuña, René. *Relaciones Geográficas novohispanas del siglo XVI*. 10 vols. México: Universidad Autónoma Nacional de México, 1982–1988.

Adams, Alice E. *Reproducing the Womb: Images of Childbirth in Science, Feminist Theory, and Literature*. Ithaca, NY: Cornell University Press, 1994.

Adorno, Rolena. "The indigenous ethnographer: the '*indio* ladino' as historian and cultural mediator." Ed. Stuart Schwartz. *Implicit Understandings*, Cambridge: Cambridge University Press, 1994. 378–402.

Aguilar Moreno, Manuel. "The *indio* ladino as a cultural mediator in the colonial society." *Estudios de cultura náhuatl* 33 (2002): 149–84.

Aguirre Beltrán, Gonzalo. *Medicina y magia: el proceso de aculturación en la estructura colonial*. México: Instituto Nacional Indigenista, 1963.

Aguirre, Félix de. *Enigmas Sacros Panegiricos, Descifrados en Tres Preciosas Ioyas, que se sirvieron al Gloriosissimo Proto-Martir de los Apostoles […]*. Zaragoza: Gaspar Tomás Martínez, 1689.

———. *Mesa soberana del sol, y de las aves. Tripode firme, y constante de la verdad, Oraculo de la Enseñaza Evangélica […]*. Zaragoza: Manuel Roman, 1690.

Albarracín Teulón, Agustín. *La medicina en el teatro de Lope de Vega*. Madrid: Consejo Superior de Investigaciones Científicas, Instituto Arnaldo de Vilanova, 1954.

Alberro, Solange. *Inquisición y sociedad en México, 1571–1700*. México: Fondo de Cultura Económica, 1998.

Albertus, Magnus. *De animalibus*. Mantua: Paulus de Butzbach, 1479.

Aldrovandi, Ulisse. *Monstrorum historia. Cum Paralipomenis historiae omnium animalium*. Bologna: Marco Antonio Bernia and Nicolò Tebaldini, 1642.

Alexander, Dorothy, and Walter L. Strauss. *The German Single-Leaf Woodcut, 1600–1700: A Pictorial Catalogue*. Vol. 1: A–N. New York: Abaris Books, 1977.

Alfaro, Gustavo A. "La anti-picaresca en *El Periquillo* de Francisco Santos." *Kentucky Romance Quarterly* 14 (1967): 321–7.

Allen, Michael J. B., Valery Rees, and Martin Davies eds. *Marsilio Ficino: His Theology, His Philosophy, His Legacy*. Leiden: Brill, 2001.

Altamirano, Fernando, and José Ramírez. "El peyote." *Anales del Instituto Médico Nacional* 7 (1914): 209–10.

Álvarez Peláez, Raquel. *La conquista de la naturaleza americana*. Madrid: CSIC, 1993.

Amelang, James S. "Exchanges between Italy and Spain: Culture and Religion." *Spain in Italy: Politics, Society, and Religion 1500–1700*. Ed. Thomas J. Dandelet and John A. Marino. Leiden: Brill, 2007. 433–55.

Andrés, Gregorio de. "31 cartas inéditas de Juan Páez de Castro, cronista de Carlos V." *Boletín de la Real Academia de la Historia* 158.3 (1971): 515–71.

Andretta, Elisa and Sabina Brevaglieri. "Storie naturali a Roma fra Antichi e Nuovi Mondi. Il 'Dioscoride' di Andrés Laguna (1555) e gli 'Animalia Mexicana' di Johannes Faber (1628)." *Quaderni Storici* 48.1 (2013): 43–87.

Antonini, Ancilla Maria. "De Auxiliis aspetti teologici di una controversia nell opera tirsiana." *Atti del Convegno di Roma: 15–16 Marzo 1995*. Ed. Associazione Ispanisti Italiani. Vol. 1. Roma: Bulzoni, 1996. 65–80.

Antonio Hernández Morejón, *Historia Bibliográfica de la Medicina Española*. Vols. 1, 2, 3, 4, and 5. Madrid: Viuda de Jordán e Hijos, 1842, 1843, 1843, 1846, 1847; Vols. 6 and 7, Madrid: Celestino G. Alvarez, 1850, 1852.

Aquinas, Thomas. *New English Translation of St. Thomas Aquinas's Summa Theologiae (Summa Theologica)*. Trans. Alfred J. Freddoso. Notre Dame, IN: University of Notre Dame. Web. Oct. 22, 2012. <http://www3.nd.edu/~afreddos/summa-translation/TOC-part1.htm>.

Arata, Stefano. Introducción. *El acero de Madrid*. By Lope de Vega. Madrid: Castalia, 2000.

Ardila, J. A. G. *The Cervantean Heritage: Reception and Influence of Cervantes in Britain*. London, UK: Legenda, 2009.

Arellano, Ignacio. "El entremés de *Las visiones* de Bances Candamo." *Criticón* 37 (1987): 11–35.

———. "El sabio y melancólico Rogerio: interpretación de un personaje de Tirso." *Criticón* 25 (1984): 5–18.

———. *Estructuras dramáticas y alegóricas en los autos de Calderón*. Kassel: Reichenberger, 2001.

Arellano, Ignacio and María Carmen Pinillos. Introducción. *El segundo blasón del Austria*. By Pedro Calderón de la Barca. Ed. Ignacio Arellano and María Carmen Pinillos. Kassel: Reichenberger, 1997. 6–84.

Arizpe, Víctor. "Francisco Santos: aclaraciones crítico-bibliográficas a las *Obras* en prosa y en verso." *Hispania: A Journal Devoted to the Teaching of Spanish and Portuguese* 74. 2 (1991): 457–8.

Arnaud, Emile. *La Vie et l'oeuvre de Alonso Jerónimo de Salas Barbadillo: contribution à l'étude du roman en Espagne au début du XVIIe siècle*. 3 vols. Toulouse: Université de Toulouse-Le Mirail, 1977.

Arrizabalaga, Jon. "Medical Responses to the 'French Disease' in Europe at the turn of the Sixteenth Century." Ed. Kevin Siena. *Sins of the Flesh, Responding to Sexual Disease in Early Modern*. Toronto: Center for Reformation and Renaissance Studies, 2005. 33–55.

————. "Nuevas tendencias en la historia de la enfermedad: a propósito del constructivismo social." *Arbor* 142 (1992): 147–65.

Arróniz, Othón. *La influencia italiana en el nacimiento de la comedia española.* Madrid: Editorial Gredos, 1969.

Asensio, Eugenio. *Itinerario del entremés desde Lope de Rueda a Quiñones de Benavente.* Madrid: Editorial Gredos, 1965.

Asensio, Raymundo. *Sagrado enigma de tres cifras en dos letras descifrado en panegirica oracion de la Virgen Santissima de la Esperanza* [...]. Valencia: Jayme de Bordazar, 1690.

Ashworth, William. "Natural History and the Emblematic World View." Ed. Marcus Hellyer. *The Scientific Revolution. The Essential Readings.* Malden, MA: Blackwell, 2003. 132–56.

Asúa, Miguel de, and Roger French. *A New World of Animals: Early Modern Europeans on the Creatures of Iberian America.* Aldershot: Ashgate, 2005.

Atienza, Belén. *El loco en el espejo: locura y melancolía en la España de Lope de Vega.* Amsterdam: Rodopi, 2009.

Azzolini, Monica. *The Duke and the Stars: Astrology and Politics in Renaissance Milan.* Cambridge, MA: Harvard University Press, 2013.

————. "Reading Health in the Stars. Politics and Medical Astrology in Renaissance Milan." *Horoscopes and Public Spheres.* Ed. Gunther Oestmann, H. Darrel Rutkin, Kocku von Stuckrad. Berlin: Walter de Gruyter, 2005. 183–205.

Baader, Berndt Ph. *Der bayerische Renaissancehof Herzog Wilhelms V. (1568– 1579).* Leipzig: Heitz, 1943.

Bakhtin, Mikhail. *La cultura popular en la Edad Media y en el Renacimiento: el contexto de François Rabelais.* Trans. Julio Forcat and César Conroy. Madrid: Alianza Editorial, 1987.

Baldwin, Martha. "Alchemy and the Society of Jesus in the Seventeenth Century: Strange Bedfellows?" *Ambix* 40 (1993): 41–64.

Ballester, Luis García. *Medicine in a multicultural society: Christian, Jewish and Muslim practitioners in the Spanish kingdoms, 1220–1610.* Aldershot: Ashgate, 2001.

Ballester, Luis García, and Rosa María Blasco Martínez. *Los moriscos y la medicina: un capítulo de la medicina y la ciencia marginadas en la España del siglo XVI.* Barcelona: Labor, 1984.

Ballester, Rosa, Maríaluz López-Terrada, and Álvar Martínez Vidal. "La realidad de la práctica médica: el pluralismo asistencial en la monarquía hispánica (ss. XVI–XVIII)." *Dynamis* 22 (2002): 21–303.

Bances Candamo, Francisco. *Sangre, valor y fortuna.* Ed. Santiago García Castañón. Oviedo: Instituto de Estudios Asturianos, 1991.

Bannet, Eve Tavor. *Empire of Letters: Letter Manuals and Transatlantic Correspondence, 1680-1820.* Cambridge: Cambridge University Press, 2005.

Barrera-Osorio, Antonio. "Empiricism in the Spanish Atlantic World." *Science and Empire in the Atlantic World.* Ed. James Delbourgo and Nicholas Dew. New York: Routledge, 2008. 177–202.

———. *Experiencing Nature: the Spanish American Empire and the Early Scientific Revolution.* Austin, TX: The University of Texas Press, 2006.

———. "Local Herbs, Global Medicines." *Merchants and Marvels: Commerce, Science and Art in Early Modern Europe.* Comp. Pamela H. Smith and Paula Findlen. New York: Routledge, 2002. 163–81.

Barrero Pérez, Óscar. "La decadencia de la novela en el siglo XVII: el ejemplo de Francisco Santos." *Anuario de Estudios Filológicos* 13 (1990): 27–38.

Bartels, Max. "Ueber abnorme Behaarung beim Menschen I." *Zeitschrift für Ethnologie* 8 (1876): 110–29 & Plate VII.

———. "Ueber abnorme Behaarung beim Menschen II." *Zeitschrift für Ethnologie* 11 (1879): 145–94 & Plates VI–VIII.

———. "Ueber abnorme Behaarung beim Menschen III." *Zeitschrift für Ethnologie* 13 (1881): 213–33 & Plate VI.

Bartra, Roger. *Cultura y melancolía: las enfermedades del alma en la España del Siglo de Oro.* Barcelona: Editorial Anagrama, 2001.

Bataillon, Marcel. "Benedetto Varchi et le Cardinal de Burgos D. Francisco de Mendoza y Bobadilla." *Les Lettres romanes* 13 (1969): 3–62.

———. *Erasmo y el erasmismo.* Barcelona: Editorial Crítica, 1978.

———. *Le docteur Laguna auteur du "Voyage en Turquie."* Paris: Librairie des éditions espagnoles, 1958.

———. *Lección Marañón. Política y literatura en el doctor Laguna.* Madrid: Universidad de Madrid, 1970.

Bayanov, Dmitri, and Igor Bourtsev. "On Neanderthal vs. Paranthropus." *Current Anthropology* 17.2 (1976): 312–18.

Bel Bravo, M. Antonia. *La familia en la historia.* Madrid: Ediciones Encuentro, 2000.

Bergman, Hannah E. "En torno a *Lo que ha de ser.*" *Lope de Vega y los orígenes del teatro español: actas del I Congreso Internacional sobre Lope de Vega.* Ed. Manuel Criado de Val. Madrid: EDI-6, 1981. 365–77.

———. *Luis Quiñones de Benavente y sus entremeses: con un catálogo biográfico de los actores citados en sus obras.* Madrid: Editorial Castalia, 1965.

Bergmann, Emilie L. "*La dama boba:* temática folklórica y neoplatónica." *Lope de Vega y los orígenes del teatro español: actas del I Congreso Internacional sobre Lope de Vega.* Ed. Manuel Criado de Val. Madrid: EDI-6, 1981. 409–14.

———. "Monstruous Maternity in Fray Antonio de Guevara's *Relox de Príncipes.*" *Brave New Worlds: Studies in Spanish Golden Age Literature.* Ed. Edward H. Friedman and Catherine Larson. New Orleans, LA: University Press of the South, 1996. 39–49.

Berman, Judith C. "Bad Hair Days in the Paleolithic: Modern (Re)Constructions of the Cave Man." *American Anthropologist* 101.2 (1999): 288–304.

Bermúdez de Pedraza, Francisco. *Historia eucharistica y reformación de abusos* [...] [Madrid]: 1643.

Bernáldez Montalvo, José María. "Las tarascas de Madrid." *Villa de Madrid* 19.71 (1981): 25–32; 19.72 (1981): 27–32.

Bernard, Carmen. *Enfermedad, daño e ideología*. Quito: Ediciones Abya Yala, 1999.

Bernheimer, Richard. *Wild Men in the Middle Ages: A Study in Art, Sentiment, and Demonology*. Cambridge, MA: Harvard University Press, 1952.

Best, Michael R., and Frank H. Brightman, eds. *The Book of Secrets of Albertus Magnus. Of the Virtues of Herbs, Stones, and Certain Beasts, Also a Book of the Marvels of the World*. Oxford, UK: Oxford University Press, 1999.

Blankaart, Steven. *A Physical Dictionary*. London, UK: J. D., 1684.

Blécourt, Willem de, and Cornelie Usborne. "Preface: Situating 'alternative medicine' in the modern period." *Medical History* 43.3 (1999): 283–5.

Bleichmar, Daniela. "Atlantic Competitions: Botany in the Eighteenth-Century Spanish Empire." *Science and Empire in the Atlantic World*. Ed. James Delburgo and Nicholas Dew. London, UK: Routledge, 2008. 225–52.

Bleichmar, Daniela, et al. *Science in the Spanish and Portuguese Empires, 1500–1800*. Stanford, CA: Stanford University Press, 2009.

Blumenberg, Hans. *The Legitimacy of the Modern Age*. Cambridge, MA: MIT Press, 1999.

Bode, Maarten. "The Transformations of Disease in Expert and Lay Medical Cultures." *Journal of Ayurveda and Integrative Medicine* 2.1 (2011): 14–20.

Bondeson, Jan. *The Two-Headed Boy, and Other Medical Marvels*. Ithaca, NY: Cornell University Press, 2000.

Bondt, Jakob de ("Bontius"). "Historiæ naturalis & medicæ Indiæ Orientalis libri sex." [Six sections with their own title pages and pagination, within *Gulielmi Pisonis medici Amstelaedamensis De Indiæ utriusque re naturali et medica: libri quatuordecim*]. Ed. Willem Piso. Amsterdam: Apud Ludovicum et Danielem Elzevirios, 1658.

Bouché-Leclercq, Auguste. *L'astrologie grecque*. Paris: E. Leroux, 1899.

Bourdieu, Pierre. *Language and Symbolic Power*. Cambridge, MA: Harvard University Press, 1991.

Bourg, Julian. "The Rhetoric of Modal Equivocacy in Cartesian Transubstantiation." *Journal of the History of Ideas* 62.1 (2001): 121–40.

Bouza, Fernando. "De lo material en el texto." *¿Qué es un texto?* Ed. Roger Chartier. Madrid: Consorcio Círculo de Bellas Artes, 2006.

Boxer, Charles R. *Two pioneers of tropical medicine: Garcia d'Orta and Nicolás Monardes*. London, UK: The Hispanic and Luso-Brasilian Councils, 1963.

Braham, Persephone. "The Monstrous Caribbean." *The Ashgate research companion to monsters and the monstrous*. Ed. Asa Simon Mittman and Peter J. Dendle. Farnham: Ashgate, 2012. 17–47.

Bravo, María Dolores. Introduction. *Tratado de las supersticiones*. By Pedro Ciruelo. Puebla: Universidad Autónoma de Puebla, 1986. 1–15.

Breydenbach, Bernhard von. *Peregrinatio in Terram Sanctum*. Mainz: Erhard Reuwich, 1486.

Bridges, Christine M. E. "El horóscopo y el vaticinio: Dos mecanismos teatrales en La vida es sueño y en Eco y Narciso, de Calderón de la Barca." *Inti: Revista de literatura hispánica* 1.34 (1991):177-184.

Brockliss, L. W. B., and Colin Jones. *The Medical World of Early Modern France*. Oxford, UK: Clarendon Press, 1997.

Browne, Sir Thomas. "Pseudodoxia Epidemica." *The Works of Sir Thomas Browne*. Ed. Geoffrey Keynes. Vol. I. London, UK: Faber and Faber, 1964.

Bustamante, Jesús. "El conocimiento como necesidad de Estado: las encuestas oficiales sobre Nueva España durante el reinado de Carlos V." *Revista de Indias* 60 (2000): 35–55.

Bustos Tovar, Eugenio de. "La introducción de las teorías de Copérnico en la Universidad de Salamanca." *Revista de la Real Academia de las Ciencias Exactas, Físicas y Naturales de Madrid* 67 (1973): 235–53.

Bynum, W. F., and Roy Porter. *Medical Fringe & Medical Orthodoxy, 1750–1850*. London, UK: Croom Helm, 1987.

Cabré i Pairet, Montserrat, and Teresa Ortiz. *Sanadoras, matronas y médicas en Europa, siglos XII–XX*. Barcelona: Icaria Editorial, 2001.

Calderón de la Barca, Pedro. "De una causa dos efectos." *Verdadera quinta parte de Comedias de don Pedro Calderón de la Barca*. Madrid: Francisco Sanz, 1682.

———. "Los dos amantes del cielo." *Comedias. Vol. V: Verdadera quinta parte de comedias*. Ed. José María Ruano de la Haza. Madrid: Fundación José Antonio de Castro, 2010.

Campbell, Joseph. *El héroe de las mil caras*. México: Fondo de Cultura Económica, 1984.

Campos, Díez M. S. *El Real Tribunal del Protomedicato castellano, siglos XIV–XIX*. Cuenca: Ediciones de la Universidad de Castilla-La Mancha, 1999.

Cañizares-Esguerra, Jorge. "The Colonial Iberian Roots of the Scientific Revolution." *Nature, Empire, and Nation: Explorations of the History of Science in the Iberian World*. Stanford, CA: Stanford University Press, 2006. 14–46.

———. *How to Write the History of the New World: Histories, Epistemologies, and Identities in the Eighteenth-century Atlantic World*. Stanford, CA: Stanford University Press, 2001.

———. "Iberian Science in the Renaissance: Ignored How Much Longer?" *Perspectives on Science* 12.1 (2004): 86–124.

———. *Nature, Empire, and Nation: Explorations of the History of Science in the Iberian World*. Stanford, CA: Stanford University Press, 2006.

———. *Puritan Conquistadors: Iberianizing the Atlantic, 1550–1700*. Stanford, CA: Stanford University Press, 2006.

Cantù, Francesca, and Maria Antonietta Visceglia. *l'Italia di Carlo V: guerra, religione e politica nel primo Cinquecento: atti del Convegno internazionale di studi, Roma, 5–7 aprile 2001*. Roma: Viella, 2003.

Capp, Bernard S. *Astrology and the Popular Press: English Almanacs, 1500–1800*. London, UK: Faber, 1979.

Cárdenas, Juan de. *Problemas y secretos maravillosos de las Indias*. México: Pedro Ocharte, 1591.

Cárdenas, Juan de, and Angeles Durán. *Problemas y secretos maravillosos de Indias*. Madrid: Alianza Editorial, 1988.

Carlino, Andrea. "Medicina e politica alla corte di Enrico III." *Être médecin à la cour (France, Italie, Espagne XIV–XVIII siècles)*. Ed. E. Andretta and M. Nicoud. Florence: Sismel Edizioni del Galluzzo, 2012. 183–98.

———. "Tre piste per l'Anatomia di Juan de Valverde. Logiche d'edizione, solidarietà nazionale e cultura artistica a Roma nel Rinascimento." *Mélanges de l'École Française de Rome* 114.2 (2002): 513–41.

Caro Baroja, Julio. *Historia de la fisiognómica: el rostro y el carácter*. Madrid: Ediciones Istmo, 1988.

Carrera de la Red, Micaela. "Análisis de situaciones comunicativas en el documento indiano por excelencia: la carta." *Haciendo lingüística*. Ed. Mercedes Sedanos et. al. Caracas: Universidad Central de Venezuela, 2006.

Casiano, Juan. *Breue discurso a cerca del cometa visto en el mez de Nouiembre deste año de 1618 y sus significaciones*. Lisboa: Pedro Craesbeeck, 1618.

Casper, Jost. *Die Geschichte des Kanarischen Drachenbaumes in Wissenschaft und Kunst: vom Arbor Gadensis des Posidonius zur Dracaena draco*. Jena: Thüringische Botanische Gesellschaft, 2000.

Cassirer, Ernst. *The Individual and the Cosmos in Renaissance Philosophy*. New York: Dover, 2000.

Castro, Guillén de. *El conde de Irlos. Obras Completas*. Vol. 1. Ed. Juan Oleza. Madrid: Fundación José Antonio de Castro, 1997.

———. *El curioso impertinente*. Ed. E. Juliá. Madrid: Real Academia Española, 1926.

Cervantes, Miguel de. *Don Quixote*. Ed. Florencio Sevilla. Guanajuato: Museo Iconográfico del Quijote, 2010.

Chapman, Allan. "Astrological Medicine." *Health, Medicine, and Mortality in the Seventeenth Century*. Ed. Charles Webster. Cambridge, UK: Cambridge University Press, 1979. 275–300.

Charlesworth, James. *The good and evil serpent: how a universal symbol became Christianized*. New Haven, CT: Yale University Press, 2010.

Chartier, Roger; Alain Boureau, and Cecile Dauphin. *Correspondence: Models of Letter-writing from the Middle Ages to the Nineteenth Century*. Princeton, NJ: Princeton University Press, 1997.

Chevalier, Maxime. "Le médecin dans la littérature du Siècle d'Or." *Le Personnage dans la littérature du Siècle d'or: statut et fonction: Colloque de la Casa de Velázquez*. Paris: Editions Recherche sur les Civilisations, 1984. 21–37.

Chinchilla, Anastasio. *Anales históricos de la medicina en general, y biografico-bibliograficos de la española en particular*. Valencia: Imprenta de López y Compañía, 1841.

Ciaramitaro, Fernando. "El virrey y su gobierno en Nueva España y Sicilia. Analogías y diferencias entre periferias del imperio hispánico." *Estudios de Historia Novohispana* 39 (2008): 117–54.

Clouse, Michele L. *Medicine, Government, and Public Health in Philip II's Spain: Shared Interests, Competing Authorities*. Farnham, UK: Ashgate, 2011.

Clusius, Carolus. *Rariorum aliquot stirpium per Hispanias observatarum historiae*. Antuerpiae: Ex officina Christophori Plantini, 1576.

Cobarrubias Orozco, Sebastián de. *Tesoro de la lengua castellana o española*. Madrid: Luis Sánchez Impresor, 1611.

Columbus, Realdus. *De re anatomica libri XV*. Paris: Apud Andream Wechelum, 1562.

Company Company, Concepción. *Documentos lingüísticos de la Nueva España. Altiplano Central*. México: UNAM, 2008.

Connor, Steven. *The Book of Skin*. Ithaca, NY: Cornell University Press, 2004.

Cook, Alexandra P., and Noble D. Cook. *The Plague Files: Crisis Management in Sixteenth-Century Seville*. Baton Rouge, LA: Louisiana State University Press, 2009.

Cook, Harold J. "The Cutting Edge of a Revolution? Medicine and Natural History Near the Shores of the North Sea." *Renaissance and Revolution: Humanists, Scholars, Craftsmen, and Natural Philosophers in Early Modern Europe*. Ed. Judith Veronica Field. Cambridge, UK: Cambridge University Press, 1993. 45–62.

———. "Global Economies and Local Knowledge in the East Indies." *Colonial Botany: Science, Commerce, and Politics in the Early Modern World*. Ed. Londa L. Schiebinger and Claudia Swan. Philadelphia, PA: University of Pennsylvania, 2005. 100–118.

———. *Matters of Exchange: Commerce, Medicine, and Science in the Dutch Golden Age*. New Haven, CT: Yale University Press, 2007.

———. "Medicine." *Early Modern Science. The Cambridge History of Science. Vol. 3*. Ed. Lorraine Daston and Katharine Park. Cambridge, UK: Cambridge University Press, 2006. 407–34.

———. "Physicians and Natural History." *Cultures of Natural History*. Comp. Nicholas Jardine, James A. Secord, and E. C. Spary. Cambridge, UK: Cambridge University Press, 1996. 91–105.

Cook, Noble David. *Born to Die: Disease and New World Conquest, 1492–1650*. Cambridge, UK: Cambridge University Press, 1998.

Cook, Noble David, and George W. Lovell. *Secret Judgment of God: Old World Disease in Colonial Spanish America*. Norman, OK: University of Oklahoma Press, 1991.

Copenhaver, Brian P. "A Tale of Two Fishes: Magical Objects in Natural History from Antiquity through the Scientific Revolution." *Journal of the History of Ideas* 52.3 (1991): 373–98.

Corcuera de Mancera, Sonia. *El fraile, el indio y el pulque. Evangelización y embriaguez en la Nueva España (1523–1548)*. México: Fondo de Cultura Económica, 1991.

Corominas, Juan. *Breve diccionario etimológico de la lengua castellana*. Madrid: Gredos, 1983.

Cortés, Jerónimo. *El non plus ultra del lunario y pronostico perpetuo, general y particular para cada reyno y provincia*. Barcelona: Antonio Lacavallería, 1670.

———. *Fisonomía y varios secretos de naturaleza*. Barcelona: Jerónimo Margarit, 1610.

———. *Fisonomía y varios secretos de naturaleza*. En Valencia: Vicente Cabrera, 1595.

Cortés Ossorio, Juan. *Constancia de la Fee, y Aliento de la nobleza española, que escrive, y dedica a los gloriosos reynos de Castilla y de Leon*. Madrid: Antonio Roman, 1684.

Covarrubias Orozco, Sebastián de. *Tesoro de la lengua castellana o española, compuesto por el licenciado Don Sebastian de Cobarruvias Orozco*. Madrid: L. Sanchez, 1611.

Crawford, Patricia. "The Construction and Experience of Maternity in Seventeenth-Century England." *Women as Mothers in pre-Industrial England: Essays in Memory of Dorothy McLaren*. Ed. Valerie Fildes. London, UK: Routledge, 1990. 3–38.

Croll, Oswald. *Basilica chymica*. Genevae: Chouet, 1658.

———. *Philosophy Reformed and Improved in Four Profound Tractates* [...]. Trans. Henry Pinnell. London: M. S. for Lodowick Lloyd, 1657. 203.

Crosby, Alfred W. *The Columbian Exchange: Biological and Cultural Consequences of 1492*. Westport, CT: Greenwood Press, 1972.

Cunningham, Andrew. *The Anatomical Renaissance: The Resurrection of the Anatomical Projects of the Ancients*. Aldershot, England: Scolar Press, 1997.

———. "Fabricius and the 'Aristotle Project' in Anatomical Teaching and Research at Padua." *The Medical Renaissance of the Sixteenth Century*. Ed. A. Wear, R. K. French, and I. M. Lonie. Cambridge, UK: Cambridge University Press, 1985. 195–222.

Curry, Patrick. *Astrology, Science, and Society: Historical Essays*. Woodbridge, Suffolk: Boydell Press, 1987.

Czyzewski, Phyllis Eloys. *Picaresque and 'Costumbrista' Elements in the Prose Works of Francisco Santos*. Doctoral dissertation, University of Illinois, 1975.

D'Antuono, Nancy L. "Lope's *Bastardo Mudarra* as Scenario and Opera Tragicomica." *The Golden Age Comedia: Text, Theory, and Performance*. Ed. Howard Mancing and Charle Ganelin. West Lafayette, IN: Perdue University Press, 1994. 178–200.

Dandelet, Thomas J. *Spanish Rome, 1500–1700*. New Haven, CT: Yale University Press, 2001.

Dandelet, Thomas J., and John A. Marino. *Spain in Italy: Politics, Society, and Religion 1500–1700*. Leiden: Brill, 2007.

Daston, Lorraine. "The Factual Sensibility." *Isis* 79 (1988): 452–67.

Daston, Lorraine, and Katharine Park, eds. *Wonders and the Order of Nature, 1150–1750*. New York, NY: Zone Books, 1998.

David-Peyre, Yvonne. *Le Personnage du médecin et la relation médecin-malade dans la littérature ibérique, XVIe et XVIIe siècles*. Paris: Ediciones Iberoamericanas, 1971.

Davies, Natalie Zemon. *Society and Culture in Early Modern France: Eight Essays*. Stanford, CA: Stanford University Press, 1973.

Davis, Charles, and J. E. Varey. "Calderón in the Country: Corpus Christi Performances in Towns around Madrid, 1636–60." *Bulletin of Hispanic Studies* 77.1 (2000): 289–316.

Daza Chacón, Dionisio. *Practica y teorica de cirugía en romance y en latin que trata de todas las heridas*. Valencia: Francisco Cipres, 1673.

De Armas, Frederick. "Black Sun: Woman, Saturn and Melancholia in Claramonte's *La estrella de Sevilla*." *Journal of Interdisciplinary Approaches to Literature* 6 (1994): 19–36.

———. "'El Planeta más impío': Basilio's Role in *La vida es sueño*." *The Modern Language Review* 81.4 (1986): 900–911.

———. "El rey astrólogo en Lope de Vega y Calderón." *El teatro clásico español a través de sus monarcas*. Ed. Luciano García Lorenzo. Madrid: Editorial Fundamentos, 2006. 119–34.

———. "'El sol sale a medianoche': amor y astrología en *Las paredes oyen*." *Criticón* 59 (1993): 119–26.

———. *Heavenly Bodies: The Realms of 'La estrella de Sevilla'*. Lewisburg, PA: Bucknell University Press, 1996.

———. "Icons of Saturn: Astrologer-Kings in Calderón's Comedias." *Forum for Modern Language Studies* 23.2 (1987): 117–30.

———. "The King's Son and the Golden Dew: Alchemy in Calderón's *La vida es sueño*." *Hispanic Review* 60.3 (1992): 301–19.

———. *The Return of Astraea: An Astral-Imperial Myth in Calderón*. Lexington, KY: University Press of Kentucky, 1986.

———. "The Saturn Factor: Examples of Astrological Imagery in Lope de Vega's Works." *Studies in Honor of Everett W. Hesse*. Ed. William Carlton McCrary and José A. Madrigal. Lincoln, NE: Society of Spanish and Spanish-American Studies, 1981. 63–80.

———. "Saturn in conjunction: from Albumasar to Lope de Vega." *Saturn from Antiquity to the Renaissance*. Ed. Massimo Ciavolella and Amilcare A. Iannucci. Ottawa: Dovehouse Editions, 1992. 151–72.

———. *A Star-Crossed Golden Age: Myth and the Spanish Comedia*. Lewisburg, PA: Bucknell University Press, 1998.

De Vos, Paula Susan. "An Herbal El Dorado: The Quest for Botanical Wealth in the Spanish Empire." *Endeavour* 27.3 (2003): 117–21.

———. "The Rare, the Singular, and the Extraordinary: Natural History and the Collection of Curiosities in the Spanish Empire." *Science in the Spanish and Portuguese Empires, 1500–1800*. Ed. Daniela Bleichmar. Stanford, CA: Stanford University Press, 2009. 271–89.

———. "The Science of Spices: Empiricism and Economic Botany in the Early Spanish Empire." *Journal of World History* 17.4 (2006): 399–427.

De Vun, Leah. *Prophecy, Alchemy, and the End of Time: John of Rupescissa in the Late Middle Ages*. New York, NY: Columbia University Press, 2009.

Dean, Carolyn, and Dana Leibsohn. "Hybridity and Its Discontents: Considering Visual Culture in Colonial Spanish America." *Colonial Latin American Review* 12.1 (2003): 5–35.

Dear, Peter. *Discipline & Experience: The Mathematical Way in the Scientific Revolution*. Chicago, IL: University of Chicago Press, 1995.

Debus, Allen G. *The Chemical Philosophy: Paracelsian Science and Medicine in the Sixteenth and Seventeenth Centuries*. New York, NY: Science History Publications, 1977.

———. *Chemistry and Medical Debate*. Canton, MA: Science History Publications, 2001.

———. *The French Paracelsians: The Chemical Challenge to Medical and Scientific Tradition in Early Modern France*. Cambridge, UK: Cambridge University Press, 1991.

———. "Paracelsianism and the diffusion of the chemical philosophy in early modern Europe." *Paracelsus: the Man and His Reputation, His Ideas and Their Transformation*. Ed. Ole Peter Grell. Leiden, Boston: Brill, 1998.

Del Río Parra, Elena. *Una era de monstruos: representaciones de lo deforme en el Siglo de Oro español*. Pamplona, Frankfurt, Madrid: Universidad de Navarra, Vervuert, Iberoamericana, 2003.

Delbourgo, James, and Nicholas Dew. *Science and Empire in the Atlantic World*. New York, NY: Routledge, 2008.

Delgado de la Vera, Justo. *Defensa y Respuesta justa, y verdadera e la medicina racional y philosophica, profanada de las imposturas de la Chimia, introductora del remedio universal y agua de la vida de Alderete. Contra [...] Luis Amigo Beltran [...] que la defiende*. Madrid: Antonio Roman, 1687.

Delpech, François. "La patraña del hombre preñado: algunas versiones hispánicas." *Nueva Revista de Filología Española* 34. 2 (1985–1986): 548–98.

Díez Borque, José María. *Sociología de la comedia española del siglo XVII*. Madrid: Ediciones Cátedra, 1976.

Dioscorides of Anazarbus. *Acerca de la materia medicinal y de los venenos mortíferos. Pedacio Dioscorides Anazarbeo; traducido de lengua griega en la vulgar castellana, e ilustrado [...] por el Doctor Andres de Laguna [...]*. Valencia: a costa de Claudio Mace, 1635.

———. *Acerca de la materia medicinal, y de los venenos mortiferos: traduzido de lengua Griega, en la vulgar Castellana, & illustrado con claras y substantiales annotationes, y con las figuras de innumeras plantas exquisitas y raras*. Vol. 1. Antwerp: J. Laët, 1555.

————. *De materia medica.* Trans Lily Beck. Hildesheim, Zurich, New York: Olms-Weidmann, 2005.

————. *Pedacio Dioscórides Anazarbeo, acerca de la materia medicinal y de los venenos mortíferos.* Ed. Andrés de Laguna and Pedro Laín Entralgo. Madrid: Fundación de Ciencias de la Salud; Doce Calles, 2005.

Dioscorides of Anazarbus, César Emil Dubler, Andrés de Laguna, and Elías Terés. *La "Materia médica" de Dioscórides, transmisión medieval y renacentista.* Barcelona: Tipografía, 1953–1959.

DiPuccio, Denise. "Destiny versus Free Will in Adonis y Venus." *Communicating Myths in the Golden Age Comedia.* Ed. Denise DiPuccio. Lewisburg, PA: Bucknell University Press. 58–71.

Dobbs, Betty Jo Teeter. *The Foundations of Newton's Alchemy: or, "The Hunt for the Greene Lyon."* New York, NY and Cambridge, UK: Cambridge University Press, 1975.

Domingo Malvadi, Arantxa. *Bibliofilia humanista en tiempos de Felipe II: la biblioteca de Juan Páez de Castro.* Salamanca: Ediciones Universidad de Salamanca, Área de Publicaciónes de la Universidad de Leon, 2011.

Domingo Malvadi, Arantxa. *Disponiendo anaqueles para libros: nuevos datos sobre la biblioteca de Jerónimo Zurita.* Zaragoza: Institución Fernando el Católico, 2010.

Domingo, Xavier. "La cocina precolombina en España." *Conquista y comida: consecuencias del encuentro de dos mundos.* Ed. Janet Long. México: UNAM, Instituto de Investigaciones Históricas, 2003. 17–28.

Donato, Maria P., and Jill Kraye. *Conflicting Duties: Science, Medicine, and Religion in Rome, 1550–1750.* London, UK: Warburg Institute, 2009.

Drummond, William. *The History of Scotland, from the Year 1423 Until the Year 1542 Containing the Lives and Reigns of James the I, the II, the III, the IV, the V: with Several Memorials of State, During the Reigns of James VI & Charls I.* London: Printed by Henry Hills for Richard Tomlins and himself, 1655.

D'Urfey, Thomas. *Collin's Walk Through London and Westminster: A Poem in Burlesque.* London: Printed for Rich. Parker and Abel Roper, 1690.

Duve, Thomas. *Sonderrecht in der frühen Neuzeit: Studien zum 'ius singulare' und den 'privilegia miserabilium personarum', 'senum' und 'indorum' in Alter und Neuer Welt.* Frankfurt-am-Main: Vittorio Klostermann, 2008.

Eamon, William. "How to Read a Book of Secrets." *Secrets and Knowledge in Medicine and Science (1500–1800).* Ed. Elaine Long and Alisha Rankin. Bodmin, Cornwall: Ashgate, 2011. 23–46, p. 31.

————. "'Nuestros males no son constitucionales, sino circunstanciales': The Black Legend and the History of Early Modern Spanish Science." *The Colorado Review of Hispanic Studies* 7 (2009): 13–30.

————. *Science and the secrets of nature: books of secrets in medieval and early modern culture.* Princeton, NJ: Princeton University Press, 1994.

————. *Science as a Hunt.* Firenze: L. S. Olschki, 1994.

Egginton, William. *How the World Became a Stage: Presence, Theatricality, and the Question of Modernity.* Albany: SUNY Press, 2003.

Egido López, Teófanes, Javier Burrieza Sánchez, and Manuel Revuelta González. *Los Jesuitas en España y en el mundo hispánico.* Madrid: Marcial Pons, 2004.

Egmond, Florike, P. G. Hoftijzer, and Robert P. W. Visser. *Carolus Clusius: Towards a Cultural History of a Renaissance Naturalist.* Amsterdam: Koninklijke Nederlandse Akademie van Wetenschappen, 2007.

Eiseley, Loren C. "The Reception of the First Missing Links." *Proceedings of the American Philosophical Society* 98.6 (1954): 453–65.

Elliott, John H. "A Europe of Composite Monarchies." *Past and Present* 137 (1992): 48–71.

———. "Britain and Spain in America: Colonists and Colonised." *Spain, Europe, and the Wider World, 1500-1800.* New Haven, CT: Yale University Press, 2009. 192–210. 149–72.

———. "Illusion and Disillusionment: Spain and the Indies." *Spain, Europe, and the Wider World, 1500-1800.* New Haven, CT: Yale University Press, 2009. 131–48.

———. "The Discovery of America and the Discovery of Man." *Spain and Its World 1500-1700.* New Haven, CT: Yale University Press, 1989. 42–64.

———. *The Old World and the New 1492–1650.* Cambridge, UK: Cambridge University Press, 1970.

———. "Same World, Different Worlds." *Spain, Europe, and the Wider World, 1500-1800.* New Haven, CT: Yale University Press, 2009. 192-210.

———. "Self-Perception and Decline in Seventeenth-Century Spain." *Spain and Its World 1500-1700.* New Haven, CT: Yale University Press, 1989. 241-62.

———. *Spain and Its World, 1500–1700: Selected Essays.* New Haven, CT: Yale University Press, 1989.

———. *Spain, Europe & the Wider World, 1500–1800.* New Haven, CT: Yale University Press, 2009.

Enders, Jody. "The Devil in the Flesh of Theater." *Transformationen des Religiösen: Performativität und Textualität im geistlichen Spiel.* Ed. Ingrid Kasten and Erika Fischer-Lichte. Berlin: De Gruyter, 2007. 127–38.

Enríquez Gómez, Antonio. *La torre de Babilonia.* Ed. María Teresa de Santos Borreguero. Doctoral thesis, Universidad Autónoma de Madrid, 1989. Microfiche edition.

Escudero y Perosso, Francisco. *Tipografía Hispalense: Anales bibliográficos de la ciudad de Sevilla desde el establecimiento de la imprenta hasta fines del siglo XVIII.* Madrid: Sucesores de Rivadeneyra, 1894.

Espantoso-Foley, Augusta M. *Occult Arts and Doctrine in the Theater of Juan Ruiz de Alarcón.* Genève: Droz, 1972.

———. "The Problem of Astrology and Its Use in Ruiz de Alarcón's *El dueño de las estrellas.*" *Hispanic Review* 32.1 (1964): 1–11.

Espinosa y Malo, Félix de Lucio. *Epistolas varias que consagra a la catolica magestad del rey D. Carlos Segundo, N.S. monarca de las Españas, y del Nuevo Mundo* [...]. Madrid: Francisco Sanz, Impressor del Reyno, 1675.

Esteban Núñez, *Miropolio general y racional de botica.* Ed. Miguel López Pérez and Mar Rey Bueno. Burgos: Colegio Oficial de Farmacéuticos, 2003.

Eustasio, E. "De las cosas necesarias para escribir historia: Memorial inédito del Dr. Juan Páez de Castro al Emperador Carlos V." *La ciudad de Dios* 28 (1892): 604–10 (1893): 1–20.

Ezpeleta, Martín de. *Libro de cuentas extraordinarias.* Zaragoza: Gaspar Martínez, Impressor en el Hospital Real y General, 1704.

Falconieri, John V. "Historia de la 'Commedia dell'Arte' en España." *Revista de literatura* 12.23–24 (1957): 69–90.

Feingold, Mordechai, and Brotons V. Navarro. *Universities and Science in the Early Modern Period.* Dordrecht: Springer, 2006.

Fernández Christlieb, Federico, and Ángel Julián García Zambrano, eds. *Territorialidad y paisaje en el altepetl del siglo XVI.* México: Fondo de Cultura Económica-UNAM, 2006.

Fernández-Morera, Darío, and Michael Hanke. *Cervantes in the English-Speaking World: New Essays.* Kassel: Edition Reichenberger, 2005.

Ficino, Marsilio. *Sulla vita.* Ed. Alessandra Tarabochia Canavero. Milano: Rusconi, 1995.

———. *Three Books on Life.* Ed. Carol V. Kaske and John R. Clark. Binghamton, NY: Medieval & Renaissance Texts & Studies in conjunction with the Renaissance Society of America, 1989.

Fields, Sherry Lee. *Pestilence and Headcolds: Encountering Illness in Colonial Mexico.* New York, NY: Columbia University Press, 2008.

Figueroa, Juan de. *Opúsculo de astrología en medicina, y de los términos, y partes de la astronomía necessarias para el uso della.* Lima: [s.n.], 1660.

Findlen, Paula. "The Economy of Scientific Exchange in Early Modern Italy." *Patronage and Institutions: Science, Technology, and Medicine at the European Court, 1500–1750.* Ed. Bruce T. Moran. Rochester, NY: Boydell, 1991. 5–25.

———. *Possessing Nature: Museums, Collecting, and Scientific Culture in Early Modern Italy.* Berkeley, CA: University of California Press, 1996.

Firpo, Massimo. "Politica imperiale e vita religiosa in Italia nell'età di Carlo V." *Studi Storici* 42.2 (2001): 245–61.

FitzPatrick, P. J. *In Breaking of Bread: The Eucharist and Ritual.* Cambridge, UK: Cambridge University Press, 1993.

Flor, Fernando R. de la. *Era melancólica: figuras del imaginario barroco.* Palma de Mallorca: José J. de Olañeta, 2007.

———. "La máquina simbólica: Picinelli y el ocaso de la teología escolástica hispánica." *Esplendor y ocaso de la cultura simbólica.* Ed. Herón Pérez Martínez and Bárbara Skinfill. Zamora, Mexico: Colegio de Michoacán, 2002. 143–60.

Flores, Enrique, and Mariana Masera. *Relatos populares de la Inquisición novohispana: rito, magia y otras 'supersticiones', siglos XVII–XVIII*. Madrid: Consejo Superior de Investigaciones Científicas, 2010.

Florescano, Enrique, and Elsa Malvido. *Ensayos sobre la historia de las epidemias en México*. 2 vols. México: Instituto Mexicano del Seguro Social, 1982.

Floridi, Luciano. *Sextus Empiricus: The Transmission and Recovery of Pyrrhonism*. Oxford, UK: Oxford University Press, 2002.

Fonseca, Rodrigo da. *In Hippocratis legem commentarium, quo perfecti medici natura explicat [...]*. Rome: Titi & Pauli de Dianis fratres, 1586.

Forth, Gregory. "Hominids, Hairy Hominoids and the Science of Humanity." *Anthropology Today* 21.3 (2005): 13–17.

Fracastoro, Girolamo. *Hieronymi Fracastorii [...] De sympathia et antipathia rerum liber vnus*. Venetiis: apud heredes Lucantonii Iuntae, 1546.

Fragoso, Juan. *Cirurgia Universal [...]; y mas otros quatro tratados [...]*. Alcalá de Henares: Juan Gracián, 1610.

Francisci, Erasmus, *Ost- und West-Indischer wie auch sinesischer Lust- und Stats-Garten*. Nürnberg: 1668.

French, Roger. "Astrology in Medical Practice." *Practical Medicine from Salerno to the Black Death*. Ed. Luis García-Ballester, Roger French, Jon Arrizabalaga, and Andrew Cunningham. Cambridge, UK: Cambridge University Press, 1994. 30–59.

———. *William Harvey's Natural Philosophy*. Cambridge, UK: Cambridge University Press, 1994.

Frenk, Margit. *Nuevo corpus de la antigua lírica popular hispánica (siglos XV a XVII)*. México: El Colegio de México, 2003.

Friedman, Edward H. "A View of Tragedy and Tragicomedy in Ruiz de Alarcón's *El dueño de las estrellas* and *La crueldad por el honor*." *Kentucky Romance Quarterly* 22.4 (1975): 429–41.

Friedman, John Block. *The Monstrous Races in Medieval Art and Thought*. Syracuse, NY: Syracuse University Press, 2000.

Friesen, Ryan C. *Supernatural Fiction in Early Modern Drama and Culture*. Brighton: Sussex Academic Press, 2010.

Froissart, Jean. *Here Begynneth the Thirde and Fourthe Boke of Sir Iohn Froissart of the Cronycles of Englande, Fraunce, Spaygne, Portyngale, Scotlande, Bretayne, Flaunders, and Other Places Adioynyng [...]*. Trans. John Bourchier, Lord Berners. London: Rycharde Pynson, 1525.

Gadamer, Hans Georg. *Truth and Method*. New York, NY: The Seabury Press, 1975.

Galenus. *Therapeutica. Metodo de Galeno en lo que toca a cirugia*. Zaragoza: viuda de Bartholome de Nagera, 1572.

Gálvez Ruiz, M. Ángeles. "Las parejas imperfectas. Viajes a ultramar y ausencias de la vida maridable, siglo XVII." *Historia, género y familia en Iberoamérica (siglos XVI al XX)*. Ed. Dora Dávila-Mendoza. Caracas: Universidad Central de Venezuela, 2004. 67–101.

García, Susan Paun de, and Donald R. Larson. *The Comedia in English: Translation and Performance.* Woodbridge, UK: Tamesis, 2008.

García Acosta Virginia, et al. *Desastres agrícolas en México: Catálogo histórico, 1. Épocas prehispánica y colonial.* México: CIESAS, 2003.

García Canclini, Néstor. *Hybrid Cultures: Strategies for Entering and Leaving Modernity.* Minneapolis, MN: University of Minnesota Press, 1995.

García Cárcel, Ricardo. "¿Son creíbles las fuentes inquisitoriales?" *Grafías del imaginario: Representaciones culturales en España y América (siglos XVI–XVIII).* Ed. Carlos Alberto González Sánchez and Enriqueta Vila Vilar. México: Fondo de Cultura Económica, 2003. 96–110.

García de León, Antonio. *Tierra adentro, mar en fuera: el puerto de Veracruz y su litoral a Sotavento, 1519–1821.* México, D.F: Fondo de Cultura Económica, 2011.

García Hourcade, Juan Luis, and Juan M. Moreno Yuste. *Andrés Laguna: humanismo, ciencia y política en la Europa renacentista: Congreso Internacional, Segovia, 22–26 de noviembre de 1999.* Valladolid: Junta de Castilla y León, Consejería de Educación y Cultura, 2001.

García Lorenzo, Luciano. "Ideología y moralismo. El Padre Manuel de Guerra y Ribera y su aprobación a las comedias de Calderón." *III y IV Jornadas de teatro.* Burgos: Universidad de Burgos, 1995.

Garin, Eugenio. *Astrology in the Renaissance: The Zodiac of Life.* London: Routledge & Kegan Paul, 1983.

———. *Marsilio Ficino y el Platonismo.* Córdoba: Alcion, 1997.

Gaukroger, Stephen. *The Emergence of Scientific Culture: Science and the Shaping of Modernity, 1210–1685.* London, UK: Clarendon Press, 2006.

Geiler von Kaysersberg, Johannes. *Die Emeis.* Strassburg: J Grieninger, 1517.

Gies, David. "Dos Preguntas Regeneracionistas, 'que se debe a Espana?' y 'que es Espana?': Identidad Nacional En Forner, Moratin, Jovellanos y la Generacion del 98." *Dieciocho: Hispanic Enlightenment* 22 (1999): 307–30.

Gélis, Jacques. *History of Childbirth: Fertility, Pregnancy and Birth in Early Modern Europe.* Cambridge, UK: Cambridge University Press, 1991.

Gentilcore, David. *Healers and Healing in Early Modern Italy.* Manchester, UK: Manchester University Press, 1998.

———. "Was there a 'Popular Medicine' in Early Modern Europe?" *Folklore* 115.2 (2004): 151–66.

Gerard, John. *The Herbal or General Historie of Plantes.* London, UK: John Norton, 1597.

Gicklhorn, Renée, Walter Göpfert, Irmgard Müller, and Hans Schadewaldt, "Bemerkungen zur Geschichte und Ikonographie des Drachenbaumes." *Deutsche Apotheker Zeitung* 27 (1980): 1260–66.

Gijswijt-Hofstra, Marijke, Hilary Marland, and Hans de Waardt. *Illness and Healing Alternatives in Western Europe.* London, UK: Routledge, 1997.

Gil-Sotres, Pedro, Juan Antonio Paniagua, and Luis García-Ballester. "Estudi introductori." Arnau de Vilanova. *Regimen sanitatis ad regem aragonum.* Arnaldi de Vilanova Opera Medica Omnia, Vol. X.1. Barcelona: Universitat de Barcelona, 1996. 15–394.

Ginzburg, Carlo. *El hilo y las huellas: lo verdadero, lo falso, lo ficticio.* Buenos Aires: Fondo de Cultura Económica, 2010.

Giralt, Sebastià. "Arnau de Vilanova i les propietats ocultes, de la mágia a la medicina universitària." *Actes de les V Trobades d'Història de la Ciència i de la Tècnica: Roquetes, 11–13 desembre 1998.* Ed. Josep Batlló Ortiz, Roser Puig Aguilar, and Pere de la Fuente Collell. Barcelona: Societat Catalana d'Història de la Ciència i de la Tècnica, 2000. 393–9.

Giraud, François. "De las problemáticas europeas al caso novohispano: apuntes para una historia de la familia mexicana." *Familia y sexualidad en Nueva España: memoria del primer simposio de historia de la mentalidades: "Familia, matrimonio y sexualidad en Nueva España."* México: Fondo de Cultura Económica, 1982. 56–80.

Glanvill, Joseph. *The Vanity of Dogmatizing, Or, Confidence in Opinions Manifested in a Discourse of the Shortness and Uncertainty of Our Knowledge, and Its Causes, with Some Reflexions on Peripateticism and an Apology for Philosophy.* Ed. by E. C. for Henry Eversden. London: 1661.

Góngora y Argote, Luis de. *Letrillas.* Ed. Robert Jammes. Madrid: Castalia, 1980.

González Manjarrés, Miguel Angel. *Andrés Laguna y el humanismo médico: estudio filológico.* Valladolid: Junta de Castilla y León, Consejería de Educacin y Cultura, 2000.

González Moreno, Joaquín. *Don Fernando Enríquez de Ribera. Tercer Duque de Alcalá de los Gazules, 1583–1637.* Sevilla: Ayuntamiento de Sevilla, 1969.

González Palencia, Ángel. *Gonzalo Pérez, secretario de Felipe Segundo.* Madrid: Consejo Superior de Investigaciones Cientificas, Instituto Jerónimo Zurita, 1946.

González Palencia, Ángel, and Eugenio Mele. *Vida y obras de Don Diego Hurtado de Mendoza.* Madrid: Instituto de Valencia de Don Juan (impr. de E. Maestre), 1941.

Goodman, David. *Power and Penury: government, technology, and science in Philip II's Spain.* Cambridge, UK: Cambridge University Press, 1988.

Grafton, Anthony, and Nancy Siraisi. "Between the Election and My Hopes: Girolamo Cardano and Medical Astrology." *Secrets of Nature: Astrology and Alchemy in Early Modern Europe.* Ed. William R. Newman and Anthony Grafton. Cambridge, MA: MIT Press, 2001. 69–132.

Granjel, Luis S. *La medicina española del siglo XVII.* Salamanca: Universidad de Salamanca, 1978.

Gräße, Johann Georg Theodor. *Der Sagenschatz des Königreichs Sachsen.* Dresden: Schönfeld, 1855.

Graux, Charles. *Essai sur les origines du fonds grec de l'Escurial: épisode de l'histoire de la Renaissance des lettres en Espagne.* Paris: F. Vieweg, 1880.

Greenfield, Amy Butler. *A Perfect Red: Empire, Espionage, and the Quest for the Color of Desire.* New York, NY: HarperCollins, 2005.

Greilsammer, Myriam. "The Midwife, the Priest, and the Physician: The Subjugation of Midwives in the Low Countries at the End of the Middle Ages." *Journal of Medieval and Early Modern Studies* 21.2 (1991): 285–327.

Groebner, Valentin. "Complexio/Complexion: Categorizing Individual Natures, 1250–1600." *The Moral Authority of Nature.* Ed. Lorraine Daston and Fernando Vidal. Chicago, IL: University of Chicago Press, 2004. 361–83.

Grubbs, Anthony J. "Major Changes in 'Minor' Theater: Luis Quiñones de Benavente's Dramatization of Dramatic Theory and Its Effects on the Interlude in Early Modern Spain." *Hispanófila* 151 (2007): 1–20.

Grundmann, Martin. *Neu-eröffnete Geist- und Weltliche Geschicht-Schule.* Görlitz: Kästner, 1677.

Gruzinski, Serge. *Las cuatro partes del mundo: historia de una mundialización.* México, D.F: Fondo de Cultura Económica, 2010.

———. *The Mestizo Mind: The Intellectual Dynamics of Colonization and Globalization.* New York, NY: Routledge, 2002.

———. "Les mondes mêlés de la Monarchie catholique et autres connected histories." *Annales. Histoire, Sciences Sociales* 56.1 (2001): 85–117.

———. *La pensée métisse.* Paris: Fayard, 1999.

———. *Les Quatre parties du monde. Histoire d'une mondialisation.* Paris: Éditions de la Martinière, 2004.

Guarinonius, Hippolytus. *Die Grewel der Verwüstung menschlichen Geschlechts: In sieben unterschiedliche Bücher [...] abgetheilt.* Ingolstatt: Angermayr, 1610.

Guazzo, Francesco M. *Compendium Maleficarum: The Montague Summers Edition.* Ed. E. A. Ashwin. New York, NY: Dover, 1988.

Guerra, Francisco. *Nicolás Bautista Monardes su vida y su obra, ca. 1493–1588.* México: Compañía fundidora de hierro y acero de Monterrey, 1961.

Guevara, Antonio de. *Relox de Príncipes.* Ed. Emilio Blanco. Madrid: ABL, Confres, 1994.

Gutiérrez, Constancio. *Españoles en Trento.* Valladolid: Consejo Superior de Investigaciones Científicas, Instituto "Jerónimo Zurita," Sección de Historia Moderna "Simancas," 1951.

Guzmán Guerra, Antonio. *El Dioscórides de Laguna y el manuscrito de Paez de Castro.* Madrid: Universidad Complutense, Facultad de Filología, 1978.

Hafter, Monroe Z. "Saavedra Fajardo plagiado en *El no importa de España* de Francisco Santos." *Bulletin Hispanique* 61 (1959): 5–11.

Halstead, Frank G. "The Attitude of Lope de Vega toward Astrology and Astronomy." *Hispanic Review* 7.3 (1939): 205–19.

———. "The Attitude of Tirso de Molina toward Astrology." *Hispanic Review* 9.4 (1941): 417–39.

Hammond, John H. "Francisco Santos and Zabaleta." *Modern Language Notes* 66. 3 (1951): 166.

——. *Francisco Santos' Indebtedness to Gracián*. Austin, TX: University of Texas Press, 1950.

——. "A Plagiarium from Quevedo's *Sueños*." *Modern Language Notes* LXIV (1949): 329–31.

——. "References to Cervantes in the Works of Francisco Santos." *Cervantes Quadricentennial* (1949): 100–102.

——. "Substitutions in the Works of Francisco Santos." *South Central Bulletin* 23. 4 (1963): 41–5.

Happel, Eberhard Werner. *E[verhardus]G[uernerus] Happelii Gröste Denckwürdigkeiten der Welt: oder so genannte Relationes curiosae*, I–V. Hamburg: Gedruckt und verlegt durch Thomas von Wiering, 1683, 1685, 1687, 1689, 1691 [=*Relationes curiosae*].

——. *Relationes curiosae. Oder Denckwürdigkeiten der Welt: [...] daß also diese Arbeit gar füglich E. G. Happelii Continuation seiner [...] curieusen Relationen genannt werden könne*. Hamburg: Reumann, 1707.

Heiple, Daniel. "Profeminist Reactions to Huarte's Misogyny in Lope De Vega's *La prueba de los ingenios* and Mariá de Zayas's *Novelas amorosas y ejemplares*. "*The Perception of Women in Spanish Theater of the Golden Age*. Ed. Anita K. Stoll and Dawn L. Smith. Lewisburg, PA: Bucknell University Press, 1991.

Henke, Robert. *Pastoral Transformations: Italian Tragicomedy and Shakespeare's Late Plays*. Newark, DE: University of Delaware Press, 1997.

Henry, John. "Occult Qualities and the Experimental Philosophy: Active Principles in Pre-Newtonian Matter Theory." *History of Science* 24 (1986): 335–81.

Hernández, Francisco. *The Mexican Treasury: The Writings of Dr. Francisco Hernández*. Ed. Simon Varey. Trans. Rafael Chabrán, Cynthia L. Chamberlin, and Simon Varey. Stanford: Stanford University Press, 2000.

Hernández, Francisco, and Germán Somolinos d'Ardois. *Obras Completas*. México: Universidad Nacional de México, 1959.

Hernando Sánchez, Carlos José. *Roma y Espanña: un crisol de la cultura europea en la edad moderna*. Madrid: Sociedad estatal para la acción cultural exterior, 2007.

Hernando y Ortega, Teófilo. *Vida y labor médica del doctor Andrés Laguna*. Segovia: Instituto Diego de Colmenares, 1960.

Herr, Richard. *The Eighteenth-century Revolution in Spain*. Princeton, NJ: Princeton University Press, 1958.

Hertel, Christiane. "'Der rauch man zu Münichen': Die Porträts der Familie Gonsalus in der Kunstkammer Erzherzog Ferdinands II. von Tirol." *Sammler, Bibliophile, Exzentriker*. Ed. Aleida Assmann, Monika Gomille, and Gabriele Rippl. Tübingen: Narr, 1998. 163–91.

Herzig, Carine. "Un episodio de la controversia ética sobre la comedia de santos: en torno a la 'Aprobación' del Padre Fray Manuel de Guerra y Ribera (1682–1684)." *Homenaje a Henri Guerreiro: la hagiografía entre historia y literatura en la España de la Edad Media y del Siglo de Oro*. Ed. Marc Vitse. Frankfurt: Iberoamericana, 2006. 713–24.

———. "Fray Manuel de Guerra y Ribera, 'Aprobación a la *Verdadera Quinta Parte de Comedias de don Pedro Calderón'* (1682): estudio, edición y notas." *Criticón* 93 (2005): 95–154.

———. "La polémica en torno a la 'Aprobación' del Padre Fray Manuel de Guerra y Ribera (1682–1684) y la moralización de la Comedia." *Criticón* 103–4 (2008): 81–92.

Hesse, E.W. "Calderón's Concept of the Perfect Prince in *La vida es sueño*." Critical Essays on the Theatre of Calderón. Ed. Bruce W. Wardropper. New York, NY: New York University Press, 1965. 114–33.

Hillman, David y Carla Mazzio, eds. *The Body in Parts: Fantasies of Corporeality in Early Modern Europe*. London, UK: Routledge, 1997.

Hobson, Anthony. *Renaissance Book Collecting: Jean Grolier and Diego Hurtado de Mendoza, Their Books and Bindings*. Cambridge, UK: Cambridge University Press, 1999.

Hochman, Stanley. *McGraw-Hill Encyclopedia of World Drama*. 2nd ed. Vol. 5. New York, NY: McGraw-Hill, 1984.

Holländer, Eugen. *Wunder, Wundergeburt und Wundergestalt: in Einblattdrucken des fünfzehnten bis achtzehnten Jahrhunderts; kulturhistorische Studie*. Stuttgart: Verlag Von Ferdinand Enke, 1921.

Holloway, James E. "Lope's Neoplatonism: *La dama boba*." *Bulletin of Hispanic Studies* 49.3 (1972): 236–55.

Hontanilla, Ana. "Images of Barbaric Spain in Eighteenth-Century English Travel Writing." *Studies in Eighteenth-century Culture*. Ed. Linda Zionkowski and Downing A. Thomas. Vol. 37. Baltimore, MD: Johns Hopkins University Press, 2008.

Hornung, Erik. *The Secret Lore of Egypt: Its Impact on the West*. Ithaca, NY: Cornell University Press, 2002.

Howard, Sharon. "Imagining the Pain and Peril of Seventeenth-Century Childbirth: Danger and Deliverance in the Making of an Early Modern World." *Social History of Medicine* 16. 3 (2003): 367–82.

Huerta Calvo, Javier. "Cómico y femenil bureo. (Del amor y las mujeres en los entremeses del Siglo de Oro)." *Criticón* 24 (1983): 5–68.

Huguet-Termes, Teresa, Jon Arrizabalaga, and Harold J. Cook.*Health and Medicine in Hapsburg Spain: Agents, Practices, Representations*. London: Wellcome Trust Centre for the History of Medicine at UCL, 2009.

Hunter, Michael. "Robert Boyle and Secrecy." *Secrets and Knowledge in Medicine and Science, 1500–1800*. Ed. Elaine Leong and Alisha Rankin. Aldershot, UK: Ashgate, 2011.

Hutchison, Keith. "What Happened to Occult Qualities in the Scientific Revolution?" *Isis* 73.2 (1982): 233–53.

Iannini, Christopher. *Fatal Revolutions: Natural History, West Indian Slavery, and the Routes of Early American Literature*. Chapel Hill, NC: The University of North Carolina Press, 2012.

Iffland, James. *Quevedo and the Grotesque*. 2 vols. London, UK: Tamesis, 1978.

Iglesias, María Carmen. "Montesquieu and Spain: Iberian Identity as Seen through the Eyes of a Non-Spaniard of the Eighteenth Century." *Iberian Identity: Essays on the Nature of Identity in Portugal and Spain*. Ed. Richard Herr and John Herman Richard Polt. Berkeley, CA: Institute of International Studies, University of California, Berkeley, 1989.

"Inquisición." Archivo General de la Nación (AGN). Gobierno Mexicano. Web. <http://www.agn.gob.mx/menuprincipal/serviciospublico/servicios/fondos.html>.

Instrucción y memoria de las relaciones que se han de hacer para la descripción de las Indias [Madrid], [s.l.], 1577.

Iso, J. J. *Anales de Zurita. Buscador en Red*. Zaragoza: Institución Fernando el Católico, 2008.

Israel, Jonathan I. *Razas, clases sociales y vida política en el México colonial 1610–1670*. México: Fondo de Cultura Económica, 2005.

Jacob, François. *The Logic of Live: a history of heredity*. New York, NY: Pantheon Books, 1971.

Jaffary, Nora. "La percepción de clase y casta en las visiones de los *falsos místicos* en México colonial." *Signos históricos* 8 (2002): 61–88.

Janson, H. W. *Apes and Ape Lore in the Middle Ages and the Renaissance*. London, UK: Warburg Institute, University of London, 1952.

Jarcho, Saul. "Galen's six non-naturals." *Bulletin of the History of Medicine* 44 (1970): 372–7.

Jardine, Nicholas, James A. Secord, and E. C. Spary. *Cultures of Natural History*. Cambridge, UK: Cambridge University Press, 1996.

Jedin, Hubert. *Storia del Concilio di Trento: il primo periodo 1545–1547*. Vol. 2. Brescia, Italia: Morcelliana, 1962.

Jedin, Hubert, and Paolo Prodi. *Il Concilio di Trento come crocevia della politica europea*. Bologna: Il Mulino, 1979.

Jerónimo Zurita: su época y su escuela: IV centenario de la Universidad de Zaragoza: Congreso Nacional, Zaragoza, 16–21 de mayo de 1983. Zaragoza, Spain: "Institución Fernando el Católico," Excma Diputación Provincial de Zaragoza, 1986.

Jiménez Catalán, Manuel. *Ensayo de una tipografía zaragozana del siglo XVII*. Zaragoza: La académica, 1925.

Jiménez de la Espada, Marcos. *Relaciones geográficas de Indias*. Madrid: Tipografía de Manuel G. Hernández, 1881.

Juan de Mora. *Enigma numerico predicable, explicado en cinco tratados de numeros doctrinales* […]. Madrid: Juan García Infanzon, 1682.

Juanini, Juan Bautista. *Nueva idea. Phisica natural demonstratva; Origen de las materias que mueven las cosas. Compuestas de la porcion mas puras de los elementos, Fraguadas en el caos, purificadas y passadas de potencia a acto en los tres primeros dias de la Creacion del Mundo [...]* Zaragoza, 1685.

Jung, Carl. *Alchemical Studies*. London, UK: Routledge & Kegan Paul, 1967.

Jütte, Robert, Motzi Eklöf, and Marie C. Nelson. *Historical Aspects of Unconventional Medicine: Approaches, Concepts, Case Studies*. Sheffield, UK: European Association for the History of Medicine and Health Publications, 2001.

Kagan, Richard L. "Prescott's Paradigm: American Historical Scholarship and the Decline of Spain." *The American Historical Review* 101.2 (1996): 423–46.

Katritzky, M. A. *Healing, Performance and Ceremony in the Writings of Three Early Modern Physicians: Hippolytus Guarinonius and the Brothers Felix and Thomas Platter*. Farnham, UK: Ashgate, 2012.

———. "Images of 'monsters' and performers: J. A. Comenius's *Orbis pictus* and *Aristotle's masterpiece*." *Practicing New Editions: Transformation and Transfer of the Early Modern Book, 1450–1800*. Ed. Hiram Kümper and Vladimir Simić. Nordhausen: Bautz, 2011. 77–118.

———. "Stefanelo Botarga and Pickelhering: fishy Italian and English stage clowns in Spain and Germany." In press.

Kaufmann, Lynn Frier. *The Noble Savage: Satyrs and Satyr Families in Renaissance Art*. Ann Arbor, MI: UMI Research Press, 1984.

Kennedy, Kenneth A. R. *God-apes and Fossil Men: Paleoanthropology of South Asia*. Ann Arbor, MI: University of Michigan Press, 2000.

Kirk, Stephanie. "El parto monstruoso: creación artística y reproducción biológica en la obra de Sor Juana Inés de la Cruz." *Revista Iberoamericana* 75 (2009): 417–32.

Klestinec, Cynthia. *Theaters of Anatomy: Students, Teachers, and Traditions of Dissection in Renaissance Venice*. Baltimore, MD: Johns Hopkins University Press, 2011.

Klibansky, Raymond, Erwin Panofsky, and Fritz Saxl. *Saturn and Melancholy: Studies in the History of Natural Philosophy, Religion, and Art*. London, UK: Nelson, 1964.

Knowles, James. "'Can ye not tell a man from a marmoset?': apes and others on the early modern stage." *Renaissance Beasts: Of Animals, Humans, and Other Wonderful Creatures*. Ed. Erica Fudge. Urbana, IL: University of Illinois Press, 2004. 138–63.

Krier, Theresa M. *Birth Passages: Maternity and Nostalgia, Antiquity to Shakespeare*. Ithaca, NY: Cornell University Press, 2001.

Kuklick, Henrika and Robert E. Kohler. *Science in the Field*. Chicago, IL: University of Chicago Press, 1996.

Kurtz, Barbara E. "*El bobo del colegio* de Lope de Vega: aproximación a su sentido." *Revista Canadiense de Estudios Hispánicos* 11.1 (1986): 11–25.

Lacey, J Hubert. "Anorexia nervosa and a bearded female saint." *British Medical Journal* 285 (1982): 1816–17.

Laguna, Andrés de. *Annotationes in Dioscoridem Anazarbeum, per Andream Lacunam, [...] juxta vetustissimorum codicum fidem elaboratae.* Lugduni: apud G. Rouillium, 1554.

———. *Epitomes omnivm Galeni Pergameni opervm, vniversam illivs viri doctrinam, & methodum, quàm accuratissimè continentis.* Vol. 1. Venetiis: Apud Hieronymum Scotum, 1548.

Lanning, John Tate. *The Royal Protomedicato: The Regulation of the Medical Profession in the Spanish Empire.* Durham, NC: Duke University Press, 1985.

Lanuza-Navarro, Tayra M. C. *Astrología, ciencia y sociedad en la España de los Austrias.* Diss. Universitat de Valencia, 2005.

———. "Medical Astrology in Spain During the Seventeenth Century." *Cronos* 9 (2006): 59–83.

Lasso de la Vega y Cortezo, Javier. *Biografía y estudio critico de las obras del médico Nicolas Monardes.* Sevilla: Padilla, 1988.

Latour, Bruno. *We Have Never Been Modern.* Cambridge, MA: Harvard University Press, 1993.

Lea, Henry Charles. *A History of the Inquisition of Spain.* New York, NY: Macmillan Co., 1922.

Leitch, Stephanie. *Mapping Ethnography in Early Modern Germany: New Worlds in Print Culture.* Basingstoke, UK: Palgrave Macmillan, 2010.

León, Andrés de. *Libro primero de annathomia.* Baeza: J. B. de Montoya, 1590.

León, (Fray) Luis de. *La perfecta casada.* Ed. Mercedes Etreros. Madrid: Taurus, 1987.

Leong, Elaine, and Alisha Rankin. Introduction. *Secrets and Knowledge in Medicine and Science (1500–1800).* Ed. Elaine Long and Alisha Rankin. Bodmin, Cornwall, UK: Ashgate, 2011. 1–20.

Levin, Michael J. *Agents of Empire: Spanish Ambassadors in Sixteenth-Century Italy.* Ithaca, NY: Cornell University Press, 2005.

Levisi, Margarita. "Hieronymus Bosch y los *Sueños* de Francisco de Quevedo." *Filología* 9 (1963): 163–200.

Lewis, Laura A. *Hall of Mirrors: Power, Witchcraft, and Caste in Colonial Mexico.* Durham, NC: Duke University Press, 2003.

Lima, Robert. *Dark Prisms: Occultism in Hispanic Drama.* Lexington, KY: University Press of Kentucky, 1995.

———. *Stages of Evil: Occultism in Western Theater and Drama.* Lexington: University Press of Kentucky, 2005.

Lindemann, Mary. *Medicine and Society in Early Modern Europe.* Cambridge, UK: Cambridge University Press, 2010.

Litt, Thomas. *Les corps célestes dans l'univers de Saint Thomas d'Aquin.* Louvain: Publications Universitaires, 1963.

Livingstone, David N. *Putting Science Its Place: Geographies of Scientific Knowledge.* Chicago, IL: University of Chicago Press, 2003.

————. "The spaces of knowledge: contributions towards a historical geography of science." *Environment and Planning D: Society and Space* 13.1 (1995): 5–34.

Lockhart, James. *The Nahuas after the Conquest. A Social and Cultural History of the Indians of Central Mexico, Sixteenth through Eighteenth Centuries.* Stanford, CA: Stanford University Press, 1992.

Lockhart, James, Lisa Sousa, and Stephanie Wood, eds. *Sources and Methods for the Study of Postconquest Mesoamerican Ethnohistory.* Eugene, OR: University of Oregon, 2007.

Long, Pamela O. *Artisan/Practitioners and the Rise of the New Sciences, 1400–1600.* Corvallis, OR: Oregon State University Press, 2011.

————. *Openness, Secrecy, Authorship. Technical Arts and the Culture of Knowledge from Antiquity to the Renaissance.* Baltimore, MD: Johns Hopkins University Press, 2001.

Look, Brandon. "Leibniz and the Substance of the *Vinculum Substantiale.*" *Journal of the History of Philosophy* 38.2 (2000): 203–20.

López Austin, Alfredo. *Textos de medicina náhuatl.* México: SEP Setentas, 1971.

López Austin, Alfredo, and Leonardo López Luján. *El pasado indígena.* México: Colegio de México, Fideicomiso Historia de las Américas, 1996.

López de Mariscal, Blanca. "El viaje a la Nueva España entre 1540 y 1625: el trayecto femenino." *Historia de las mujeres en América Latina.* Ed. Juan Andreo and Sara B. Guardia. Murcia: Comunidad Autónoma de la Región de Murcia, 2002. 89–109.

López Pérez, Miguel. "Ciencia y pensamiento hermético en la Edad Moderna española." *Más allá de la leyenda negra: España y la revolución científica / Beyond the black legend: Spain and the scientific revolution.* Ed. Víctor Navarro Brotóns and William Eamon. Valencia: CSIC-Universitat de València, 2007. 57–72.

————. *Asclepio renovado: alquimia y medicina en la España Moderna (1500–1700).* Madrid: Corona Borealis, 2003.

López Pérez, Miguel, and Mar Rey Bueno. "La instrumentalización de la espagiria en el proceso de renovación: las polémicas sobre medicamentos químicos." *Los Hijos de Hermes. Alquimia y espagiria en la terapéutica española moderna.* Ed. Javier Puerto Sarmiento, Esther Alegre, Mar Rey Bueno, and Miguel López. Madrid: Corona Borealis, 2001. 281–347.

López Piñero, José María. *Ciencia y técnica en la sociedad española de los siglos XVI y XVII.* Barcelona: Labor Universitaria, 1979.

————. *El 'Dialogus' (1589) del paracelsista Llorenç Coçar y la cátedra de medicamentos químicos de Valencia (1591).* Valencia: CSIC-Universitat de València, 1977.

————. "*Paracelsus* and his Work in 16th and 17th Century Spain." *Clio Medica* 8 (1973): 119–31.

López Piñero, José María, and Maríaluz López-Terrada, eds. *La influencia española en la introducción en Europa de las plantas americanas: 1493–1623.* Valencia: CSIC-Universitat de València, 1997.

López-Terrada, Maríaluz. "El tratamiento de la sífilis en un hospital renacentista: la sala del 'mal de siment' del Hospital General de Valencia." *Asclepio* 41.2 (1989): 19–50.

———. "Los tribunales del protomedicato y el protoalbeiterato." *Historia de la ciencia y de la técnica en la corona de Castilla. Siglos XVI y XVII.* Ed. José María López Piñero. Salamanca: Junta de Castilla y León, 2002. 107–25.

———. "Medical Pluralism in the Iberian Kingdoms: The Control of Extra-Academic Practitioners in Valencia." *Health and Medicine in Hapsburg Spain: Agents, Practices, Representations.* Ed. Teresa Huguet-Termes, Jon Arrizabalaga, and Harold John Cook. London, UK: Wellcome Trust Centre for the History of Medicine at UCL, 2009. 7–25.

López-Terrada, Maríaluz, and Àlvar Martínez Vidal. "El Tribunal del Real Protomedicato en la Monarquía hispánica (1593–1808)." *Dynamis* 16 (1996): 17–19.

Lozoya, Xavier. *Los señores de las plantas: herbolaria y medicina en Mesoamérica.* México: Pangea Editores, 1990.

Lugt, Maaike van der. "The *Incubus* in Scholastic Debate: Medicine, Theology and Popular Belief." *Religion and Medicine in the Middle Ages.* Ed. Peter Biller and Joseph Ziegler. Woodbridge, Suffolk, UK: York Medieval Press, 2001. 175–200.

Luna. John Carter Brown Archive of Early American Images. "El dragón." Web. <http://jcb.lunaimaging.com/luna/servlet/detail/JCB~1~1~2178~3600006:El-dragon-?qvq=q:el%2Bdragon%2Bmonardes;lc:JCB~1~1,JCBBOOKS~1~1,J CBMAPS~1~1,JCBMAPS~2~2&mi=0&trs=1>.

Lusitanus, Zacutus. *Praxis medica admiranda.* Lugduni: Huguetan, 1637.

Lykosthenes, Konrad. *Prodigiorum ac ostentorum chronicon, quae praeter naturae ordinem, motum, et operationem, et in superioribus & his inferioribus mundi regionibus, ab exordio mundi usque ad haec nostra tempora, acciderunt.* Basileae: Per Henricum Petri, 1557.

MacKay, Ruth. *"Lazy, Improvident People": Myth and Reality in the Writing of Spanish History.* Ithaca, NY: Cornell University Press, 2006.

Madroñal Durán, Abraham. "Diferencias en *El parecido* de Agustín Moreto." *Moretiana: adversa y próspera fortuna de Agustín Moreto.* Ed. María Luisa Lobato and Juan Antonio Martínez Berbel. Madrid: Iberoamericana, 2008. 141–54.

Mahdi, Waruno. *Malay words and Malay things: lexical souvenirs from an exotic archipelago in German publications before 1700.* Wiesbaden: Harrassowitz ('Frankfurter Forschungen zu Südostasien, 3'), 2007.

Mandujano, Angélica, et al. "Historia de las epidemias en el México antiguo. Algunos aspectos biológicos y sociales." *Casa del Tiempo* 5 (2003): 9–21.

Manlius, Johannes Jacobus. *Locorvm Commvnivm Der Erste Theil. Schöne ordentliche Gatteirung allerley alten und newen Exempel [...] aus des Herrn Philippi Melanthonis / und anderer gelehrten / fürtrefflichen Menner.* Trans. Johann Huldreich Ragor. Frankfurt: Peter Schmidt, 1566.

Marini, Gaetano Luigi. *Degli archiatri pontifici.* Vol. 1. Rome: V. Pagliarini, 1784.

Martín Martín, Teodoro, and Juan Páez de Castro. *Vida y obra de Juan Páez de Castro.* Guadalajara: Institución Provincial de Cultura Marqués de Santillana, 1990.

Martin, Vincent. *El concepto de "representación" en los autos sacramentales de Calderón.* Kassel: Reichenberger, 2002.

Martinengo, Alessandro. *La astrología en la obra de Quevedo: una clave de lectura.* Pamplona: Ediciones Universidad de Navarra, 1992.

Martínez, Enrico. *Reportorio de los tiempos y historia natural de esta Nueva España.* México: Enrico Martínez, 1606.

Martínez, José Luis. *Pasajeros de Indias. Viajes trasatlánticos en el siglo XVI.* México: Fondo de Cultura Económica, 1999.

Martínez Hernández, Gerardo. *La medicina en la nueva España. Siglos XVI–XVII.* Diss. Universidad de Salamanca, 2010. *Repositorio Documental de la Universidad de Salamanca.* Web. Jan. 15, 2013. <http://hdl.handle.net/10366/83189>.

Mason, Paul H. and Roger V. Short. "Neanderthal-human hybrids." *Hypothesis* 9.1 (2011): 1–5.

Mason, Peter. "A dragon tree in the Garden of Eden." *Journal of the History of Collections* 18 (2006): 169–85.

Mazzoni, Cristina. *Maternal Impressions: Pregnancy and Childbirth in Literature and Theory.* Ithaca, NY: Cornell University Press, 2002.

McGuire, Robert A., and Philip R. P. Coelho. *Parasites, Pathogens, and Progress: Diseases and Economic Development.* Cambridge, MA: MIT Press, 2011.

McKendrick, Melveena. *Woman and Society in the Spanish Drama of the Golden Age: A Study of the Mujer Varonil.* London, UK: Cambridge University Press, 1974.

Melero Jiménez, Elisa Isabel. *La tarasca de parto en el mesón del infierno, y días de fiesta por la noche. Su autor Francisco Santos, criado del Rey Nuestro Señor, y natural de Madrid. Dedicada a Juan Díaz Rodero.* Edición y estudio de los preliminares y del libro primero. Presentado en el Departamento de Filología Hispánica, Facultad de Filosofía y Letras, de la Universidad de Extremadura, el día 25 de septiembre de 2004.

Melis, Chantal, and Agustín Rivero Franyutti. *Documentos lingüísticos de la Nueva España. Golfo de México.* México: UNAM, 2008.

Mello e Souza, Laura de. *The Devil and the Land of the Holy Cross: Witchcraft, Slavery, and Popular Religion in Colonial Brazil.* Austin, TX: University of Texas Press, Teresa Lozano Long Institute of Latin American Studies, 2003.

Memarzadeh, Maher. *Medical Practitioners in Early Colonial Mexico.* Diss. University of California, Los Angeles, 2005.

Méndez, Sigmund. "Del Barroco como el ocaso de la concepción alegórica del mundo." *Andamios: revista de investigación social* 4 (2006): 147–80.

Merkle, Sebastian. *Concilium Tridentinum: [diariorum, actorum, epistularum, tractatuum nova collectio] [Tomus primus]*. Concilium Tridentinum. Friburgi Brisgoviae [i.e. Freiburg im Breisgau]: Herder, 1901.

Miguel Alonso, Aurora. "Las ediciones de la obra de Dioscórides en el siglo XVI. Fuentes textuales e iconográficas." *Pedacio Dioscórides Anazarbeo, acerca de la materia medicinal y de los venenos mortíferos*. Ed. Andrés de Laguna and Pedro Laín Entralgo. Madrid: Fundación de Ciencias de la Salud; Doce Calles, 2005.

Mobley, Gregory. "The Wild Man in the Bible and the Ancient Near East." *Journal of Biblical Literature* 116.2 (1997): 217–33.

Mochón Castro, Montserrat. *El intelecto femenino en las tablas áureas: contexto y escenificación*. Madrid: Iberoamericana, 2012.

Molina, Tirso de. *Amazonas en las Indias. Trilogía de los Pizarros*. Ed. Miguel Zugasti. Vol. 3. Kassel: Ed. Reichenberger, 1993.

———. *Don Gil de las calzas verdes*. Ed. Enrique García Santo-Tomás. Madrid: Cátedra, 2009.

———. *El amor médico*. Ed. Blanca Oteiza. Madrid-Pamplona: Instituto de Estudios Tirsianos, 1997.

———. *El melancólico. Obras completas. Doce comedias nuevas*. Ed. María del Pilar Palomo and Isabel Prieto. Vol. 3. Madrid: Fundación José Antonio de Castro, 1997.

———. *Obras Completas: Cuarta parte de comedias I*. Ed. Ignacio Arellano. Navarra: Instituto de Estudios Tirsianos, 1999.

Monardes, Nicolás. *Diálogo del hierro y sus grandezas*. Sevilla: Alonso Escrivano, 1574.

———. *Dos libros: El vno trata de todas las cosas q[ue] trae[n] de n[uest]ras Indias Occide[n]tales, que sirven al vso de medicina [...] El otro libro, trata de dos medicinas marauillosas q[ue] son co[n]tra todo veneno [...] con la cura delos venenados [...]*. Sevilla: Sebastian Trugillo, 1565.

———. *Historia medicinal de las cosas que se traen de nuestras Indias occidentales que sirven en medicina*. Sevilla: Padilla, 1988.

———. *Segunda parte del libro, de las cosas que se traen de nuestras Indias Occidentales, que sirven al uso de medicina*. Sevilla: Alonso Escriuano, impressor, 1571.

Moncó Rebollo, Beatriz. "Demonio y mujeres: historia de una transgresión." *El Diablo en la Edad Moderna*. Ed. María Tausiet and James S. Amelang. Madrid: Marcial Pons, 2004. 187–210.

———. *Mujer y demonio: una pareja barroca*. Madrid: Instituto de Sociología Aplicada, 1989.

Montaigne, Michel de. *The Complete Essays of Montaigne*. Trans. Donald Murdoch Frame. Stanford, CA: Stanford University Press, 1958.

————. *Essayes*. Trans. John Florio. London: Printed by Melch. Bradwood for Edward Blount and William Barret, 1613.

Montesquieu, Baron de. *The Spirit of the Laws*. Trans. Thomas Nugent. 2 vols. New York, NY: Hafner, 1949.

Morant, Isabel. *Discursos de la vida buena: matrimonio, mujer y sexualidad en la literatura humanista*. Madrid: Cátedra, 2002.

More, Ellen S., Elizabeth Fee, and Manon Parry. *Women Physicians and the Cultures of Medicine*. Baltimore: Johns Hopkins University Press, 2009.

Moreno, Cristóbal. *Jornadas para el Cielo*. Alcalá: Juan Íñiguez de Lequerica, 1596.

Moreto, Agustín. *El parecido*. Ed. Lluisa Castillo Roselló. Valencia: Imprenta de Benito Macé, 1676. *Moretianos*. Web. Jan. 17, 2013. <http://www.moretianos. com/pormoreto.php>.

————. *El parecido de la Corte*. Ed. D. Luis Fernández-Guerra y Orbe. Alicante: Biblioteca Virtual Miguel de Cervantes, 1999. *Biblioteca Virtual Miguel de Cervantes*. Web. <http://www.cervantesvirtual.com/obra/el-parecido-en-la-corte--0/>.

Morley, S. Griswold. "El acero de Madrid." *Hispanic Review* 13.2 (1945): 166–9.

Motolinía, Toribio. *Historia de los indios de la Nueva España*. México: Editorial Porrúa, 2007.

Murdoch, John. "The Analytical Character of Medieval Learning: Natural Philosophy Without Nature." *Approaches to Nature in the Middle Ages: Papers of the Tenth Annual Conference of the Center for Medieval & Early Renaissance Studies*. Vol. 16. Ed. Lawrence D. Roberts. Binghamton, NY: Center for Medieval & Early Renaissance Studies, 1982. 171–213.

Myers, Kathleen Ann, and Nina M. Scott. *Fernández De Oviedo's Chronicle of America: A New History for a New World*. Austin, TX: University of Texas, 2007.

Nadeau, Carolyn. "Authorizing the Wife/Mother in Sixteenth-Century Advice Manuals." *Women in the Discourse of Early Modern Spain*. Ed. Joan Cammarata. Gainesville, FL: University Press of Florida, 2003. 19–34.

————. "Blood Mother/Milk Mother: Breastfeeding, the Family, and the State in Antonio de Guevara's *Relox de Príncipes* (*Dial of Princes*)." *Hispanic Review* 69. 2 (2001): 153–74.

————. "Star-Crossed Love: Spheres of Reality in Ruiz de Alarcón's *La verdad sospechosa*." *A Star-Crossed Golden Age: Myth and the Spanish Comedia*. Ed. Frederick De Armas. London, UK: Associated University Presses, 1998.

Navarrete, Ignacio Enrique. *Orphans of Petrarch: Poetry and Theory in the Spanish Renaissance*. Berkeley, CA: University of California Press, 1994.

Navarro Brotóns, Víctor. "Aguilera, Juan (¿–1560)." *La web de las Biografías*. Web. Jan. 23, 2013. <http://www.mcnbiografias.com/app-bio/do/show?key= aguilera-juan>.

————. "La actividad astronómica en la España del siglo XVI: perspectivas historiográficas." *Arbor* 142 (1992): 185–216.

————. "The Reception of Copernicus in Sixteenth-Century Spain: The Case of Diego de Zúñiga." *Isis* 86.1 (1995): 52–78.

Navarro Brotons, Víctor, and William Eamon. *Mas allá de la Leyenda Negra: España y la revolución científica. Beyond the Black Legend: Spain and the Scientific Revolution.* Valencia: Instituto de Historia de la Ciencia y Documentación López Piñero, 2007.

Navarro Pérez, Milagros. "Bibliografía crítica de la obra de Francisco Santos." *Cuadernos bibliográficos* 30 (1973): 148–9.

————. *Francisco Santos, un costumbrista del siglo XVII.* Madrid: Consejo Superior de Investigaciones Científicas, 1975.

Navarro Santos, Milagros. "Bibliografía crítica de la obra de Francisco Santos." *Cuadernos bibliográficos* 30 (1973): 148–9.

Nelson Novoa, James W. "Andrés Laguna in Papal Rome. The Documents of the Mozoncillo Ecclesiastical Benefice." *Minerva* 25 (2012): 211–32.

Newman, William. *Atoms and Alchemy: Chymistry and the Experimental Origins of the Scientific Revolution.* Chicago, IL: University of Chicago Press, 2006.

————. *The Summa perfectionis of Pseudo-Geber: a critical edition, translation and study.* Leiden-New York: Brill, 1991.

Newman, William and Lawrence M. Principe. *Alchemy Tried in the Fire: Starkey, Boyle, and the Fate of Helmontian Chymistry.* Chicago, IL: University of Chicago Press, 2002.

Newson, Linda A. "Medical Practice in Early Colonial Spanish America: A Prospectus." *Bulletin of Latin American Research* 25 (2006): 367–91.

Nieremberg, Juan Eusebio. *Curiosa y oculta filosofia. Primera y segunda parte de las marauillas de la naturaleza, examinadas en varias questiones naturales.* Alcalá: Imprenta de María Fernandez, 1649.

Nieto-Galán, Agustí. "The Images of Science in Modern Spain. Rethinking the 'Polémica'." *The Sciences in the European Periphery during the Enlightenment.* Ed. Kostas Gavroglu. Dordrecht: Kluwer Acadademic Publishers, 1999. 73–94.

Niseno, Diego. *Asuntos predicables para todos los domingos despues de Pentecostes* […]. Barcelona: Sebastian de Cormellas, 1631.

Norton, Marcy. *Sacred Gifts and Profane Pleasures: A History of Tobacco and Chocolate in the Atlantic World.* Ithaca, NY: Cornell University Press, 2008.

Nummedal, Tara. *Alchemy and Authority in the Holy Roman Empire.* Chicago, IL: University of Chicago Press, 2007.

Obendorf, Peter J., Charles E. Oxnard, and Ben J. Kefford. "Are the Small Human-like Fossils Found on Flores Human Endemic Cretins?" *Proceedings of the Royal Society: Biological Sciences* 275.1640 (2008): 1287–96.

Oberman, Heiko Augustinus. *'Contra vanam curiositatem'. Ein Kapitel der Theologie zwischen Seelenwinkel und Weltall.* Zürich: Theologischer Verlag, 1974.

Obregón, Diana, ed. *Culturas científicas y saberes locales: asimilación, hibridación, resistencia.* Santafé de Bogotá: Universidad Nacional de Colombia, 2000.

Ogilvie, Brian W. *The Science of Describing: Natural History in Renaissance Europe*. Chicago, IL: University of Chicago Press, 2006.

Ojeda Calvo, María del Valle. "Nuevas aportaciones al estudio de la *Commedia dell'arte* en España: el *zibaldone* de Stefanello Bottarga." *Criticón* 63 (1995): 119–38.

———. *Stefanelo Botarga e Zan Ganassa. Scenari e zibaldoni di comici italiani nella Spagna del cinquecento*. Rome: Bulzoni, 2007.

Oleza, Juan. "Hipótesis sobre la génesis de a comedia barroca y la historia teatral del XVI." *Teatros y prácticas escénicas I: El Quinientos valenciano*. Ed. Juan Oleza and Manuel V. Diago. Valencia: Institució Alfons el Magnànim, 1984. 9–41.

Oliva, César. "Tipología de los 'Lazzi' en los pasos de Lope de Rueda." *Criticón* 42 (1988): 65–79.

Olmi, Giuseppe. *L'inventario del mondo. Catalogazione della natura e luoghi del sapere nella prima età moderna*. Bologna: Il Mulino, 1992.

Ongaro, G. "Girolamo Fracastoro e lo Studio di Padova." *Girolamo Fracastoro: fra medicina, filosofia e scienze della natura*. Ed. Alessandro Pastore and Enrico Peruzzi. Firenze: L. S. Olschki, 2006. 31–54.

"Orang Pendek." *Wikipedia*. Wikimedia Foundation, Jan. 15, 2013. Web. Sept. 5, 2012. <http://en.wikipedia.org/wiki/Orang_Pendek>.

Orta, García de. *Colóquios dos simples e drogas he cousas medicinais da Índia*. Goa: Ioannes de Endem, 1563.

Ortega Gato, Esteban. "Los Enriquez, almirantes de Castilla." *Publicaciones de la Institución Tella Téllez de Meneses* 70 (1999): 23–65.

Ortiz de Moncada, Pedro. *Practica de la comunion puramente espiritual, ilustrada con muchos exemplos y autoridades* […]. Madrid: Diego Martinez Abad, 1695.

Ortiz, Teresa. "La educación de las matronas en la Europa Moderna: ¿liberación o subordinación?" *De leer a escribir: la educación de las mujeres, ¿libertad o subordinación?* Ed. Cristina Segura Graiño. Granada: Asociación Cultural Al-Mudayna, 1996. 155–70.

———. "From Hegemony to Subordination: Midwives in Early Modern Spain." *The Art of Midwifery: Early Modern Midwives in Europe*. Ed. Hilary Marland. London, UK: Routledge, 1993. 99–106.

Otte, Enrique. *Cartas privadas de emigrantes a Indias: 1540–1616*. México: Fondo de Cultura Económica, 1993.

Oviedo, Luis de. *Methodo de la colección y reposicion de las medicinas simples, y de su corrección y preparación*. Madrid: Luis Sánchez, 1595.

Padrón, Ricardo. *The Spacious Word: Cartography, Literature, and Empire in Early Modern Spain*. Chicago, IL: University of Chicago Press, 2004.

Pagden, Anthony. *European Encounters with the New World: From Renaissance to Romanticism*. New Haven, CT: Yale University Press, 1993.

———. *The Fall of Natural Man: The American Indian and the Origins of Comparative Ethnology*. Cambridge, UK: Cambridge University Press, 1982.

———. *Lords of All the World: Ideologies of Empire in Spain, Britain and France c. 1500–c. 1800*. New Haven, CT: Yale University Press, 1995.

———. *Spanish Imperialism and the Political Imagination: Studies in European and Spanish-American Social and Political Theory, 1513–1830*. New Haven, CT: Yale University Press, 1990.

Pagel, Walter. *Joan Baptista Van Helmont: Reformer of Science and Medicine*. Cambridge, UK: Cambridge University Press, 1982. 62.

———. *Paracelsus: an introduction to philosophical medicine in the era of the Renaissance*. Basel/New York: Palter, 1982.

Pallarés, Berta. "La melancolía como enfermedad en la obra de Tirso de Molina (contribución a su estudio)." *Tirso de Molina: textos e intertextos*. Ed. Laura Dolfi and Eva Galar. Pamplona, Spain: Instituto de Estudios Tirsianos, 2001. 125–78.

———. "La melancolía en la comedia palatina de Tirso de Molina (contribución al estudio del tema en su obra)." *El sustento de los discretos: la dramaturgia áulica de Tirso de Molina*. Ed. Eva Galar and Blanca Oteiza. Madrid: Instituto de Estudios Tirsianos, 2003. 91–123.

Pan, James A. "On Fate, Suicide and Free Will in Alarcón's *El dueño de las estrellas*." *Hispanic Review* 42 (1974): 199–207.

Paravicino y Arteaga, Hortensio Félix. *Oracion evangelica del maestro Fray Hortensio Felix Paravicino [...] al patronato de España, de la Santa Madre Teresa de Iesus [...] en febrero de 1628*. Madrid: Juan Gonzalez, 1628.

Pardo-Tomás, José. "Andrés Laguna y la medicina europea del Renacimiento." *Los orígenes de la ciencia moderna. Seminario 'Orotava' de la Historia de la Ciencia. Actas XI y XII*. La Orotava: Consejería de Educación, cultura y deportes del Gobierno de Canarias, 2002. 45–68.

———. *Ciencia y censura: la Inquisición española y los libros científicos en los siglos XVI y XVII*. Madrid: Consejo Superior de Investigaciones Científicas, 1991.

———. "Conversion Medicine: Communication and Circulation of Knowledge in the Franciscan Convent and College of Tlatelolco, 1527–1577." *Quaderni Storici* 48 (2013): 28–42.

———. "Natural Knowledge and Medical Remedies in the Book of Secrets: Uses and Appropriations in Juan De Cárdenas's Problemas Y Secretos Maravillosos De Las Indias (Mexico, 1591)." *A Passion for Plants: Materia Medica and Botany in Scientific Networks from the 16th to 18th Centuries*. By Sabine Anagnostou, Florike Egmond, and Christoph Friedrich. Stuttgart: Wissenschaftliche Verlagsgesellschaft, 2011. 1–16.

———. *Oviedo, Monardes, Hernández: el tesoro natural de América: colonialismo y ciencia en el siglo XVI*. Madrid: Nivola, 2002.

Pardo-Tomás, José, and Maríaluz López-Terrada. *Las primeras noticias sobre plantas americanas en las relaciones de viajes y crónicas de Indias, 1493–1553*. Valencia: CSIC-Universitat de València, 1993.

Paré, Ambroise. *The workes of that famous chirugion Ambrose Parey translated out of Latine*. London: Th Cotes & R Young, 1634.

Paster, Gail Kern. *The Body Embarrassed: Drama and the Disciplines of Shame in Early Modern England*. Ithaca, NY: Cornell University Press, 1993.

Pastore, Alessandro. "Il consulto di Girolamo Fracastoro sul tifo petecchiale (Trento, 1547)." *Girolamo Fracastoro: fra medicina, filosofia e scienze della natura*. Ed. Alessandro Pastore and Enrico Peruzzi. Firenze: L. S. Olschki, 2006. 91–101.

Pastore, Alessandro and Enrico Peruzzi. *Girolamo Fracastoro: fra medicina, filosofia e scienze della natura: atti del convegno internazionale di studi in occasione del 450° anniversario della morte: Verona-Padova 9–11 ottobre 2003*. Firenze: L. S. Olschki, 2006.

Pastore, Stefania. "Una Spagna anti-papale? Gli anni italiani di Diego Hurtado de Mendoza." *Roma moderna e contemporanea* 15 (2007): 63–94.

Pavia, Mario N. *Drama of the Siglo de Oro: A Study of Magic, Witchcraft, and Other Occult Beliefs*. New York, NY: Hispanic Institute in the United States, 1959.

Pelling, Margaret, and Scott Mandelbrote. *The Practice of Reform in Health, Medicine, and Science, 1500–2000: Essays for Charles Webster*. Aldershot, Hampshire, UK: Ashgate, 2005.

Peña, Margarita. "Los hermanos de Juan Ruiz de Alarcón: ortodoxia y judaísmo. " *Elementos* 43 (2001): 48.

Pennuto, Concetta. *Simpatia, fantasia e contagio: il pensiero medico e il pensiero filosofico di Girolamo Fracastoro*. Roma: Edizioni di storia e letteratura, 2008.

Pepys, Samuel. *The Diary of Samuel Pepys*. <http://ebooks.adelaide.edu.au/p/pepys/samuel/wheatley>. Accessed 16 July 2013.

Perdiguero Gil, Enrique. "'Con medios humanos y divinos': la lucha contra la enfermedad y la muerte en el Alicante del siglo XVIII." *Dynamis* 22 (2002): 121–50.

———. "The Popularization of Medicine during the Spanish Englightenment." *The Popularization of Medicine: 1650–1850*. Ed. Roy Porter. London, UK: Routledge, 1992. 160–93.

Pérez Bautista, Florencio L. "La medicina y los médicos en el teatro de Calderón de la Barca." *Cuadernos de Historia de la Medicina Española* 7 (1968): 149–245.

Pérez de Montalbán, Juan. *A lo hecho no hay remedio y El príncipe de los montes. Primero tomo de las Comedias*. Alcala: Antonio Vazquez, Impressor de la Universidad, 1638.

———. *Doze comedias las mas famosas que asta aora han salido de los meiores y mas insignes poetas : tercera parte* ... Lisboa: Antonio Alvarez ..., [1649?].

———. *Don Florisel de Niquea. Segundo tomo de las Comedias*. En Madrid: En la Impr[enta]. del Reyno, a costa de Alonso Pérez de Montalván, Librero de su Magestad, y padre del autor, 1638.

———. *El valiente más dichoso, Don Pedro Guiral. Segundo tomo de las Comedias*. En Madrid: En la Impr[enta]. del Reyno, a costa de Alonso Pérez de Montalván, Librero de su Magestad, y padre del autor, 1638.

Perry, Mary Elizabeth. "Finding Fatima, a Slave Woman of Early Modern Spain." *Contesting Archives: Finding Women in the Sources*. Ed. Nupur Chaudhuri, Sherry J. Katz, and Mary Elizabeth Perry. Urbana, IL: University of Illinois, 2010. 3–19.

Peset Reig, José Luis. *Las melancolías de Sancho: humores y pasiones entre Huarte y Pinel*. Madrid: Asociación Española de Neuropsiquiatría, 2010.

Peset y Vidal, Juan Bautista. "Bosquejo de historia de la medicina valenciana. Quarta época, siglo XVII. Continuación." *Boletín del IMV* 9 (1867): 198–9.

Pesic, Peter. "Wrestling with Proteus: Francis Bacon and the 'torture' of nature." *Isis* 90 (1999): 81–94.

Peyton, Myron A. *Alonso Jerónimo de Salas Barbadillo*. New York, NY: Twayne, 1973.

Picatoste y Rodríguez, Felipe. "Concepto de la naturaleza deducido de las obras de don Pedro Calderón de la Barca [...]." *Calderón y la crítica, historia y antología*. Ed. Manuel Durán and Roberto González Echevarría. Madrid: Editorial Gredos, 1976. 166–248.

Pimentel, Juan. "The Iberian Vision: Science and Empire in the Framework of a Universal Monarchy, 1500–1800." *Osiris* 15 (2000): 17–21.

Pinto Crespo, Virgilio. *Inquisición y control ideológico en la España del siglo XVI*. Madrid: Taurus, 1983.

Platter, Felix, Nicholas Culpeper, and Abdiah Cole. *Platerus Histories and Observations Upon Most Diseases Offending the Body and Mind*. London: Peter Cole, 1664.

Platter, Thomas, d. J. *Beschreibung der Reisen durch Frankreich, Spanien, England und die Niederlande 1595–1600*. Ed. Rut Keiser. Basel: Schwabe, 1968.

Plutarch. *The Third Volume of Plutarch's Lives. Translated from the Greek, by Several Hands*. Ed. M. Burghers. London: Printed by R. E. for Jacob Tonson, at the Judges-Head in Chancery-Lane, near Fleet-street, 1693.

Porshnev, B. F., Dmitri Bayanov, and Igor Bourtsev. "Ideas for Discussion: The Troglodytidae and the Hominidae in the Taxonomy and Evolution of Higher Primates." *Current Anthropology* 15.4 (1974): 449–56.

Portuondo, Maria. *Secret Science. Spanish Cosmography and the New World*. Chicago, IL: University of Chicago Press, 2006.

Prieto, Andrés. *Missionary Scientists: Jesuit Science in Spanish South America, 1570–1810*. Nashville, TN: Vanderbilt University Press, 2011.

Principe, Lawrence M. *The Aspiring Adept: Robert Boyle and his Alchemical Quest*. Princeton, NJ: Princeton University Press, 1998.

Puerto Sarmiento, Francisco Javier. *La leyenda verde: naturaleza, sanidad y ciencia en la corte de Felipe II (1527–1598)*. Valladolid: Consejería de Educación y Cultura, 2003.

———. "La panacea áurea. Alquimia y destilación en la corte de Felipe II (1527–1598)." *Dynamis* 17 (1997): 107–40.

Puerto Sarmiento, Francisco Javier, et al., eds. *Los hijos de Hermes: alquimia y espagiria en la terapéutica española moderna.* Madrid: Corona Borealis, 2001.

Pueyo y Abadía, Luis. "Aprobación." *Primera parte de Medicina y Cirugia racional y espagirica* […]. By Juan de Vidós y Miró. Zaragoza: Gaspar Tomas Martinez, 1691.

———. *Dialectica economica, politica, moral: en la publica alegria, y festiuos aplausos, con que la [...] Escuela de la [...] Ciudad de Zaragoza, celebrò la entrada feliz de su [...] Retor [...] D. Miguel Marta y Mendoza [...] / por [...] Fray Luis Puero y Abadia.* Zaragoza: Diego Dormer, n.d.

———. *Proporciones predicables en fiestas de Maria Santissima, y del Patriarca San Ioseph* […]. Zaragoza: Herederos de Diego Dormer, 1694.

Quevedo, Francisco de. *Los sueños.* Ed. Ignacio Arellano. Madrid: Cátedra, 2007.

Quezada, Noemí. *Amor y magia entre los aztecas: supervivencia en el México colonial.* México: Universidad Nacional Autónoma, 1996.

Quiñones de Benavente, Luis. *Entremeses completos I. Jocoseria.* Ed. Ignacio Arellano, Juan Manuel Escudero, and Abraham Madroñal Durán. Pamplona: Universidad de Navarra, 2001.

Quiroga, Gaspar. *Index et catalogus librorum prohibitorum.* Madriti: apud Alphonsum Gomezium, 1583.

Ramírez de Arellano, Juan Bautista. *Cirugía, ciencia y método racional.* Madrid: Antonio González de Reyes, 1680.

Ramírez Ruiz, Marcelo, and Federico Fernández Christlieb. "La policía de los *indios* y la urbanización del *altepetl*. Ed. F. Fernández Christlieb and A. J. García Zambrano. *Territorialidad y paisaje en el altepetl del siglo XVI.* México: Fondo de Cultura Económica-UNAM, 2006. 114–62.

Respuesta a las razones del advogado Doctor Manuel Urbina […] n.p.: n.p., n.d.

Rey Bueno, Mar. "El debate entre ciencia y religión en l literatura médica de los novatores." *Silos, un milenio: actas del Congreso Internacional sobre la Abadía de Santo Domingo de Silos.* Vol. 3. Burgos: Universidad de Burgos, 2003. 347–66.

———. "El informe Valles: los desdibujados límites del arte de boticarios a finales del siglo XVI (1589–1594)." *Asclepio* 56 (2004): 243–68.

———. "Juntas de herbolarios y tertulias espagíricas: el círculo cortesano de Diego de Cortavila (1597–1657)." *Dynamis* 24 (2004): 243–67.

———. "La Mayson pour Distiller des Eaües at El Escorial: Alchemy and Medicine at the Court of Philip II, 1556–1598." Ed. Teresa Huguet-Termes, Jon Arrizabalaga, and Harold J. Cook. *Heallth and Medicine in Hapsburg Spain: Agents, Practices, Representations.* London, UK: The Wellcome Trust Centre for the History of Medicine at UCL, 2009. 26–39.

———. "Los paracelsistas españoles: medicina química en la España Moderna." *Más allá de la leyenda negra: España y la revolución científica / Beyond the black legend: Spain and the scientific revolution*. Ed. Víctor Navarro Brotóns and William Eamon. Valencia: CSIC-Universitat de València, 2007. 41–56.

———. *Los señores del fuego. Destiladores y espagiricos en la corte de los Austrias*. Madrid: Corona Borealis, 2002.

Rey Bueno Mar, and M. Esther Alegre Pérez, "Los destiladores de su majestad. Destilación, espagiria y paracelsismo en la corte de Felipe II." *Dynamis* 21 (2001): 323–50.

Ricard, Robert. *The Spiritual Conquest of Mexico: An Essay on the Apostolate and the Evangelizing Methods of the Mendicant Order in New Spain*. Berkeley, CA: University of California Press, 1966.

Risse, Gunter. "Medicine in New Spain." *Medicine in the New World*. Ed. Ronald L. Numbers. Knoxville, TN: University of Tennessee Press, 1987. 12–63.

———. "Transcending Cultural Barriers." *Botanical Drugs of the Americas in the Old and New Worlds*. Ed. Wolfgang Hagen Hein. Stuttgart: Wissenschaftliche Verlagsgesellschaft, 1984. 31–42.

Rodríguez Delgado, Adriana. "El estudio del procedimiento inquisitorial a través de los documentos del Santo Oficio Novohispano." *De sendas, brechas y atajos: Contexto y crítica de las fuentes eclesiásticas, siglos XVI–XVIII*. Ed. Doris Bieñko de Peralta and Berenise Bravo Rubio. México: Escuela Nacional de Antropología e Historia, 2008.

Rodríguez de Monforte, Pedro. *Sueños mysteriosos de la escritura en discursos sagrados, politicos y morales*. Madrid: Imprenta de Antonio Roman, 1687.

Rodríguez Marín, Francisco. *La verdadera biografía del doctor Nicolás de Monardes*. Sevilla: Padilla, 1988.

Rodríguez-Guerrero, José. "La Primera Gran Red Comercial de un Medicamento *chymico*: Vittorio Algarotti y su Quintaesencia del Oro Medicinal." *Azogue* 6 (2008–2009): 12–67.

Rodríguez-Puértolas, Julio. "Francisco Santos y los mitos del casticismo hispano." *Studia Hispanica in Honorem Rafael Lapesa*. Vol. III. Ed. Dámaso Alonso. Madrid: Cátedra, 1975. 419–30.

———. "Introducción." *El no importa de España*. London, UK: Támesis, 1974.

Rojas Zorrilla, Francisco de. *Santa Isabel, reina de Portugal*. Ed. Elena Arenas. *Obras completes III: Primera parte de comedias*. Ed. Felipe B. Pedraza Jiménez, Rafael González Cañal, and Gema Gómez Rubio. Cuenca: Ediciones de la Universidad de Castilla-La Mancha, 2011.

Romano, Antonella. *Rome et la science moderne: entre Renaissance et Lumières*. Rome: École française de Rome, 2008.

———. "Rome, un chantier pour les savoirs de la catholicité post-tridentine." *Revue d'histoire moderne et contemporaine* 55.2 (2008): 101–20.

Roodenburg, Herman. "The Maternal Imagination: The Fears of Pregnant Women in Seventeenth-Century Holland." *Journal of Social History* 21. 2 (1988): 701–16.

Roos, Anne Marie. "Luminaries in Medicine: Richard Mead, James Gibbs, and Solar and Lunar Effects on the Human Body in Early Modern England." *Bulletin of the History of Medicine* 74.3 (2000): 433–57.

Rossi, Paolo. "The Aristotelians and the 'Moderns': Hypothesis and Nature." *Annali dell'Istituto e Museo di Storia della Scienza di Firenze* 7 (1982): 3–28.

———. *Philosophy, Technology, and the Arts in the Early Modern Era*. New York, NY: Harper & Row, 1970.

Rublack, Ulinka. "Pregnancy, Childbirth and the Female Body in Early Modern Germany." *Past & Present* 150.1 (1996): 84–110.

Ruiz de Alarcón, Hernando, and María Elena de la Garza Sánchez. *Tratado de las supersticiones y costumbres gentílicas que hoy viven entre los indios naturales desta Nueva España: escrito en 1629*. México, D.F: Secretaría de Educación Pública, 1988.

Ruiz de Alarcón, Juan. *La cueva de Salamanca. Comedias de Don Juan Ruiz de Alarcón y Mendoza*. Ed. Juan Eugenio Hartzenbusch. Madrid: Ediciones Atlas, 1946.

Ruiz, Javier. "Los alquimistas de Felipe II." *Historia 16* 12 (1977): 49–55.

Ryan, Michael T. "Assimilating New Worlds in the Sixteenth and Seventeenth Centuries." *Comparative Studies in Society and History* 23 (1981): 519-38.

Sabik, Kazimierz. "La problemática de la libertad-destino en el teatro cortesano español de la segunda mitad del siglo XVII." *Actas del XIII Congreso de la Asociación Internacional de Hispanistas*. Ed. Florencio Sevilla Arroyo and Carlos Alvar. Vol. 1. Madrid: Editorial Castalia, 2000. 714–19.

Safier, Niel. "Global Knowledge on the Move: Itineraries, Amerindian Narratives, and Deep Histories of Science." *Isis* 101 (2010): 133–45.

———. "Itineraries of Atlantic science: New questions, new approaches, new directions." *Atlantic Studies* 7 (2010): 357–64.

Sahagún, Bernardino de. *General History of the Things of New Spain*. Sacramento, CA: California State Library, 1985.

———. *Historia general de las cosas de la Nueva España [...] nueva edición, con numeración, anotaciones y apéndices Angel María Garibay*. 3 vols. México: Porrúa, 1969.

———. *Historia general de las cosas de la Nueva España*. Barcelona: Tusquets, 1985.

Salas, Xavier de. *El Bosco en la literatura española*. Barcelona: J. Sabater, 1943.

Salomon, Noël. "Sur les représentations théâtrales dans les pueblos des provinces de Madrid et Tolède, 1589–1640." *Bulletin Hispanique* 62.4 (1960): 398–427.

———. *La vida rural castellana en tiempos de Felipe II*. Barcelona: Editorial Ariel, 1988.

Sánchez del Castellar y Arbustante, Manuel. *Gramatica consagrada, Celestial Literatura, Misterio Plato, en la Mesa Soberana del Altar* ... Zaragoza: Herederos de Juan de Ybar, 1676.

———. *Sacro enigma en la santisima imagen del Santo Cristo de la parroquia de S. Salvador de la ciudad de Valencia* ... Valencia: por Vicente Cabrera , 1679.

————. *Triangulo de Perfecciones ... Su centro el Angelico Dotor S. Tomas de Aquino.* Valencia: Francisco Mestre, 1691.

Sánchez Jiménez, Antonio. *El pincel y el Fénix: pintura y literatura en la obra de Lope de Vega Carpio.* Preface by Javier Portús Pérez. Pamplona, Madrid, Frankfurt: Universidad de Navarra, Iberoamericana, Vervuert, 2011.

Sancho de San Román, R. *La medicina y los médicos en la obra de Tirso de Molina.* Salamanca: Libr. Cervantes, 1960.

Sanders, Julie. "Midwifery and the New Science in the Seventeenth Century: Language, Print, and the Theater." *At the Borders of the Human: Beasts, Bodies, and Natural Philosophy in the Early Modern Period.* Ed. Erica Fudge, Ruth Gilbert, and Susan Wiseman. New York, NY: Palgrave, 2002, 74–90.

————. *The Cultural Geography of Early Modern Drama, 1620–1650.* Cambridge, UK: Cambridge University Press, 2011.

Santos, Francisco. *Día y noche de Madrid. Obras selectas.* 2 vols. Ed. Milagros Navarro Pérez. Madrid: Instituto de Estudios Madrileños, 1976.

————. *El rey Gallo y discursos de la Hormiga.* Ed. Víctor Arizpe. London: Tamesis, 1991.

————. *La Tarasca de parto en el Mesón del Infierno y días de fiesta por la noche.* Madrid: Domingo García Morrás, 1672.

Sato, Masayuki. "Imagined Peripheries: the world and its peoples in Japanese cartographic imagination." *Facing Each Other: The World's Perception of Europe and Europe's Perception of the World.* 2 vols. Ed. Anthony Pagden. Vol 2. Aldershot, UK: Ashgate, 2000. 367–93.

Sawday, Jonathan. *The Body Emblazoned: Dissection and the Human Body in Renaissance Culture.* London, UK: Routledge, 1995.

Scaligero, Giulio Caesare. *Exotericarvm Exercitationvm Liber quintus decimus. De Subtilitate, Ad Hieronymvm Cardanvm.* Paris: Michaelis Vascasani, 1557.

Scarry, Elaine. *The Body in Pain: The Making and Unmaking of the World.* New York, NY: Oxford University Press, 1985.

Schiebinger, Londa, and Claudia Swan, eds. *Colonial Botany: Science, Commerce, and Politics in the Early Modern World.* Philadelphia, PA: University of Pennsylvania, 2005.

Schmitt, Charles B. "Aristotle Among the Physicians." *The Medical Renaissance of the Sixteenth Century.* Ed. A. Wear, R. K. French, and I. M. Lonie. Cambridge, UK: Cambridge University Press, 1985. 1–15.

Schock, Flemming. *Die Text-Kunstkammer: populäre Wissenssammlungen des Barock am Beispiel der 'Relationes Curiosae' von E W Happel.* Cologne: Böhlau, 2011.

Schultes, Richard E., Albert Hofmann, Alberto Blanco, Gastón Guzmán, and Salvador Acosta. *Plantas de los dioses: Orígenes del uso de los alucinógenos.* México: Fondo de Cultura Económica, 1993.

Serrano Perdices, Laura. "*La Tarasca de Parto*: Mayas, moralistas e infancia en el Madrid del siglo XVII." *Las edades de las mujeres.* Ed. Pilar Pérez Cantó and Margarita Ortega López. Madrid: Universidad Autónoma de Madrid, 2002. 81–93.

Shergold, Norman D. "Ganassa and the *Commedia dell'arte* in Sixteenth-Century Spain." *The Modern Language Review* 51.3 (1956): 359–68.

———., and John E. Varey. *Representaciones palaciegas: 1603–1699, estudio y documentos*. London, UK: Tamesis, 1982.

Signorotto, G. V. "Papato e principi italiani nell'ultima fase del conflitto tra Asburgo e Valois." *Carlos V y la quiebra del humanismo político en Europa, 1530–1558: congreso internacional: Madrid 3–6 de julio de 2000*. Ed. José Martínez Millán. Vol. 1. Madrid: Sociedad Estatal para la Conmemoración de los Centenarios de Felipe II y Carlos V, 2001. 259–80.

Simón Díaz, José. *Bibliografía de la literatura hispánica*. Vol. XVI. Madrid: CSIC, 1993.

Simón Palmer, María del Carmen. "Hipócrates y Galeno en el teatro del Siglo de Oro." *Tes Philies Tade Dora: Miscelánea léxica en memoria de Conchita Serrano*. Madrid: C.S.I.C., 1999, 523–34.

Simón Palmer, María del Carmen. "La Cuaresma en el Palacio Real de Madrid." *Revista de Dialectología y Tradiciones Populares* 43 (1988): 579–84.

Siraisi, Nancy G. "Life Sciences and Medicine in the Renaissance World." *Rome Reborn. The Vatican Library and Renaissance Culture*. Ed. Anthony Grafton. Washington, DC: Library of Congress, 1993: 169–98.

———. *Medieval & Early Renaissance Medicine: An Introduction to Knowledge and Practice*. Chicago, IL: University of Chicago Press, 1990.

Sixtus V. *Coeli et Terrae*. 1585.

Skafari, Janne et. al., *Opening Windows on Texts and Discourses of the Past*. Philadelphia, PA: John Benjamins, 2005.

Slater, John. "Rereading Cabriada's Carta: Alchemy and Rhetoric in Baroque Spain." *Colorado Review of Hispanic Studies* 7 (2009): 67–80.

———. *Todos son hojas: literatura e historia natural en el barroco español*. Madrid: Consejo Superior de Investigaciones Científicas, 2010.

———. "The Green Gold Falacies: Myth and Reality in the Transatlantic Trade in Medicinal Plants (1493-1663). *Geografías médicas: Orillas y fronteras culturales de la medicina (siglos XVI y XVII)*. Ed. José Pardo-Tomás and Mauricio Sánchez Menchero. Mexico: UNAM, 2014.99–122.

Slater, John, and Maríaluz López-Terrada. "Scenes of Mediation: Staging Medicine in the Spanish Interludes." *Social History of Medicine* 24.2 (2011): 226–43.

Smith, Miles, and Thomas Bilson. *The Holy Bible: Conteyning the Old Testament, and the New: Newly Translated Out of the Originall Tongues: & with the Former Translations Diligently Compared and Reuised, by His Maiesties Speciall Comandement: Appointed to Be Read in Churches*. London, UK: Robert Barker, 1611.

Smith, Pamela. *The Body of the Artisan: Art and Experience in the Scientific Revolution*. Chicago, IL: University of Chicago Press, 2004.

———. *The Business of Alchemy: Science and Culture in the Holy Roman Empire*. Princeton, NJ: Princeton University Press, 1994.

———. "Vermilion, Mercury, Blood, and Lizards: Matter and Meaning in Metalworking." *Materials and Expertise in Early Modern Europe: Between Market and Laboratory*. Ed. Ursula Klein and Emma Spary. Chicago, IL: University of Chicago Press, 2010.

———. "What is a Secret? Secrets and Craft Knowledge in Early Modern Europe." Ed. Elaine Leong and Alisha Rankin. *Secrets and Knowledge in Medicine and Science, 1500–1800*. Aldershot, UK: Ashgate, 2011.

Smith, Pamela H., and Paula Findlen. *Merchants and Marvels: Commerce, Science, and Art in Early Modern Europe*. New York, NY: Routledge, 2002.

Smith, Paul Julian. *The Body Hispanic: Gender and Sexuality in Spanish and Spanish-American Literature*. Oxford, UK: Clarendon, 1988.

Sorapán de Rieros, Juan. *Medicina Española*. Granada: Juan Muñoz, 1615.

Soufas, Teresa Scott. *Melancholy and the Secular Mind in Spanish Golden Age Literature*. Columbia, MO: University of Missouri Press, 1990.

Spain. Archivo del Reino de Valencia. *Papeles de Real Audiencia*. 1590.

Spinks, Jennifer S. *Monstrous Births and Visual Culture in Sixteenth-Century Germany: Religious Cultures in the Early Modern World*. London, UK: Pickering & Chatto Publishers, 2009.

Spivakovsky, Erika. *Son of the Alhambra: Don Diego Hurtado de Mendoza, 1504–1575*. Austin, TX: University of Texas Press, 1970.

Stannard, Jerry. "Dioscorides and Renaissance Materia Medica." Ed. Marcel Florkin. *Analecta Medico-Historica I: Materia Medica in the XVIth Century*. Oxford, UK: Oxford University Press, 1966.

Stearns, Raymond. *Science in the British Colonies of America*, Urbana, IL: University of Illinois Press, 1970.

Stephenson, Marcia. "From Marvelous Antidote to the Poison of Idolatry: the transatlantic role of Andean Bezoar Stones during the late sixteenth and early seventeenth centuries." *Hispanic American Historical Review* 90 (2009): 3–39.

Stern, Steve J. *La historia secreta del género: mujeres, hombres y poder en México en las postrimerías del periodo colonial*. México: Fondo de Cultura Económica, 1999.

Strauss, Walter L. *The German Single-Leaf Woodcut, 1550–1600: A Pictorial Catalogue*. Vol. 3: S–Z. New York, NY: Abaris Books, 1975.

Strumia, Renata. "Skin signs in anorexia nervosa." *Dermato-endocrinology* 1.5 (2009): 268–70.

Suárez de Figueroa, Cristóbal. *Plaza universal de todas las ciencias y artes [...]*. Madrid: Luis Sánchez, 1615.

Tarabochia Canavero, Alessandra. "Il De Triplici Vita di Marsilio Ficino: una strana vicenda ermeneutica." *Rivista di filosofia neoscolastica* 69 (1977): 697–717.

Tarifa y arancel de medicinas para la ciudad de Zaragoza, terminos y barrios. Zaragoza: Herederos de Diego Dormer, 1679.

Tenorio, Antonio. "El peyote. Anhalonium lewinii y Anhalonium williamsii. Cactáceas." *Anales del Instituto Médico Nacional* 4 (1900): 233–49.

Thomas, Keith. *Religion and the Decline of Magic: Studies in Popular Beliefs in Sixteenth and Seventeenth Century England.* Harmondsworth, UK: Penguin Group, 1973.

Thompson, Peter. *The Triumphant Juan Rana: A Gay Actor in Spanish Golden Age Theatre.* Toronto: University of Toronto Press, 2006.

Torquemada, Antonio de. *The Spanish Mandeuile of Miracles, or the Garden of Curious Flowers.* Trans. Lewis Lewkenor and Ferdinand Walker. London: I[ames] R[oberts] for Edmund Matts, 1600.

Torre Revello, José. *El sevillano Nicolás Monardes y sus libros de medicina americana.* [Madrid]: [Publicaciones de la Cátedra de Historia de la Medicina], [1940].

Trevor-Roper, Hugh. "The Paracelsian Movement." *Renaissance Essays.* Chicago, IL: University of Chicago Press, 1985. 149–99.

Tulp, Nicolaes. *Observationes Medicæ.* Amsterdam: Apud Ludovicum Elzevirium, 1652.

Turnbull, Colin M. *The Forest People.* New York, NY: Simon and Schuster, 1961.

Tutino, John. *De la insurrección a la revolución en México: las bases sociales de la violencia agraria 1750–1940.* México, D. F: Ediciones Era, 1990.

Uztarroz, Juan Francisco Andrés de, and Diego José Dormer. *Progresos de la historia de Aragón y vida de sus cronistas, desde que se instituyó este cargo hasta su extinción: primera parte, que comprende la biografía de Gerónimo Zurita.* Zaragoza: Impr. del Hospicio Provincial, 1878.

Valbuena Briones, A. J. "El concepto del hado en el teatro de Calderón." *Bulletin Hispanique* 63.1–2 (1961): 48–53.

Valle, Bartolomé del. *Explicación y pronóstico de los dos cometas.* Granada: Franciso Heylán y Pedro de la Cuesta, 1619.

Valverde de Amusco, Juan. *Anatomia del corpo humano.* In Roma: Per Ant. Salamanca, et Antonio Lafrerj, 1559.

Van Nouhuys, T. *The Age of Two-Faced Janus. The Comets of 1577 and 1618 and the Decline of the Aristotelian World View in the Netherlands.* Leiden: Brill, 1998.

Vanden Broecke, Steven. *The Limits of Influence: Pico, Louvain, and the Crisis of Renaissance Astrology.* Leiden: Brill, 2003.

Varey, Simon, Rafael Chabrán, and Dora Weiner, eds. *Searching for the Secrets of Nature: the life and works of Dr. Francisco Hernández.* Stanford, CA: Stanford University Press, 2000.

Vega, Felix Arturo Lope de. *El amigo por fuerza.* Ed. Gonzalo Pontón and José Enrique Laplana. *Comedias de Lope de Vega: Parte IV.* Ed. Alberto Blecua, Guillermo Serés, Luigi Giuliani, and Ramón Valdés. Vol. 2. Lleida: Editorial Milenio, 2002.

———. *El acero de Madrid.* Ed. Stefano Arata. Madrid: Castalia, 2000.

———. *Barlaán y Josafat.* Ed. José F. Montesinos. Madrid: Junta para la Ampliación de Estudios, 1935.

————. *Las bizarrías de Belisa.* Ed. Enrique García Santo-Tomás. Madrid: Cátedra, 2004.

————. *El bobo del colegio.* Ed. J. San José Lera. Salamanca: Ediciones Universidad de Salamanca, 2001.

————. *La dama boba. Comedias de Lope de Vega: Parte IX.* Ed. Alberto Blecua, Guillermo Serés, and Marco Presotto. Vol. 3. Lleida: Editorial Milenio, 2007.

————. *Décima séptima parte de las comedias de Lope de Vega Carpio procurador Fiscal de la Cámara Apostólica y Familiar del Santo Oficio de la Inquisición.* Madrid: Fernando Correa de Montenegro, 1621.

————. *La Dorotea.* Ed. Edwin S. Morby. Madrid: Editorial Castalia, 1968.

————. *El hidalgo Abencerraje. Decima séptima parte de las comedia.* Madrid: Fernando Correa de Montenegro, 1621.

————. *Fuenteovejuna.* Ed. Donald McGrady and Noel Salomon. Barcelona: Critica, 1993.

————. *La prueba de los ingenios.* Ed. Julián Molina. *Comedias de Lope de Vega: Parte IX.* Ed. Alberto Blecua, Guillermo Serés, and Marco Presotto. Lleida: Editorial Milenio, 1997.

————. *Lo que ha de ser. Obras de Lope de Vega: Obras dramáticas.* Ed. Emilio Cotarelo y Mori. Vol. 12. Madrid: Real Academia Española, 1930.

————. *La resistencia honrada y condesa Matilde.* Ed. Miguel Marón García Bermejo. *Comedias de Lope de Vega: Parte II.* Ed. Alberto Blecua, Guillermo Serés, and Silvia Iriso. Vol. 2. Lleida: Editorial Milenio, 1998.

Velasco, Sherry. *Male Delivery: Reproduction, Effeminacy, and Pregnant Men in Early Modern Spain.* Nashville, TN: Vanderbilt University Press, 2006.

Vélez de Guevara, Luis. *El diablo cojuelo.* Ed. Ramón Valdés. Barcelona: Crítica, 1999.

Vesalius, Andreas. *The epitome of* Andreas Vesalius, *translated from the Latin with preface and introduction by L. R. Lind, with anatomical notes by C. W. Asling. Foreword by Logan Clendening.* Cambridge, MA: MIT Press, 1969.

Vicente, Zamora. Introduction. *Don Gil de las calzas verdes.* By Tirso de Molina. Madrid: Castalia, 1999.

Vidós y Miró, Juan de. *Manifiesto del Licenciado Juan de Vidós: en su defensa* [...] n.p.: n.p., n.d.

————. *Primera parte de Medicina y Cirugia racional y espagirica* [...]. Zaragoza: Gaspar Tomas Martinez, 1691.

————.*Memorial y manifiesto a la Augusta y Imperial Ciudad de Zaragoza...* Zaragoza: Tomás Gaspar Martínez, 1683.

————. *Súplica de Juan de Vidós al Justicia de Aragón, para que le permita hacer y administrar medicamentos en la Ciudad de Zaragoza, lo cual le prohibía el Colegio de Médicos y Cirujanos de la misma.* n.p.: n.p. [after 1681?].

Viesca Treviño, Carlos. "Hechizos y hierbas mágicas en la obra de Juan de Cárdenas." *Estudios de Historia Novohispana* 9 (1987): 37–50.

Vilches, Elvira. *New World Gold: Cultural Anxiety and Monetary Disorder in Early Modern Spain.* Chicago, IL: Chicago University Press, 2010.

Villani, Matteo. *Cronica di Matteo Villani*. Florence: Per Il Magheri, 1825.

Villaseñor Black, Charlene. "The Moralized Breast in Early Modern Spain." *The Material Culture of Sex, Procreation, and Marriage in Early Modern Europe*. Ed. Anne L. McClanan and Karen Rosoff Encarnación. New York, NY: Palgrave, 2002, 191–219.

Visceglia, Maria Antonietta. *Roma papale e Spagna: diplomatici, nobili e religiosi tra due corti*. Roma: Bulzoni, 2010.

Vivalda, Nicolás M. "Basilio o el ocaso del monarca-astrólogo: juegos de la similitud e inconveniencias políticas en *La vida es sueño*." *Hacia la tragedia áurea: lecturas para un nuevo milenio*. Ed. Frederick Alfred de Armas, Luciano García Lorenzo, and Enrique García Santo-Tomás. Madrid: Iberoamericana, 2008. 383–96.

Vives, Juan Luis. *Vives on Education: a translation of the* De tradendis disciplinis *of Juan Luis Vives*. Totowa, NJ: Rowman and Littlefield, 1971.

Walton, Michael T. *Genesis and the Chymical Philosophy: True Christian Science in the Sixteenth and Seventeenth Centuries*. New York, NY: AMS Press, 2011.

Wardropper, Bruce. "Lope's *La dama boba* and Baroque Comedy." *Bulletin of the Comediantes* 13 (1961): 1–3.

Webster, Charles. *Paracelsus: Medicine, Magic, and Mission at the End of Time*. New Haven, CT: Yale University Press, 2008.

Wesenigk, Georg. *Das Spiel-süchtige, sieben-fächtige Polysigma der Bösen Spiel-Sieben*. Dresden: Zimmermann, 1702.

Whaley, Leigh. *Women and the Practice of Medical Care in Early Modern Europe, 1400–1800*. Houndmills, Basingstoke, UK: Palgrave Macmillan, 2011.

Whicker, Jules. "Los magos neoestoicos de *La cueva de Salamanca* y *La prueba de las promesas* de Ruiz de Alarcón." *El escritor y la escena V: estudios sobre teatro español y novohispano de los Siglos de Oro: homenaje a Marc Vitse*. Ed. Ysla Campbell. Ciudad Juárez, Chihuahua, México: Universidad Autónoma de Ciudad Juárez, 2000. 211–19.

White, Michael. *Isaac Newton: the last sorcerer*. Reading, MA: Addison-Wesley, 1997.

Wiesner-Hanks, Merry E. *The Marvelous Hairy Girls: The Gonzales Sisters and Their Worlds*. New Haven, CT: Yale University Press, 2009.

Williams, Charles Allyn. *The German Legends of the Hairy Anchorite*. Urbana, IL: University of Illinois, 1935.

Wilson, Adrian. "The Ceremony of Childbirth and Its Interpretation." *Women as Mothers in Pre-Industrial England: Essays in Memory of Dorothy McLaren*. Ed. Valerie Fildes. London, UK: Routledge, 1990, 68–107.

Wilson, Edward M. Introduction. *Fieras afemina amor.* By Pedro Calderón de la Barca. Ed. Edward M. Wilson. Kassel: Reichemberger, 1984.

———. "The Four Elements in the Imagery of Calderón." *Spanish and English Literature of the 16th and 17th Centuries: Studies in Discretion, Illusion, and Mutability*. By Edward M. Wilson and Don William Cruickshank. Cambridge, UK: Cambridge University Press, 1980. 1–14.

Winter, Calvert J. "Notes on the Works of Francisco Santos." *Hispania: A Journal Devoted to the Teaching of Spanish and Portuguese* 12.5 (1929): 457–64.

Young, Robert J. C. *Colonial Desire. Hybridity in Theory, Culture and Race.* London, UK: Routledge, 1995.

Yule, Henry, ed. and trans. "Recollections of travel in the East, by John de Marignolli, Papal Legate to the court of the Great Khan and afterwards Bishop of Bisignano." *Cathay and the Way Thither: Being a Collection of Medieval Notices of China.* 2 vols. London, UK: Hakluyt Society, 1866. Vol. II. 335–94.

Zanier, G. *La medicina astrologica e la sua teoria: Marsilio Ficino e i suoi critici contemporanei.* Rome: Edizioni dell'Ateneo e Bizzarri, 1977.

Zapperi, Roberto. *Der wilde Mann von Teneriffa: Die wundersame Geschichte des Pedro Gonzalez und seiner Kinder.* Munchen: C. H. Beck, 2004.

Zarzoso, Alfons. "El pluralismo médico a través de la correspondencia privada en la Cataluña del siglo XVIII." *Dynamis* 21 (2001): 409–33.

Ziller, Camenietzki. "Jesuits and Alchemy in the early seventeenth century: Father Johannes Roberti and the Weapon-Salve controversy." *Ambix* 48 (2001): 83–101.

Zilsel, Edgar. *The Sociological Roots of Science.* Chicago, IL: University of Chicago Press, 1942.

Index

Page numbers in bold indicate illustrations.